ATLAS
OF
GASTROINTESTINAL
PATHOLOGY

ATLASES IN
DIAGNOSTIC SURGICAL PATHOLOGY

Published:

WOLD, McLEOD, SIM, and UNNI:
ATLAS OF ORTHOPEDIC PATHOLOGY

COLBY, LOMBARD, YOUSEM AND KITAICHI:
ATLAS OF PULMONARY SURGICAL PATHOLOGY

KANEL AND KORULA:
ATLAS OF LIVER PATHOLOGY

WENIG:
ATLAS OF HEAD AND NECK PATHOLOGY

Forthcoming:

DEMETRIS:
ATLAS OF TRANSPLANTATION PATHOLOGY

RO, GRIGNON, AMIN, AND AYALA:
ATLAS OF SURGICAL PATHOLOGY OF THE MALE REPRODUCTIVE TRACT

ATLAS OF GASTROINTESTINAL PATHOLOGY

David A. Owen, M.B.
Head, Division of Anatomical Pathology
Vancouver General Hospital

Professor of Pathology
University of British Columbia
Vancouver, British Columbia
Canada

James K. Kelly, M.B., F.R.C.P.
Pathologist
Greater Victoria Hospital Society

Department of Laboratories
Victoria General Hospital
Victoria, British Columbia
Canada

W.B. SAUNDERS COMPANY
A Division of Harcourt Brace & Company
Philadelphia ■ London ■ Toronto ■ Montreal ■ Sydney ■ Tokyo

W.B. SAUNDERS COMPANY
A Division of Harcourt Brace & Company

The Curtis Center
Independence Square West
Philadelphia, Pennsylvania 19106

Library of Congress Cataloging-in-Publication Data

Owen, David A.
    Atlas of gastrointestinal pathology / David A. Owen, James K. Kelly.
        p.   cm.
    ISBN 0–7216–6730–9
    1. Gastrointestinal system—Diseases—Atlases.
I. Kelly, James K.   II. Title.
    [DNLM: 1. Gastrointestinal Diseases—pathology—atlases.
WI 17 097a 1994]
    RC802.9.094   1994   616.3′307—dc20
DNLM/DLC   94-989

Atlas of Gastrointestinal Pathology   ISBN 0–7216–6730–9

Printed in the United States of America

Last digit is the print number: 9   8   7   6   5   4   3   2   1

DEDICATION

To Elizabeth, Gary, and Daniel and
to my father and mother who have always
encouraged and supported me. *DAO*
To Mary, John, Sarah, Fearghal,
and Anne and to my father who gave
me a love of learning. *JKK*

ACKNOWLEDGMENT

We wish to thank all of the
colleagues and friends who gave us
transparencies and microscope slides.
JKK wishes to thank Dr. Sandy McColl for
constructive criticism of the text.

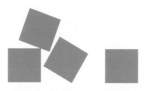

PREFACE

This Atlas of Gastrointestinal Pathology is intended primarily as an introduction to the subject, rather than a comprehensive text in which all diseases, common and rare, are described in minute detail. It offers a starting point for pathology residents, surgery residents, and gastroenterology residents who wish to learn more about bowel diseases. We believe that it will also serve as a concise and easily utilized reference book for hospital-based and non–hospital-based pathologists who do not practice as subspecialists in this area.

The atlas is organized along traditional lines, with most diseases grouped according to the principal part of the gastrointestinal tract involved. Some conditions, for example, ischemia, stromal neoplasms, and lymphoreticular diseases, which may affect the stomach or bowel at any level, are illustrated and described in separate sections. We think that this approach avoids unnecessary duplication.

Because the text information is intended to be practical and pertinent to clinical practice, it is provided in a summary or list format. The format is uniform for all conditions, containing sections on biology of the disease, clinical presentation, gross and microscopic pathology, differential diagnosis, and references. Once familiar with this format, the reader will be able to locate specific information relevant to any disease without a prolonged search. The format also facilitates comparisons between sections on different diseases.

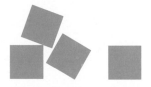

CONTENTS

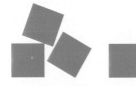

CHAPTER ■ 1

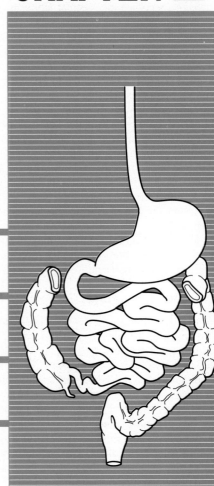

DISEASES
OF THE
ESOPHAGUS

NORMAL APPEARANCES

Gross Anatomy

- The upper border of the esophagus is the cricopharyngeal muscle. Its lower border is that point where the tubular esophagus becomes the saccular stomach.
- The average esophagus measures 25 cm in length.
- Endoscopically, the esophagus starts 15 cm from the incisor teeth and extends to 40 cm from the incisor teeth. Esophageal length varies from individual to individual, however, according to height and presence or absence of a sliding hiatus hernia.
- The squamocolumnar junction at the lower esophagus (Z line) is commonly irregular and may be up to 2.5 cm proximal to the anatomical gastroesophageal junction.
- For clinicopathologic purposes, the esophagus may be divided into upper, middle, and lower thirds. The lymphatic drainage of the upper third is to the cervical nodes, of the middle third to the paraesophageal and paratracheal nodes, and the lower third to the para-aortic nodes and celiac nodes.
- The lower esophageal sphincter may be appreciated endoscopically by observing the location of the proximal margin of gastric mucosal folds.

Microscopic Appearances

- The mucosal lining consists of a nonkeratinizing squamous epithelium, which may be divided into basal, prickle cell, and functional layers.
- The basal layer is 1 to 4 cells thick (up to 15% of the total epithelium) and contains cells with nonglycogenated cytoplasm. The upper margin of the basal zone may be identified as the level where nuclei are separated by at least one nuclear diameter.
- The basal layer contains occasional mitoses and endocrine cells. In some individuals, melanocytes are also present.
- The lamina propria of the esophagus is similar to that found elsewhere in the gastrointestinal (GI) tract and contains small numbers of inflammatory cells, particularly lymphocytes. Fingerlike upward extensions of lamina propria are termed *papillae*. Normally, these are not longer than two thirds of the epithelial thickness.
- Isolated lymphocytes may be present between epithelial cells, usually in the suprabasal region. These may be convoluted and have been referred to as "squiggle cells." They are OKT3 and OKT8 positive, indicating a suppressor-cytotoxic function.
- Occasionally, the suprabasal squamous cells contain focal accumulations of excess glycogen and may appear endoscopically as pearly gray plaques. This finding is considered a variant of normal and has been termed *glycogenic acanthosis*.
- Isolated mucous glands may be present in the lamina propria and submucosa. They are connected to the surface by a duct lined proximally by cuboidal epithelium and distally by squamous epithelium. They resemble pyloric and Brunner's glands.
- The muscularis mucosae, submucosa, and muscularis propria of the esophagus are similar to those layers elsewhere in the bowel.
- The lower 2.5 cm of esophagus may be lined by cardiac-type gastric epithelium. If this epithelium extends further up the esophagus or shows metaplasia with the presence of acid mucin, it is considered to be Barrett's esophagus.

References

Bender MD, Allison J, Cuartas F, Montgomery C. Glycogenic acanthosis of the esophagus: a form of benign epithelial hyperplasia. Gastroenterology 1973;65:373–380.

De Nardi FG, Riddell RH. The normal esophagus. Am J Surg Pathol 1991;15:296–309.

Hopwood D, Logan KR, Bouchier IA. The electron microscopy of normal human esophageal epithelium. Virchows Archiv [B] 1978;26:345–358.

Stern Z, Sharon P, Ligumsky M, Levij IS, et al. Glycogenic acanthosis of the esophagus. A benign, but confusing endoscopic lesion. Am J Gastroenterol 1980;74:261–263.

Tateishi R, Taniguchi H, Wada A, Horai T, et al. Argyrophil cells and melanocytes in esophageal mucosa. Arch Pathol 1974;98:87–89.

Weinstein WM, Bogoch ER, Bowes KL. The normal human esophageal mucosa: a histologic reappraisal. Gastroenterology 1975;68:40–44.

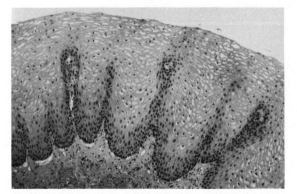

Figure 1–1. Low power view of normal esophagus to show the thickness of the basal layer and the height of papillae.

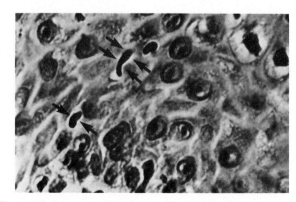

Figure 1–2. Intramucosal lymphocytes ("squiggle" cells).

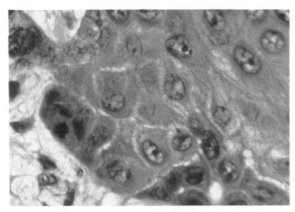

Figure 1–3. Desmosomes present between adjacent squamous cells. In this example, the epithelium is mildly inflamed and edematous. Under these circumstances, desmosomes are more easily identified.

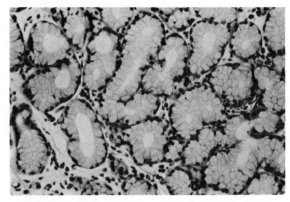

Figure 1–4. Mucous glands in the esophageal submucosa. They are virtually identical to Brunner's glands.

HETEROTOPIAS

Biology of Disease

■ Two types of heterotopia are described. Gastric heterotopia, present at endoscopy in 4% of individuals, is usually located just below the upper esophageal sphincter as an "inlet patch."

■ Heterotopic sebaceous glands are present in 2% of individuals. The lesions may be solitary or may be present at multiple sites along the length of the esophagus.

Clinical Findings

■ Heterotopic gastric mucosa may secrete acid. Patients may complain of a burning retrosternal pain. Complications include peptic ulceration, stricture formation, and adenocarcinoma.

■ The presence of sebaceous glands in the esophagus is usually a chance finding on endoscopy. They have no clinical significance.

Gross Pathology

■ Heterotopic gastric mucosa is a pinkish red patch, usually 1 to 2 cm in diameter but occasionally larger. It rarely extends around the esophageal circumference.

■ Heterotopic sebaceous glands appear as single or multiple yellowish papules 1 to 2 mm in diameter.

Microscopic Pathology

■ Heterotopic gastric mucosa has a variety of appearances. It may consist of a mixture of normal cardiac and normal fundic mucosa or may be cardiac mucosa alone. Secondary inflammation and metaplasia may occur, but they are in no way related to Barrett's mucosa.

■ Sebaceous glands in the esophagus closely resemble cutaneous sebaceous glands. No true hair follicles are present.

Differential Diagnosis

Barrett's esophagus.

Heterotopic gastric mucosa usually occurs in the upper esophagus in patients without evidence of reflux, whereas Barrett's esophagus occurs in the lower esophagus and is due to reflux. Histologically, heterotopia may be identical to Barrett's mucosa, and making the differential diagnosis may be impossible without proper clinical information.

References

Bogomoletz WV, Geboes K, Feydy P, et al. Mucin histochemistry of heterotopic gastric mucosa of the upper esophagus in adults. Hum Pathol 1988;19:1301–1306.

de la Pava S, Pickren JW. Ectopic sebaceous glands in the esophagus. Arch Pathol 1962;72:397–399.

Jabbari M, Goresky CA, Lough J, et al. The inlet patch: heterotopic gastric mucosa in the upper esophagus. Gastroenterology 1985; 89:252–256.

Merino MJ, Brand M, LiVolsi VA, et al. Sebaceous glands in the esophagus. Arch Pathol Lab Med 1981;106:47–48.

Shah KK, De Ridder PH. Ectopic gastric mucosa in proximal esophagus: its clinical significance and hormonal profile. J Clin Gastroenterol 1986;8:509–513.

Truong LD, Strohlein JR, McKechnie JC. Gastric heterotopia of the proximal esophagus: a report of four cases and a review of the literature. Am J Gastroenterol 1986;81:1162–1166.

Zak FG, Lawson W. Sebaceous glands in the esophagus. Arch Dermatol 1976;112:1153–1154.

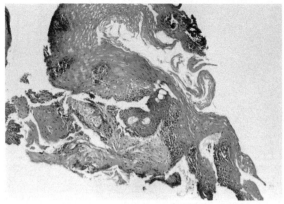

Figure 1–5. Esophageal sebaceous glands. They are present in an intraepithelial location rather than as discrete submucosal structures.

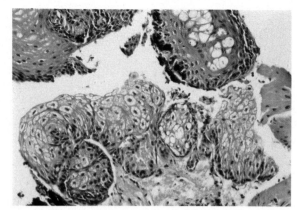

Figure 1–6. Sebaceous glands showing bubbly cytoplasm containing lipid. This cytoplasm stains negatively for mucin.

CYSTS AND DUPLICATIONS

Biology of Disease

■ The vast majority of cysts are congenital in origin. Duplications are always congenital.

■ Most (60%) of these lesions occur in the lower third of the esophagus.

■ The morphologic distinction between a cyst and a duplication is not clear-cut in every case.

Clinical Findings

■ Patients commonly present in childhood with respiratory distress or a feeding problem.

■ A mass in the mediastinum may be discovered, either through investigation of symptoms or incidentally on routine chest radiograph.

■ Bleeding and carcinoma are recognized complications but are exceedingly uncommon.

■ In a majority of patients, there are abnormalities (spina bifida, hemivertebrae) of the dorsal spinal column. These are generally occult, being discovered only radiologically.

Gross Pathology

■ Cysts measure on average 5.0 cm in diameter. They are always attached to the esophagus and protrude into the posterior mediastinum.

■ Duplications may be communicating or noncommunicating.

Microscopic Pathology

■ A duplication is located within the esophageal wall and has two muscle layers in its coating (inner circular and outer longitudinal). The lining epithelium is similar to the types that may occur in the embryologic esophagus.

■ The lining epithelium of both cysts and duplications may be squamous, simple cuboidal-columnar, or ciliated.

■ Cysts are of three major types: bronchogenic, enteric, and retention cysts.

■ Bronchogenic cysts have cartilage in their walls.

■ Enteric cysts may be signified by the presence of gastric mucosa in their lining.

■ Retention cysts (pseudodiverticula) originate from dilated submucosal mucus glands and are lined by a simple mucus-secreting epithelium. Retention cyst is the only type of acquired cyst.

Differential Diagnosis

Diverticula.

Diverticula are acquired lesions that usually occur in adults. They are always communicating, with a large mouth, and are lined by squamous epithelium.

References

Arbona JL, Fazzi JG, Mayoral J. Congenital esophageal cysts: case report and review of the literature. Am J Gastroenterol 1984;79:177–182.

Kaneko E, Kohda A, Honda N, Kino I. Incomplete tubular duplication of the esophagus with heterotopic gastric mucosa. Dig Dis Sci 1989;34:948–951.

Ratan ML, Anand R, Mittal SK, Taneja S. Communicating oesophageal duplication: a report of two cases. Gut 1988;29:254–256.

Salyer DC, Salyer WR, Eggleston JC. Benign developmental cysts of the mediastinum. Arch Pathol Lab Med 1977;101:136–139.

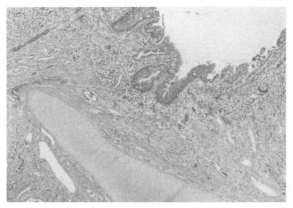

Figure 1–7. Low-power view of an esophageal duplication cyst of bronchogenic type. Note the presence of cartilage.

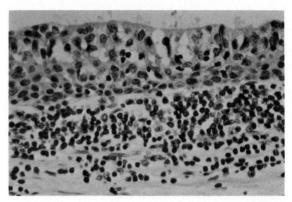

Figure 1–8. Cyst lining showing the presence of a ciliated epithelium.

DIVERTICULA

Biology of Disease

- A diverticulum represents an outpouching of the mucosa through the wall. There are two major types.
- Zenker's diverticulum occurs in the upper esophagus in a posterior or posterolateral location, between the inferior constrictor muscle of the pharynx and the cricopharyngeus. Originally, it was thought to be the result of muscular incoordination in swallowing, but this explanation is now not generally accepted. It is an acquired true diverticulum.
- Middle and lower esophageal diverticula are usually the result of muscular disorders such as achalasia. They may be multiple and large.

Clinical Findings

- Zenker's diverticulum presents with a gurgling sound on swallowing. There may be a mass in the neck.
- Middle and lower esophageal diverticula present with dysphagia.
- All diverticula may result in halitosis and regurgitation of undigested food.

Gross Pathology

- Gross pathology is most easily appreciated on barium examination.
- Both types of diverticula are saccular and have a smooth lining.
- The size is variable, ranging from a few centimeters to a large mass.

Microscopic Pathology

- All esophageal diverticula are lined by squamous epithelium, which may be inflamed or ulcerated when stasis is present.
- Most are true diverticula with the usual bowel wall layers in their coat. With large diverticula, the muscularis propria may be severely attenuated, making it difficult to recognize the normal layers.

Differential Diagnosis

Pseudodiverticulum (retention cyst).

  Pseudodiverticula are multiple, dilated cystic structures originating from dilated ducts of submucosal mucus glands. The etiology of pseudodiverticula is unknown. These lesions are almost always multiple and small. They are located in the esophageal submucosa. Duct openings may be visible radiologically. These openings may narrow the esophageal lumen but do not impinge on the muscularis propria.

References

Castillo S, Aburashad A, Kimmelman J, Alexander LC. Diffuse intramural pseudodiverticulosis: new cases and review. Gastroenterology 1977;72:541–545.

Debas HT, Payne WS, Cameron AJ, Carlson HC. Pathophysiology of lower esophageal diverticulum and its implications for treatment. Surg Gynecol Obstet 1980;151:593–600.

Knuff TE, Benjamin SB, Castell DO. Pharyngeo-esophageal (Zenker's) diverticulum: a reappraisal. Gastroenterology 1982;82:734–736.

Medeiros LJ, Doos WG, Balogh K. Esophageal intramural pseudodiverticulosis: a report of two cases with analysis of similar, less extensive changes in "normal" autopsy esophagi. Hum Pathol 1988;19:928–931.

Umlas J, Sakhuja R. The pathology of esophageal intramural pseudodiverticulosis. Am J Clin Pathol 1976;65:314–320.

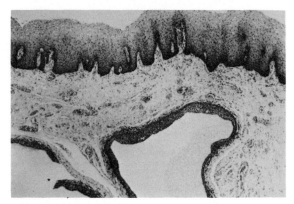

Figure 1–9. Esophageal pseudodiverticulum.

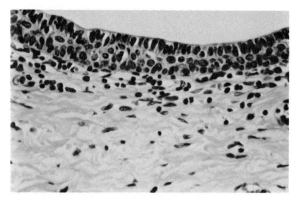

Figure 1–10. Lining of pseudodiverticulum, showing epithelium that resembles the normal mucosal gland duct.

ESOPHAGEAL VARICES

Biology of Disease

■ Almost all varices are secondary to portal hypertension, which in most cases is due to cirrhosis of the liver.
■ The varices are fed by a branch of the left gastric vein and drain into the azygos (systemic) system.
■ Varices involve intramucosal (lamina propria) veins, submucosal veins, perforating veins, and adventitial veins.

Clinical Findings

■ Esophageal varices are generally asymptomatic until bleeding occurs.
■ Most bleeding veins are in the distal 5.0 cm of the esophagus.
■ At endoscopy, bleeding veins are easily identified, but the actual mucosal rupture may be difficult to define.

Gross Pathology

■ At autopsy, the varicose veins collapse and the blood drains once the esophagus is opened.
■ Submucosal and lamina propria veins may be visible through the mucosa as tortuous channels.
■ In life, varicose veins may be so engorged that they occlude the esophageal lumen.

Microscopic Pathology

■ Dilated veins are present in the wall of the esophagus. They may be thick or thin walled.
■ Thrombosis is usually not present unless sclerotherapy has been performed.
■ Often it is difficult to identify the exact point at which bleeding has occurred.

Special Techniques

■ Injection techniques are available but are time consuming and not suitable for routine use.

References

Kitano S, Terblanche J, Kahn D, Bornman PC. Venous anatomy of the lower esophagus in portal hypertension: practical limitations. Br J Surg 1986;73:525–531.

Spence RA, Sloan JM, Johnston GW, Greenfield A. Oesophageal mucosal changes in patients with varices. Gut 1983;24:1024–1029.

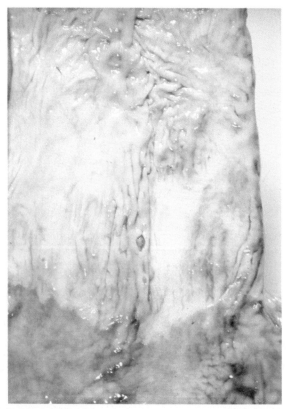

Figure 1–11. Esophageal varices. Note the clear demarcation between gastric and esophageal epithelium. One of the varices has a surface erosion that was considered to be the source of a fatal hemorrhage.

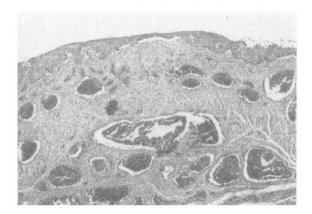

Figure 1–12. Dilated veins located immediately below the esophageal mucosa.

ACHALASIA

Biology of Disease

■ Achalasia should be considered along with two closely related conditions (vigorous achalasia and diffuse esophageal spasm) that probably represent different phases of the same clinicopathologic entity.

■ The clinical and esophageal manometric findings in these three conditions are different, but the pathologies are similar.

■ Classically, achalasia consists of esophageal aperistalsis, incomplete lower esophageal sphincter (LES) relaxation, and increased resting LES pressure.

■ In vigorous achalasia, there are vigorous nonpropagative contractions of the esophagus and noncoordinated relaxation of the LES.

■ In diffuse spasm, there are nonpropagative contractions of the esophagus with normal rhythmic relaxation of the LES.

■ The presumed etiology in all three conditions is an acquired loss of ganglion cells secondary to a ganglionitis that may be virally induced.

■ *Idiopathic hypertrophy* is an asymptomatic enlargement of the lower esophageal sphincter. Descriptions of this condition have been confined to autopsy series. It probably represents part of the spectrum of diffuse spasm—possibly a forme fruste.

Clinical Findings

■ Patients with this group of disorders typically present between ages 20 to 40 years. Sex incidences are equal.

■ Patients with achalasia present with dysphagia and regurgitation of undigested food. It is rarely painful. Barium swallow shows a megaesophagus.

■ Vigorous achalasia and diffuse spasm manifest as substernal pain accompanied by dysphagia. Barium swallow shows a corkscrew esophagus.

■ Patients with achalasia have a risk of developing squamous carcinoma that is 2.5 to 14 times that in the general population.

Gross Pathology

■ The main feature of achalasia is esophageal dilation—sometimes producing megaesophagus. The muscle, particularly the circular layer, may be thickened but can be normal or even thinned. Mucosal inflammation or even ulceration may be present where food is retained.

■ In diffuse spasm, (1) either the esophagus is normal or (2) there is a fusiform thickening, sometimes up to 1 cm, at the lower end of the esophagus.

Microscopic Pathology

■ In achalasia, there is virtually complete loss of ganglion cells in the dilated portion of the esophagus and diminution in number at the site of the LES.

■ The normal esophagus has two types of ganglion cells: argyrophilic cells, whose axons remain with the nerve plexuses, and argyrophobic cells, whose axons innervate smooth muscle fibers. In achalasia, it is the argyrophilic cells that are destroyed.

■ In diffuse spasm, the ganglion cells are mainly preserved, although there may be a ganglionitis consisting of a perigangliar infiltration of lymphocytes.

■ The histologic changes of vigorous achalasia are poorly described.

■ Changes in the muscle (fibrosis) and mucosa (inflammation and ulceration) are secondary.

Differential Diagnosis

Chagas's disease.

The pathologic features of chronic Chagas's disease may be identical to those of achalasia. Parasites are rarely seen within the tissues at this chronic stage, and the diagnosis may have to be inferred from the clinical history and associated clinical findings (travel to or residence in South America and cardiomyopathy).

Special Techniques

■ The silver impregnation methods used to demonstrate argyrophilic and argyrophobic ganglion cells are complex and suitable for research laboratories only.

References

Casella RR, Brown AL, Sayre GP, Ellis FM. Achalasia of the esophagus: pathology and etiologic considerations. Ann Surg 1964;160:474–487.

Castell DO. Achalasia and diffuse esophageal spasm. Arch Intern Med 1976;136:571–579.

Cohen S. Motor disorders of the esophagus. N Engl J Med 1979; 301:184–192.

Deminan SD, Varges-Cortes F. Idiopathic muscular hypertrophy of the esophagus: post-mortem incidental finding in 6 cases and a review of the literature. Chest 1978;73:28–32.

Leonardi HK, Shea JA, Crozier RE, Ellis FH. Diffuse spasm of the esophagus. Clinical, manometric and surgical considerations. J Thorac Cardiovasc Surg 1977;74:736–743.

Smith B. The neurologic lesion of achalasia of the esophagus. Gut 1970;11:388–391.

Vantrappen G, Janssens J, Hellemans J, Coremans G. Achalasia, diffuse spasm and related motility disorders. Gastroenterology 1979;76: 450–457.

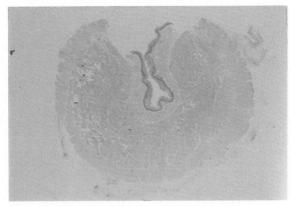

Figure 1–14. Diffuse spasm of the esophagus showing a marked muscular thickening at the lower end.

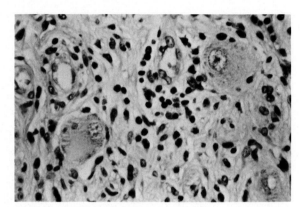

Figure 1–15. Ganglionitis, characteristic of diffuse spasm.

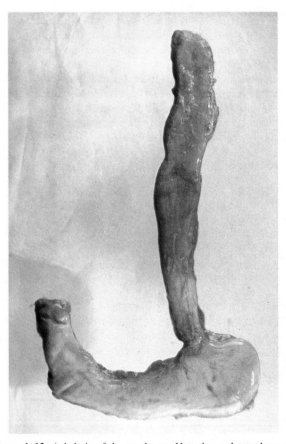

Figure 1–13. Achalasia of the esophagus. Note the moderate degree of proximal dilatation in this individual, who died of unrelated causes.

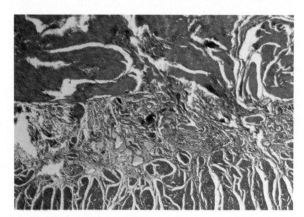

Figure 1–16. Scarring of the muscle in a case of diffuse spasm (Trichrome).

REFLUX ESOPHAGITIS

Biology of Disease

- Reflux esophagitis is inflammation due to the reflux of stomach contents, particularly acid into the esophagus.
- Factors promoting reflux esophagitis include defects of lower esophageal sphincter, diminished esophageal peristalsis leading to reduced clearance, and impaired esophageal mucosal resistance.
- A certain amount of reflux is considered normal, and there is no clear-cut point at which normal reflux becomes abnormal. Symptomatology is not always a reliable indicator of significant reflux.

Clinical Findings

- There is a considerable range of severity of reflux, with a corresponding variation in extent of symptomatology.
- Symptoms include dysphagia, regurgitation, and chest pain (sometimes mimicking cardiac pain).
- Complications include aspiration pneumonia, Barrett's esophagus, and peptic ulceration, leading to bleeding or stricture formation.
- A number of tests are available to assess the presence of reflux. The most reliable of these is endoscopic examination.

Gross Pathology

- In up to 30% of cases, the mucosa may look normal at endoscopy.
- Mucosal erythema and friability are common but are subjective criteria.
- The only reliable criterion for the gross diagnosis of reflux is the presence of erosions, ulcers, or strictures.

Microscopic Pathology

- Epithelial hyperplasia, in the form of basal cell hyperplasia and elongated epithelial papillae, is present in 80% or more of patients. Basal cell hyperplasia is present when the basal cells exceed 15% of the mucosal thickness. The papillae are taller than the normal 60% of the mucosal thickness.
- Infiltration of the squamous epithelium by neutrophils or eosinophils is present in 20 to 50% of cases.
- Dilated vessels may be present in the lamina propria; this, however, is a subjective finding.
- In more severe disease, erosions or ulcers are present. An *erosion* is an epithelial defect that does not penetrate the full thickness of the mucosa. Disease of this severity is usually accompanied by a heavy infiltrate of chronic inflammatory cells in the submucosa. A marked degree of reactive epithelial hyperplasia may be present at the edge of an ulcer; it may be hard to distinguish from squamous carcinoma. In problem cases, the patient should be treated with antacids, and a biopsy should be repeated.
- The end result of chronic ulceration is stricture formation. The situation is analogous to pyloric stenosis complicating duodenal ulceration.

Differential Diagnosis

Esophageal candidiasis, herpes.

In candidiasis, there may be intense neutrophilic infiltration of the epithelium. Spores and hyphae are usually identifiable on hematoxylin & eosin (H&E) sections, but occasionally can be sparse. Periodic acid–Schiff (PAS) or silver stains should be used routinely if there is a clinical suspicion of candidal infection.

In herpes esophagitis, the epithelium is inflamed, and erosions may be present. Infected squamous cells typically may have multilobulated nuclei with a ground-glass appearance.

References

Brown LF, Goldman H, Antonioli DA. Intraepithelial eosinophils in endoscopic biopsies of adults with reflux esophagitis. Am J Surg Pathol 1984;8:899–905.
Collins BJ, Elliott H, Sloan JM, McFarland RS, Love AH. Oesophageal histology in reflux oesophagitis. J Clin Pathol 1985;38:1265–1272.
Eastwood GL. Histologic changes in gastroesophageal reflux. J Clin Gastroenterol 1986;8:45–51.
Ismail-Beigi F, Pope CE. Distribution of the histological changes of esophageal reflux in the distal esophagus of man. Gastroenterology 1974;66:1109–1113.
Ismail-Beigi F, Horton PF, Pope CE. Histological consequences of gastroesophageal reflux in man. Gastroenterology 1970;58:163–174.
Lee RG. Marked eosinophilia in esophageal mucosal biopsies. Am J Surg Pathol 1985;9:475–479.
Wesdorp IC. Reflux esophagitis: a review. Postgrad J Med 1986;62:43–55.
Winter HS, Madara JL, Stafford RJ, et al. Intraepithelial eosinophils: a new diagnostic criterion for reflux esophagitis. Gastroenterology 1982;83:818–823.

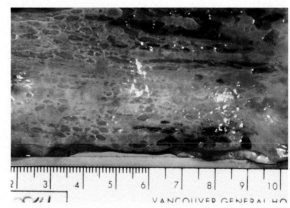

Figure 1–17. Multiple esophageal erosions from a case of persistent severe reflux.

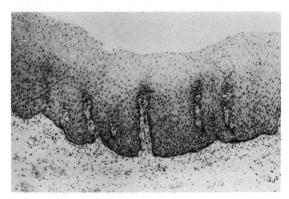

Figure 1–18. Mild reflux, identified only on the presence of basal cell hyperplasia.

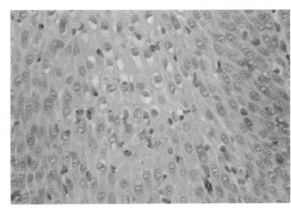

Figure 1–21. Eosinophils in mucosa.

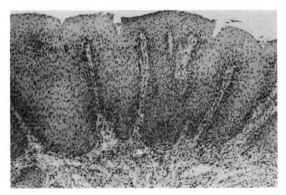

Figure 1–19. Moderately severe reflux showing elongation of papillae, basal cell hyperplasia, and an inflammatory infiltrate.

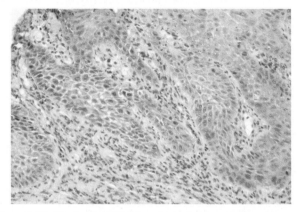

Figure 1–22. Basal cell proliferation of a marked degree adjacent to an ulcer. This is an example of pseudoepitheliomatous hyperplasia.

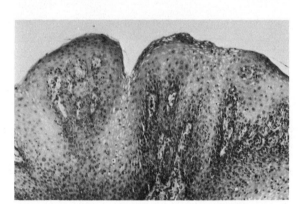

Figure 1–20. Many esophageal biopsies may not be perfectly oriented, but even in this example, the elongation of papillae is apparent.

BARRETT'S ESOPHAGUS

Biology of Disease

- *Barrett's esophagus* may be defined as the presence of metaplastic glandular epithelium above the normal squamocolumnar junction.
- The normal squamocolumnar junction is never more than 2.5 cm proximal to the point at which the tubular esophagus becomes the saccular stomach.
- Barrett's esophagus is due to reflux of gastric contents, which may be promoted by smoking and by excessive consumption of alcohol.
- As measured in an autopsy series of unselected cases, the prevalence of Barrett's esophagus is 0.49%. In patients with symptoms of reflux, the prevalence is between 8% and 20%; in patients with a peptic stricture, it is 40%.
- The incidence of adenocarcinoma in Barrett's esophagus is between 1 in 81 and 1 in 440 cases per person years (30- to 40-fold above the general population)

Clinical Findings

- Many cases are asymptomatic.
- The symptoms may be the same as for patients who have reflux not complicated by Barrett's esophagus: heartburn, regurgitation, and dysphagia.
- Endoscopically, Barrett's esophagus must be distinguished from a sliding hiatus hernia.
- At endoscopy, the squamocolumnar junction is more irregular than usual, frequently with islands of squamous epithelium surrounded by glandular epithelium.

Gross Pathology

- The squamocolumnar junction is displaced proximally at least 2.5 cm from the anatomic gastroesophageal junction.
- There is greater irregularity of the squamocolumnar junction, often with islands of one type of mucosa surrounded by another type.

Microscopic Pathology

- Specialized (intestinal metaplastic) epithelium is the hallmark of Barrett's esophagus. It is present in the proximal esophagus. Mucosa resembling normal cardiac and fundic gastric mucosa may be found in the distal esophagus in 50% of cases. Without the presence of specialized epithelium, however, a diagnosis of Barrett's esophagus should be made with caution, because of possible confusion with a sliding hiatus hernia.
- Specialized mucosa consists of a simplified crypt-bearing mucosa. Primitive intervening villi may be present. Glands are usually not prominent, although there may be occasional mucus-secreting glands.
- The epithelium consists of a mixture of columnar cells and goblet cells. The columnar cells may resemble either gastric surface epithelial cells or small intestinal absorptive cells with a brush border. The goblet cells resemble those of the large and small bowel.
- Inflammation is a variable feature. It may be active (neu-

trophils infiltrating the epithelium) or chronic (lymphocytes and plasma cells within the lamina propria).
- The criteria for the diagnosis of dysplasia in Barrett's mucosa are similar to those for gastric dysplasia.
- The concept of "short-segment Barrett's esophagus" has been advanced. In these cases, specialized mucosa is confined to a 3-cm zone above the lower end of the esophagus. This lesion can best be demonstrated histologically, by showing the presence of epithelial cells containing acid mucin. It may be presumed that short-segment Barrett's esophagus is also premalignant and accounts for some cases of adenocarcinoma arising in the lower esophagus and gastric cardia.

Special Techniques

- Some authorities recommend the use of an Alcian blue stain (pH 2.5), either alone or in combination with H&E. This method stains acidic mucins and helps to highlight the presence of goblet cells. Acidic mucin may be present in columnar cells also, representing a form of incomplete metaplasia (see Chapter 2).

References

Cameron AJ, Ott BJ, Payne WS. The incidence of adenocarcinoma in columnar lined (Barrett's) esophagus. N Engl J Med 1985;313:857–859.
Cameron AJ, Zinsmeister AR, Ballard DJ, Carney JA. Prevalence of columnar lined (Barrett's) esophagus. Gastroenterology 1990;99:918–922.
Hamilton SR, Smith RR. The relationship between columnar epithelial dysplasia and invasive adenocarcinoma arising in Barrett's esophagus. Am J Clin Pathol 1987;87:301–312.
Paull A, Trier JS, Dalton MD, et al. The histologic spectrum of Barrett's esophagus. N Engl J Med 1976;295:476–480.
Rothery GA, Patterson JE, Stoddard CJ, Day DW. Histological and histochemical changes in the columnar lined (Barrett's) esophagus. Gut 1986;27:1062–1068.
Spechler SJ, Goyal RK. Barrett's esophagus. N Engl J Med 1986;315:362–371.
Spechler SJ, Robbins AH, Rubins HB, et al. Adenocarcinoma and Barrett's esophagus: an overrated risk. Gastroenterology 1984;87:927–933.
Spechler SJ, Sperber H, Doos WG, Schimmel EM. The prevalence of Barrett's esophagus in patients with chronic peptic esophageal strictures. Dig Dis Sci 1983;28:769–774.
Weinstein W, Marin-Sorensen K, Lewin K, et al. Short segment Barrett's esophagus and cardiac mucosa in gastro-esophageal reflux disease have a similar prevalence of specialized epithelium. Gastroenterology 1991;100:A72.
Winters C, Sparling TJ, Chobanian SJ, et al. Barrett's esophagus: a prevalent, occult complication of gastro-esophageal reflux disease. Gastroenterology 1987;92:118–124.

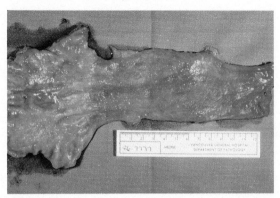

Figure 1–23. Barrett's esophagus. The site of the normal squamocolumnar junction is evident, but columnar epithelium now extends proximally for several centimeters.

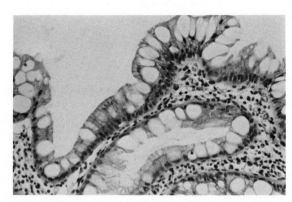

Figure 1–25. Barrett's esophagus, showing complete intestinalization without inflammation.

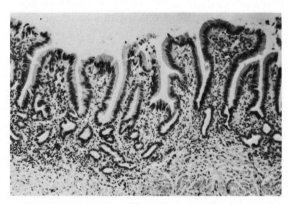

Figure 1–24. Low-power view of Barrett's mucosa, showing an early papillary appearance.

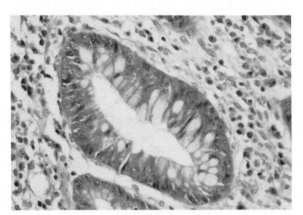

Figure 1–26. Regenerative changes at the base of a crypt. This is not dysplasia. This change is confined to the crypt, and the epithelium becomes less reactive in appearance as it matures toward the surface.

SQUAMOUS PAPILLOMA

Biology of Disease

- Squamous papilloma is a rare lesion, usually occurring in the mid-esophagus.
- It is most common in infants and young children.
- In the majority of cases, there is a direct or presumptive relationship with human papillomavirus (HPV) infection.

Clinical Findings

- Squamous papillomas are often multiple and may also involve the larynx and trachea.
- They usually manifest as an incidental finding, although larger examples can produce dysphagia.
- Spontaneous resolution is not uncommon.

Gross Pathology

- Lesion size varies from a few millimeters to 1.5 cm.
- Endoscopically, squamous papillomas appear as pale, broad-based excrescences.

Microscopic Pathology

- Squamous papillomas have a fibrovascular core of lamina propria.
- The overlying epithelium is hyperplastic but nondysplastic and nonkeratinizing.
- Koilocytes may or may not be present.

Special Techniques

- HPV can be demonstrated in some cases by immunostaining.

References

Colina F, Solis JA, Munoz MT. Squamous papilloma of the esophagus; report of three cases and a review of the literature. Am J Gastroenterol 1980;74:410–414.

Javdan P, Pitman ER. Squamous papilloma of esophagus. Dig Dis Sci 1984;29:317–320.

Politoske EJ. Squamous papilloma of the esophagus associated with human papilloma virus. Gastroenterology 1991;102:668–673.

Quitadamo M, Benson J. Squamous papilloma of the esophagus. A case report and review of the literature. Am J Gastroenterol 1988;83:194–201.

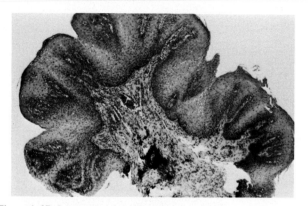

Figure 1–27. Low-power view of squamous papilloma.

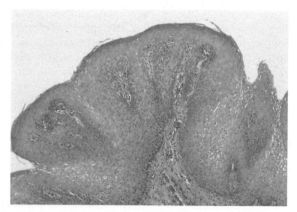

Figure 1–28. At high power, the epithelium is hyperplastic but fully mature. Koilocytes are not present in this example.

SQUAMOUS CELL CARCINOMA

Biology of Disease

■ Squamous cell carcinoma accounts for 90% of all esophageal malignancies.
■ In North America, the incidence is approximately 10 per 100,000 per year.
■ Squamous cell carcinoma is most common in individuals over 50 years of age, and the ratio of males to females is 6:1.
■ The associated etiologic factors include smoking, alcohol consumption, and geographic variables. High-incidence areas include northern China, Iran, and parts of South Africa, where the incidence may reach 200 per 100,000 per year.
■ For epidemiologic and clinical purposes, squamous cell carcinoma may be divided into tumors involving the upper, middle, and lower thirds of the esophagus.
■ Cancer of the upper esophagus is rare (5% of all squamous cell carcinomas) and is much more common in women. It has been associated with Plummer-Vinson syndrome (esophageal webs).

Clinical Findings

■ The major symptom is dysphagia, which is often accompanied by anorexia and weight loss.
■ The radiologic and endoscopic appearances vary. In half the cases, there is a circumferential stricture with a smooth surface, which is sometimes difficult to separate from a benign stricture. The remaining cases are characterized by an exophytic lesion.
■ Multiple tumors may be encountered in 15% of patients.

Gross Pathology

■ In the early stages of the disease, some patients may have a completely flat lesion, and the biopsy histology may show various grades of dysplasia or carcinoma in situ. Microinvasion may be difficult to demonstrate.
■ Most tumors are advanced at the time of diagnosis, and manifest as strictures, fungating growths, polyps, or ulcers.

Microscopic Pathology

■ Most squamous cell carcinomas are moderately differentiated and show identifiable early keratinization and/or desmosomes. Many cells have a clear cytoplasm owing to the presence of glycogen.
■ Poorly differentiated squamous cell carcinomas may be hard to distinguish from poorly differentiated adenocarcinomas.
■ Spindle cell carcinoma is a variant of squamous cell carcinoma that typically has a polypoid appearance and histologically shows either a pure spindle cell component (pseudosarcoma) or mixed spindle and epithelial (carcinosarcoma) components.
■ Invasive tumors in which the neoplasm is confined to the lamina propria and submucosa are referred to as *superficial* carcinomas; they have a 5-year survival rate of more than 60%.
■ Verrucous carcinoma is another rare histologic variant. This tumor is papillary and is exceedingly well differentiated. Initially, it shows superficial invasion with mild atypia, which is usually confined to the basal layer.

Differential Diagnosis

Regenerative changes.
Regenerative changes may take the form of pseudoepitheliomatous hyperplasia, in which long tongues of nondysplastic epithelium extend down to the deep margin of the biopsy specimen. The cells are regular but have enlarged nuclei. Maturation proceeds normally.

Regeneration may also produce basal cell hyperplasia. On low-power magnification, this may appear worrisome. High power, examination, however, shows no dysplasia.

Most examples of regenerative change mimicking carcinoma occur in the presence of severe inflammation, usually at the edges of ulcers. In cases in which the differential diagnosis is difficult, the biopsy may be repeated after a course of antiulcer therapy.

References

Bogomoletz WV, Molas G, Gaget B, Potet F. Superficial squamous carcinoma of the esophagus: a report of 76 cases and review of the literature. Am J Surg Pathol 1989;13:535–546.

Du Boulay CE, Isaacson P. Carcinoma of the oesophagus with spindle cell features. Histopathology 1981;5:403–414.

Kahajda FP, Sun TT, Mendelsohn G. Polypoid squamous carcinoma of the esophagus. Am J Surg Pathol 1983;7:495–499.

Minelly JA, Harrison EG, Fontana RS, Payne WS. Verrucous squamous cell carcinoma of the esophagus. Cancer 1967;20:2078–2087.

Norton GA, Postlethwaite RW, Thompson WM. Esophageal carcinoma: a survey of populations at risk. South Med J 1980;73:25–27.

Osamura RY, Shinamura K, Hata J, et al. Polypoid carcinoma of the esophagus. A unifying term for "carcinosarcoma" and "pseudosarcoma." Am J Surg Pathol 1978;2:201–208.

Schmidt LW, Dean PJ, Wilson RT. Superficially invasive squamous cell carcinoma of the esophagus. Gastroenterology 1987;91:1456–1461.

Wynder EL, Bross IJ. A study of etiological factors in cancer of the esophagus. Cancer 1961;14:389–413.

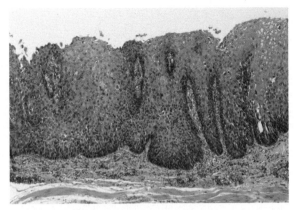

Figure 1–31. Squamous cell carcinoma in situ.

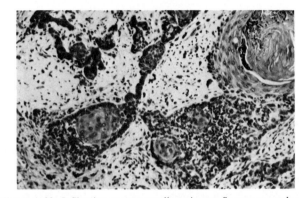

Figure 1–32. Infiltrating squamous cell carcinoma. Squamous pearls can be identified in the centers of the epithelial islands.

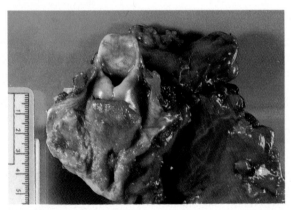

Figure 1–29. Postcricoid squamous cell carcinoma.

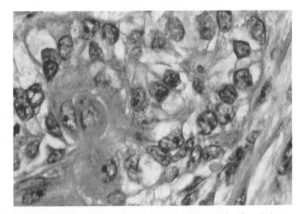

Figure 1–33. Clear cell areas are not uncommonly found in many esophageal squamous carcinomas.

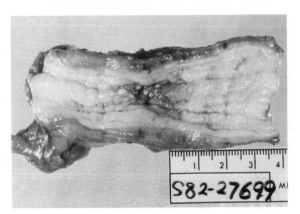

Figure 1–30. Ulcerated carcinoma of mid-esophagus.

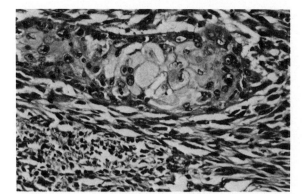

Figure 1–34. Squamous cell carcinoma with spindle cell areas (so-called carcinosarcoma).

ADENOCARCINOMA

Biology of Disease

- The vast majority of esophageal adenocarcinomas arise in Barrett's esophagus (probably greater than 95%). A small minority arise in the ducts or acini of submucosal glands.
- Adenocarcinoma constitutes approximately 10% of esophageal neoplasms.
- Adenocarcinoma of the esophagus shares clinical, epidemiologic, and possibly etiologic features with adenocarcinoma of the gastric cardia.
- In many cases, a carcinoma develops in preexisting patches of dysplasia.
- The disease affects patients of all ages, but predominately individuals 60 years or more. Male preponderance is marked (ratio 3:1). The condition is uncommon in blacks.

Clinical Findings

- The symptoms may not be materially different from Barrett's esophagus without a carcinoma.
- Some patients have no history suggestive of preexisting Barrett's esophagus.
- The endoscopic findings are virtually indistinguishable from those of squamous cell carcinoma and carcinoma of the gastric cardia.

Gross Pathology

- Adenocarcinoma is similar to squamous cell carcinoma in most respects.
- Lesions may be exophytic, ulcerated, or cause a stricture.
- If the tumor reaches a large size, determining whether it has arisen in the esophagus or stomach may be impossible.
- If Barrett's esophagus is extensive, it may be seen alongside the tumor.

Microscopic Pathology

- Adenocarcinoma of the esophagus is virtually identical to gastric cardiac cancer.
- Usually, the tumor is a gland-forming, moderately or poorly differentiated intestinal adenocarcinoma.
- Diffuse cancer (signet-ring type) is uncommon.
- Occasional tumors may have glandular and squamous differentiation.
- Carcinomas arising from submucosal glands are usually well differentiated and may have mucoepidermoid or adenoid cystic features.

Differential Diagnosis

Dysplasia, trapped glands.

Severe dysplasia and early invasive carcinoma can be difficult to separate on small biopsy specimens. If doubt persists, repeat biopsy is indicated. The principle of this distinction lies in the presence of invasion of the lamina propria or submucosa. Such invasion is recognized by finding glandular budding and irregularity with infiltration of the muscularis mucosae.

Trapped glands in the esophagus are analogous to colitis cystica profunda (see Chapter 5).

References

Bosch A, Frais Z, Caldwell WL. Adenocarcinoma of the esophagus. Cancer 1979;43:1557–1561.

De Baecque C, Potet F, Molas G, et al. Superficial adenocarcinoma of the esophagus arising in Barrett's mucosa with dysplasia: a clinicopathologic study of 12 patients. Histopathology 1990;16:213–220.

Kalish RJ, Clancy PE, Orringer MB, Appelman HD. Clinical, epidemiologic and morphologic comparison between carcinomas arising in Barrett's esophageal mucosa and in the gastric cardia. Gastroenterology 1984;86:461–467.

MacDonald WC, MacDonald JB. Adenocarcinoma of the esophagus and/or gastric cardia. Cancer 1987;60:1094–1098.

Smith RR, Hamilton SR, Boitnott JK, Rodgers EL. The spectrum of carcinoma arising in Barrett's esophagus. Am J Surg Pathol 1984; 8:563–573.

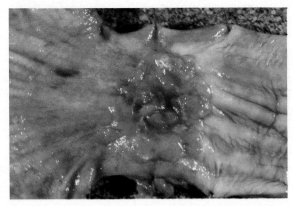

Figure 1–35. Adenocarcinoma of the esophagus arising in a relatively short segment of Barrett's mucosa.

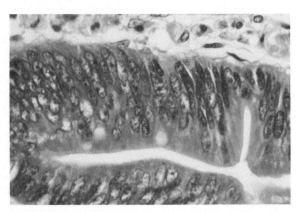

Figure 1–38. Severe dysplasia. Note the nuclear crowding and pseudostratification.

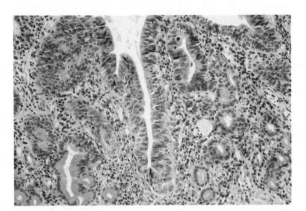

Figure 1–36. Dysplasia in Barrett's esophagus. Note that the atypical epithelium extends to the mucosal surface.

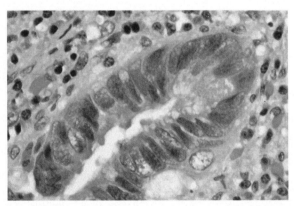

Figure 1–39. Severe dysplasia. Typically, dysplastic epithelium is non–mucus-secreting.

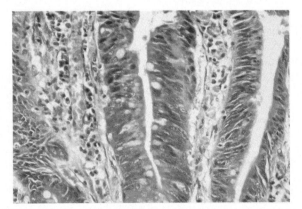

Figure 1–37. Severe dysplasia.

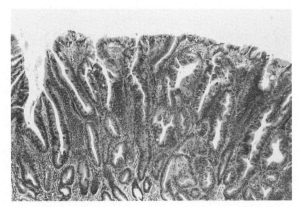

Figure 1–40. Intramucosal adenocarcinoma. The gland crowding and architectural complexity indicate early invasion of the lamina propria.

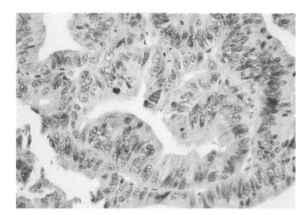

Figure 1–41. Well-differentiated adenocarcinoma.

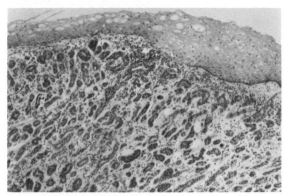

Figure 1–43. Adenocarcinoma of esophageal gland origin infiltrating beneath intact squamous epithelium.

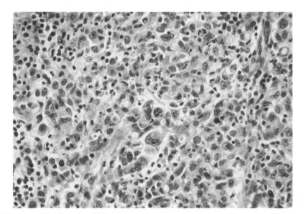

Figure 1–42. Poorly differentiated adenocarcinoma.

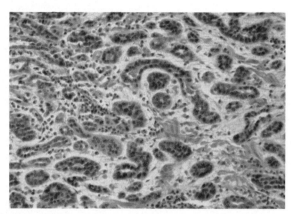

Figure 1–44. Well-differentiated esophageal gland adenocarcinoma.

CHAPTER 2

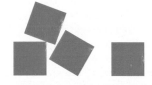

DISEASES
OF THE
STOMACH

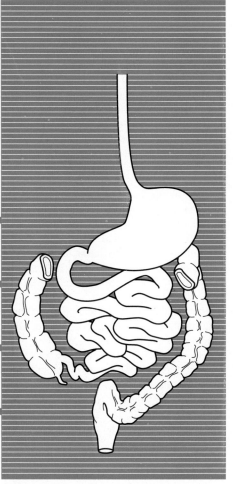

NORMAL APPEARANCES

Gross Anatomy

■ Three zones are recognized: cardia, fundus (also called corpus or body), and antrum. These are not fixed by rigid anatomical landmarks, and their extent varies between individuals and with age.

■ The cardia is a small ill-defined zone lying just distal to the lower end of the esophagus.

■ The antrum comprises the distal third of the stomach proximal to the pylorus.

■ The remainder of the stomach is termed the fundus.

■ Mucosal folds, called rugae, are present when the stomach is empty but are flattened out when it is full of food.

■ The gastric incisura is not a landmark that can be identified at autopsy or in surgically resected stomachs.

Microscopic Appearances

■ The mucosa is divided into pits and glands. The glands are coiled and empty into the base of the pits.

■ Throughout the stomach, the surface and the pit-lining epithelium are identical, consisting of a single layer of tall columnar cells with basal nuclei and cytoplasm that on its luminal aspect is stuffed with multiple small mucous vacuoles. This neutral mucin is PAS positive and Alcian blue negative.

■ The glands vary in different parts of the stomach. The histologic zones are similar to, but not identical to, the gross anatomic zones.

■ The pyloric gland zone differs slightly from the gross antrum and extends more proximally along the lesser curvature than it does along the greater curvature.

■ In the cardiac and pyloric gland zones, the glands are loosely packed. They are mucus secreting and occupy about one half of the mucosal thickness.

■ In the fundic gland zone, the glands are tightly packed and occupy about three quarters of the mucosal thickness. The base of the glands contains mainly chief cells, which stain bluish-gray on H&E sections. The isthmic portion of the glands contains mainly parietal cells, which are brightly eosinophilic on H&E sections. The neck portion of the glands contains a mixture of chief and parietal cells together with a third type, the mucus neck cells. It is the mucus neck cells that act as stem cells and are responsible for mucosal regeneration. They contain a mixture of neutral and acid mucins.

■ The lamina propria contains a fine meshwork of reticulin fibers that provide structural support for the mucosa. It also contains small numbers of fibroblasts, histiocytes, plasma cells, and lymphocytes.

■ Endocrine cells are present within the gastric glands and at the base of the pits. The granules are located between the nucleus and the basement membrane. In the antrum, 50% of endocrine cells secrete gastrin, 30% are enterochromaffin (serotonin secreting), and 15% secrete somatostatin. In the fundic mucosa, the majority are enterochromaffin-like (ECL) cells (histamine secreting). Of these, only the enterochromaffin cells are argentaffin positive. All the cells, however, are positive with argyrophil stains (Grimelius) and with immunostains for chromogranin.

Biopsy Artifacts

■ Crush artifact may result in an apparent focal hypercellularity of the lamina propria, simulating a cellular infiltrate.

■ Crush artifact may herniate epithelial cells into the pit lumina.

■ Stretching artifact may produce a spurious appearance of mucosal edema.

■ Pools of blood in the lamina propria, occurring in patients without vascular abnormality, are usually a biopsy artifact.

References

Owen DA. Normal histology of the stomach. Am J Surg Pathol 1986;10:48–61.

Rubin W, Ross LL, Sleisenger MH, Jeffries GH. The normal human gastric epithelia. A fine ultrastructural study. Lab Invest 1968;19:598–626.

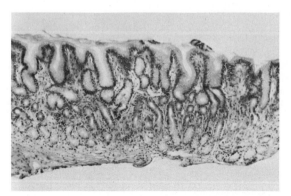

Figure 2–1. Low-power view of gastric antrum. Note that the glands are loosely packed and that the pits occupy about half of the mucosal thickness.

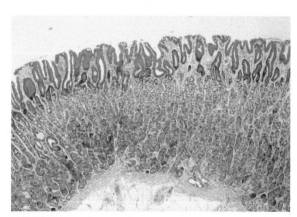

Figure 2–2. Fundic mucosa. The glands are tightly packed and the pits are short.

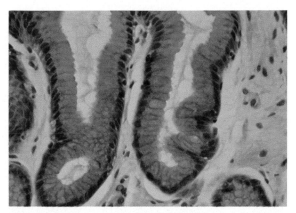

Figure 2–3. The gastric pits and surface are lined by a tall, columnar, mucus-secreting epithelium.

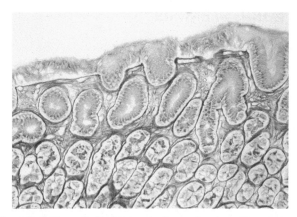

Figure 2–6. Fine reticulin framework of normal, nonatrophic mucosa.

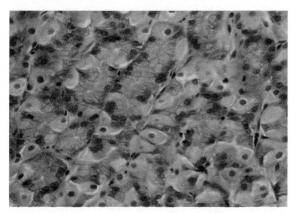

Figure 2–4. The fundic glands contain chief cells (purplish cytoplasm) and parietal cells (pinkish cytoplasm).

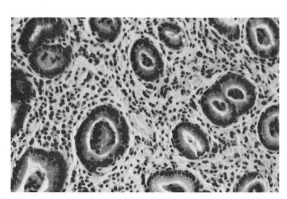

Figure 2–7. Crush artifact in gastric mucosa. The telescoping of mucosa into pits is commonly observed.

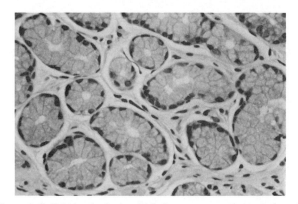

Figure 2–5. Pyloric glands, in which the mucus-secreting cytoplasm is bubbly in appearance.

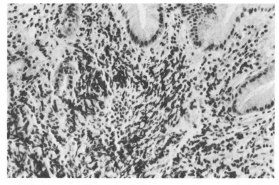

Figure 2–8. Crush artifact giving a spurious appearance of hypercellularity.

PYLORIC STENOSIS

Biology of Disease

- This is predominately a disease of infants, although rarely adults may be affected.
- Pyloric stenosis mainly affects males.
- It has a high familial incidence.
- The cause is unknown but the underlying abnormality is hypertrophy of the pyloric muscle mass which develops shortly after birth.
- It has recently been postulated that a lack of nitric oxide synthase in pyloric muscle tissue is responsible for pylorospasm.
- Pyloric stenosis has been associated with prostaglandin therapy in neonates.
- Adult pyloric stenosis may be due to persistence of an abnormality that has been present since infancy.
- No abnormality of nerves or ganglia is present.
- If untreated, death may occur due to persistent vomiting and dehydration.

Clinical Features

- Particularly in infants, projectile vomiting may occur.
- A firm, 2- to 3-cm epigastric mass may be palpated.
- Epigastric peristaltic waves may be observed.

Gross Pathology

- In childhood cases, the mass is a fusiform swelling at the pylorus. It has an abrupt distal termination and looks pale on cross-section.
- In adults, the swelling may be fusiform as in children, but can also be focal or multinodular.

Microscopic Pathology

- The lesion mainly involves the circular layer of the muscularis propria as an irregular hypertrophy of fibers.
- Increased fibrous tissue may be present between the muscle fibers.
- The surface mucosa may be inflamed and ulcerated.
- A light lymphocytic infiltrate may be present in the main lesion.

Differential Diagnosis

Leiomyoma, pyloric stenosis secondary to pyloric peptic ulcer.

Leiomyomas are sharply circumscribed lesions that are eccentrically (not circumferentially) located in relation to the pylorus.

Stenosis secondary to peptic ulceration is characterized by proliferation of scar tissue with only a minor increase in smooth muscle. There is usually no distinct mass.

References

Benson DC. Infantile pyloric stenosis. Prog Pediatr Surg 1970;1:63–89.

Peled N, Dagan O, Babyn P, et al. Gastric outlet obstruction induced by prostaglandin therapy in neonates. N Engl J Med 1992;327:505–510.

Spicer RD. Infantile hypertrophic pyloric stenosis: a review. Br J Surg 1982;69:128–135.

Wellman IKF, Kagan A, Fang H. Hypertrophic pyloric stenosis in adults. Survey of the literature and report of a case of the localized form. Gastroenterology 1964;46:601–608.

Vanderwinden J-M, Mailleux P, Schiffman SN, Vanderhaeghen J-J, et al. Nitric oxide synthase activity in infantile hypertrophic pyloric stenosis. N Engl J Med 1992;327:511–515.

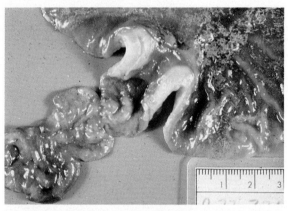

Figure 2–9. Neonatal pyloric stenosis. Note the marked thickening of the muscle, which is producing a narrowed canal. (Courtesy of Intellipath Inc., Santa Monica, CA.)

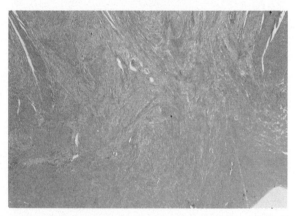

Figure 2–10. Adult pyloric stenosis. There is hypertrophy of the fibers with muscle bundles running in various directions.

XANTHELASMA (XANTHOMA, LIPID ISLAND)

Biology of Disease

- These lesions are present in up to 50% of stomachs at autopsy and in 4% of endoscopic biopsy specimens.
- They consist of aggregates of foam cells containing neutral fat and cholesterol.
- There is no relationship with any type of hyperlipidemia.
- In most instances, the cause is unknown and they are not related to chronic gastritis.
- They occur more frequently in situations in which there is increased bile reflux into the stomach.
- In occasional cases, there is an association with cholestasis. The xanthelasmas may disappear when the cholestasis is relieved.

Clinical Features

- Xanthelasmas are an incidental finding at gastroscopy, where they appear as yellowish nodules. They are asymptomatic.

Gross Pathology

- They occur mainly along the lesser curvature.
- Endoscopically, they appear as cream colored plaques, usually less than 5 mm in diameter.
- They may be multiple.

Microscopic Pathology

- The lesions consist of a loosely organized aggregate of foamy histiocytes in the superficial lamina propria.
- The nuclei are bland.
- Associated nonspecific inflammation may be present if there is a coincidental *Helicobacter pylori* infection.

Differential Diagnosis

Diffuse adenocarcinoma, Whipple's disease, *Mycobacterium avium-intracellulare* infection.

In all these diseases, the clear cytoplasm is due to the presence of Diastase/PAS-positive material. In xanthelasma, the cytoplasm is not positive with this stain.

In diffuse adenocarcinoma, the nuclei may appear cytologically bland but are usually much larger than in xanthelasmas.

References

Coates AG, Nostrant TT, Wilson JA, et al. Gastric xanthomatosis and cholestasis: a causal relationship. Dig Dis Sci 1986;31:925–928.

Domellof L, Eriksson S, Helander HF, Janvger KG. Lipid islands in the gastric mucosa after resection for benign ulcer disease. Gastroenterology 1977;72:14–18.

Kimura K, Hiramoto T, Buncher CR. Gastric xanthelasma. Arch Pathol 1969;87:110–117.

Pieterse AS, Rowland R, Labrooy JT. Gastric xanthomas. Pathology 1985;17:455–457.

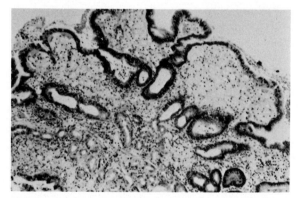

Figure 2–11. Xanthoma showing marked expansion of the lamina propria by foam cells.

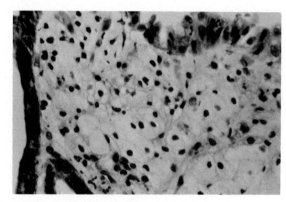

Figure 2–12. Foam cells with bland nuclear features.

GASTRIC ANTRAL VASCULAR ECTASIA

Biology of Disease

- Gastric antral vascular ectasia (GAVE) is an acquired abnormality of the antral gastric mucosa, typically affecting elderly women.
- Some cases may be related to mucosal trauma or prolapse, but in most instances the cause is unknown.
- The basic abnormality is dilatation and bleeding of superficial mucosal capillaries.

Clinical Features

- Iron deficiency anemia due to chronic bleeding is the most common presentation.
- Rarely massive bleeding requiring transfusion may occur.
- Endoscopically, the typical appearance is of linear broad erythematous stripes traversing the antral mucosa. This appearance has been termed *watermelon stomach*.

Gross Pathology

■ Usually, there is no obvious gross abnormality seen on antral resection specimens because any dilated vessels collapse when transected.

Microscopic Pathology

■ Dilated capillaries are present in the superficial lamina propria immediately below the surface epithelium. These changes are often subtle and are difficult to distinguish from normal capillaries, which may also appear engorged with blood.
■ The capillaries are usually larger in diameter than normal lamina propria capillaries.
■ The capillaries may contain fibrin thrombi.
■ There may be fibromuscular hyperplasia of the lamina propria.

Differential Diagnosis

Osler-Weber-Rendu (OWR) disease, arteriovenous malformations, vascular ectasia secondary to portal hypertension, normal dilated congested capillaries.

The endoscopic appearance of GAVE (linear erythema radiating from the pylorus) is characteristic. Other ectasias are in the form of circular patches.

In OWR disease, telangiectasias are present in the mouth and on the face.

Portal hypertension produces lesions in the gastric fundus, rather than the antrum.

Arteriovenous malformations usually involve larger caliber vessels than GAVE.

GAVE has a characteristic associated fibromuscular hyperplasia of the lamina propria.

Capillaries in GAVE are larger than those found in normal gastric mucosal biopsy specimens.

References

Jabbari M, Cherry R, Lough JO, et al. Gastric antral vascular ectasia: the watermelon stomach. Gastroenterology 1984;87:1165–1170.

Quintero E, Pique JM, Bombi JA, et al. Gastric mucosal vascular ectasias causing bleeding in cirrhosis. Gastroenterology 1987;93:1054–1061.

Suit PF, Petras RE, Bauer TW, Petrini JL. Gastric antral vascular ectasia. A histologic and morphometric study of "the watermelon stomach." Am J Surg Pathol 1987;11:750–757.

Vase P, Grove O. Gastrointestinal lesions in hereditary hemorrhagic telangiectasia. Gastroenterology 1986;91:1079–1083.

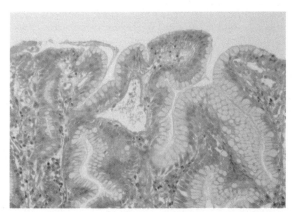

Figure 2–13. Dilated vessel in the superficial lamina propria. Normal mucosa does not have vessels of this caliber located so superficially.

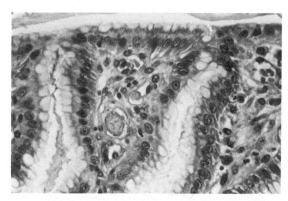

Figure 2–15. Fibrin thrombus in a superficial capillary.

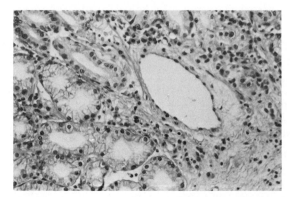

Figure 2–14. Large-caliber, thin-walled vessel in the lower portion of the mucosa.

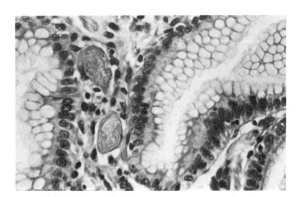

Figure 2–16. Prominent fibrin thrombi.

ACUTE EROSIVE GASTRITIS

Biology of Disease

- This is a relatively common cause of upper gastrointestinal (GI) bleeding that can occur in patients of all ages.
- It develops as a result of damage to the gastric mucosal barrier, which produces back diffusion of gastric acid into the mucosa.
- The causes include alcohol, nonsteroidal anti-inflammatory drugs (NSAIDs), and stress (shock, sepsis, and hypoxia).
- In some cases focal erosions may be secondary to the presence of nasogastric tubes.
- An erosion is defined as a superficial ulcer that involves only part of the mucosal thickness and has not penetrated more deeply than the muscularis mucosae.
- Because the damage is acute and superficial, it may heal rapidly, with complete restoration of the normal mucosal architecture.

Clinical Features

- This condition may have a variable extent and severity.
- Mild forms can be confined to a small number of localized erosions that are asymptomatic and discovered incidentally.
- Severe forms of the disease are accompanied by widespread intense hemorrhage into the lamina propria with multiple bleeding erosions.

Gross Pathology

- The basic lesion is a mucosal erosion that grossly appears as a 1- to 2-mm spot with a white base surrounded by a ring of erythema.
- With more severe disease, the mucosa between erosions becomes intensely hemorrhagic and oozes blood.
- The antrum and fundus may be involved.

Microscopic Pathology

- The surface of the erosion consists of a layer of serum and necrotic tissue. It is frequently hyalinized, eosinophilic, and amorphic.
- At the base of the erosion, there is usually vascular ectasia with a light infiltrate of acute inflammatory cells.
- Glands at the base of and surrounding the erosion are not distorted.
- Mucin depletion is present in epithelium immediately adjacent to the erosions.
- Mucosa between erosions may show intense hemorrhage into the superficial lamina propria.

Differential Diagnosis

Hemorrhage due to biopsy artifact, lymphocytic gastritis, chronic erosions.

Based purely on biopsy findings, it may be impossible to distinguish hemorrhage due to biopsy artifact from hemorrhagic gastritis. The endoscopic appearance of the mucosa prior to biopsy is a key distinguishing criterion. In hemorrhagic gastritis, there is generally a more dense and widespread hemorrhage than there is in biopsy artifact. Erosions are not present as a result of biopsy artifact.

Erosions may occasionally be seen in lymphocytic gastritis. However, they are not accompanied by hemorrhage, and the adjacent epithelium and lamina propria are heavily infiltrated by lymphocytes.

Chronic erosions frequently occur in patients taking NSAIDs. Morphologically, these are very similar to acute erosions, except that hemorrhage in the lamina propria is not present. Temporally there is evidence of chronicity.

References

Aabakken L. NSAIDs and the gastrointestinal tract—case closed? Scand J Gastroenterol 1991;26:801–805.

Cheung LY. Pathogenesis, prophylaxis and treatment of stress gastritis. Am J Surg 1988;156:437–440.

Laine L, Weinstein WM. Subepithelial hemorrhages and erosions of human stomach. Dig Dis Sci 1988;33:490–503.

Laine L, Weinstein WM. The histology of erosive "gastritis" in alcoholic patients: a prospective study. Gastroenterology 1988;94:1254–1262.

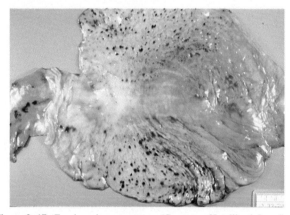

Figure 2–17. Focal erosions at autopsy. (Courtesy of Intellipath Inc., Santa Monica, CA.)

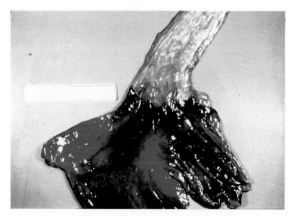

Figure 2–18. Dramatic widespread hemorrhagic gastritis. (Courtesy of Intellipath Inc., Santa Monica, CA.)

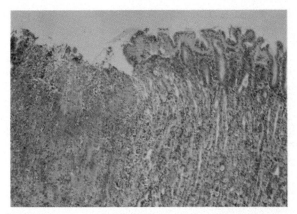

Figure 2–19. Edge of an erosion. Note that it is very sharply demarcated.

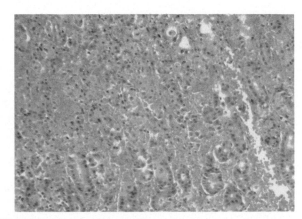

Figure 2–21. Hemorrhagic gastritis.

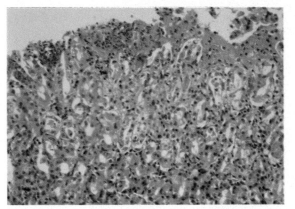

Figure 2–20. Very superficial erosion. It is easy to overlook lesions of this size.

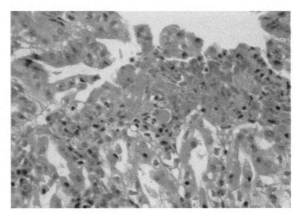

Figure 2–22. Erosion with a small amount of surface slough.

SUPPURATIVE GASTRITIS AND DUODENITIS

Biology of Disease

■ This rare disease is a bacterial cellulitis involving the submucosa of the stomach and/or duodenum.

■ *Streptococcus pyogenes* (alpha-hemolytic) is the organism most frequently isolated. Other common bacteria include *Escherichia coli* and *Haemophilus influenzae*.

■ Two thirds of cases are fatal and first diagnosed at autopsy.

■ If a gas-forming organism is responsible, bubbles may form in the wall of the viscus.

■ Predisposing conditions include alcoholism, cirrhosis, chronic renal failure, immunodeficiency states, mucosal ulceration, hypochlorhydria, and recent polypectomy.

■ In most instances, the route of infection is hematogenous.

Clinical Features

■ The onset is sudden with rigor, fever, prostration, and abdominal pain.

■ On endoscopic examination, the mucosa is edematous and hemorrhagic.

■ Superficial biopsies may not reveal the diagnosis, since the disease is mainly confined to the submucosa, with a normal overlying mucosa.

■ Ultrasound examination may show thickening of the wall of the viscus.

Gross Pathology

■ The serosal surface of the viscus shows a fibropurulent exudate.

■ The wall shows brawny thickening, which on sectioning exudes frank pus or serosanguineous fluid.

■ The overlying mucosa is usually intact, although the mucosal folds may be less prominent.

Microscopic Pathology

■ There is massive submucosal edema, which may be hemorrhagic.

■ Large numbers of neutrophils are present in the submucosa and, to a lesser extent, within the muscularis propria.

■ The mucosa is usually normal.

Special Techniques

■ The responsible organism often can be identified by Gram staining.

Differential Diagnosis

Eosinophilic gastroenteritis, ischemia.

The gross and microscopic findings can be very similar to those in eosinophilic gastroenteritis, except that in suppurative gastritis a neutrophil infiltrate is present.

Ischemia can produce edema and a neutrophil infiltrate, but usually there is also mucosal necrosis present. In ischemia, the inflammatory infiltrate tends to be bandlike at the junction of infarcted and viable tissue.

References

Bron BA, Deyhle P, Pelloni S, at al. Phlegmonous gastritis diagnosed by endoscopic snare biopsy. Am J Dig Dis 1977;22:729–733.

Kneafsey PA, Kelly JK, Church DL, et al. Phlegmonous duodenitis complicating multiple myeloma: a successfully treated case. Am J Gastroenterol 1987;82:1322–1325.

Miller AI, Smith B, Rogers AI. Phlegmonous gastritis. Gastroenterology 1975;68:231–238.

Mittleman RE, Suarez RV. Phlegmonous gastritis associated with the acquired immunodeficiency syndrome. Arch Pathol Lab Med 1985;109:765–767.

O'Toole PA, Morris JA. Acute phlegmonous gastritis. Postgrad Med J 1988;64:315–316.

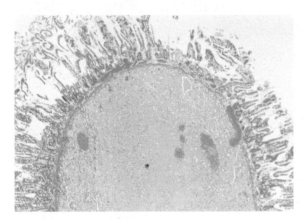

Figure 2–23. Low-power view to show swelling of the mucosal folds from a case of suppurative duodenitis.

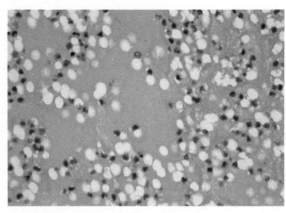

Figure 2–24. Submucosal exudate rich in neutrophils.

HELICOBACTER PYLORI GASTRITIS

Biology of Disease

■ This condition is due to infection of the stomach by *Helicobacter pylori*, a gram-negative, slender, curved rod. The organism is a potent source of urease, which may be an important mediator of mucosal damage.

■ The disease can affect individuals of all ages, including children, although infection rates are higher in more elderly populations.

■ The disease is common in all populations but particularly affects individuals from undeveloped countries and those in the lower socioeconomic classes.

■ Organisms are presumed to gain entrance to the stomach by the oral route, but the source and reservoir of infection have not yet been identified.

■ It is stated in the literature that in up to 10% of cases, *H. pylori* may be present in the stomach without evidence of inflammatory changes. It has been our experience, however, that a thorough examination of *Helicobacter*-positive biopsies will always disclose an increase in lymphocytes and plasma cells within the lamina propria.

Clinical Features

■ At the time of first infection, some patients develop epigastric pain, vomiting, and transient hypochlorhydria. However, many patients are asymptomatic.

■ In cases of ongoing *H. pylori* gastritis, the symptomatology is not specific and there may or may not be a history of dyspepsia.

Gross Pathology

■ Endoscopic appearances correlate poorly with histologic findings. In some individuals with very active disease, there may be red streaks in the antral mucosa.

Microscopic Pathology

■ Usually, the bacteria are readily identified on H&E sections as slender curved spirals in the superficial mucous layer and in the pits. Typically, they are attached to the mucosa in the region of the intercellular junctions.

■ Inflammation is most pronounced in the antrum, although organisms may be identified in both antral and fundic zones.

- The presence of organisms is associated with a neutrophilic infiltrate in the superficial and pit-lining epithelium. Collections of neutrophils (pit abscesses) may be present within the pit lumen. The greater the number of neutrophils present, the more numerous the bacteria.
- When large numbers of organisms are present, the epithelium may show a loss of apical mucus and a tufted appearance with intervening microerosions.
- The lamina propria contains an inflammatory infiltrate in which plasma cells are particularly prominent. These may be present in the superficial portion of the mucosa (chronic superficial gastritis) or may involve the full thickness (diffuse antral gastritis or panmucosal gastritis).
- The presence of lymphoid follicles in the stomach strongly correlates with the presence of *H. pylori*.
- Reactive changes in the pit-lining cells include cytoplasmic mucin loss and nuclear enlargement with hyperchromasia and prominent nucleoli.
- Intestinal metaplasia, xanthelasma, carcinoma, and other abnormalities may be seen coincidentally with *H. pylori* gastritis. At present, controversy exists as to whether intestinal metaplasia is the end result of "burned out" *H. pylori* gastritis or is due to other factors. However, although organisms and intestinal metaplasia may be present in the same biopsy, the organisms are invariably found on nonmetaplastic mucosa.

Special Diagnostic Techniques

- *H. pylori* organisms may be demonstrated by a variety of special stains, including modified Giemsa stains, Warthin-Starry silver stains, and immunostains. However, routine use of these is not recommended since the bacteria are readily seen on H&E sections.
- Serologic methods (particularly ELISA) will demonstrate antibodies to *H. pylori* in instances in which the organism is not readily identifiable in biopsy material.

Differential Diagnosis

Drug-induced gastritis, multifocal atrophic gastritis, autoimmune gastritis, gastritis due to organisms other than *H. pylori*.

At present, *H. pylori* gastritis should be diagnosed only when the organisms are demonstrated. However, when only a small number of organisms are present, they may be hard to find on H&E sections; in this situation, if the biopsy is otherwise compatible, a special stain should be performed.

There are rare cases of gastric infection by a tightly coiled spiral organism provisionally labeled *Gastrospirillum hominis*. This can satisfactorily be identified only with special stains.

References

Blaser MJ. Hypotheses on the pathogenesis and natural history of *Helicobacter* induced inflammation. Gastroenterology 1992;102:720–727.

Blaser MJ. Epidemiology and pathophysiology of *Campylobacter pylori* infections. Rev Infect Dis 1990;12:S99–106.

Correa P, Yardley JH. Grading and classification of chronic gastritis: one American response to the Sydney system. Gastroenterology 1992;102:355–359.

Heilmann KL, Borchard F. Gastritis due to spiral shaped bacteria other than *Helicobacter pylori*: clinical, histological and ultrastructural findings. Gut 1991;32:137–140.

Hui PK, Chan WY, Cheung PS, et al. Pathologic changes of gastric mucosa colonized by *Helicobacter pylori*. Hum Pathol 1992;23:548–556.

Morris A, Nicholson G. Ingestion of *Campylobacter pyloridis* causes gastritis and raised fasting gastric pH. Am J Gastroenterol 1987;82:192–199.

Peterson WL. *Helicobacter pylori* and peptic ulcer disease. N Engl J Med 1991;324:1042–1048.

Siurala M, Sipponen P, Kekki M. Campylobacter pylori in a sample of Finnish population: Relations to morphology and functions of the gastric mucosa. Gut 1988;29:909–915.

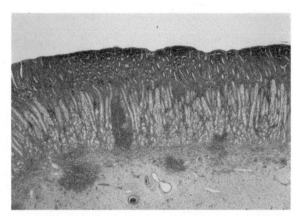

Figure 2–25. Antral mucosa showing a superficial gastritis with lymphoid follicles.

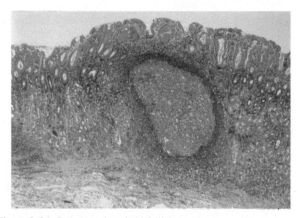

Figure 2–26. Prominent lymphoid follicles.

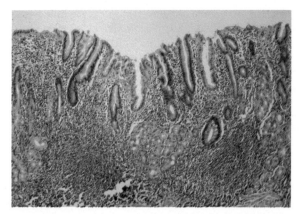

Figure 2–27. Full-thickness chronic inflammatory infiltrate in the lamina propria.

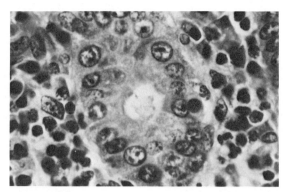

Figure 2–30. Reactive changes in the epithelium. Note the vesicular nuclei with prominent nucleoli.

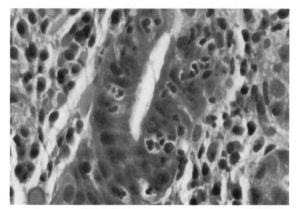

Figure 2–28. Neutrophil infiltration of gastric pits.

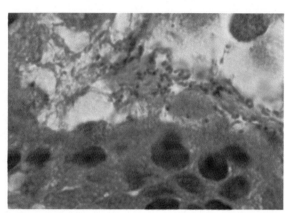

Figure 2–31. *Helicobacter* in superficial mucus layer (oil immersion).

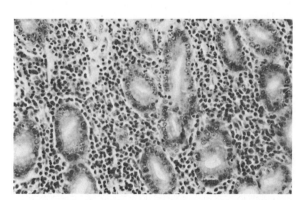

Figure 2–29. Chronic inflammatory infiltrate in lamina propria.

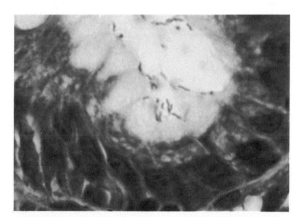

Figure 2–32. *Helicobacter* stained by a modified Giemsa stain.

MULTIFOCAL ATROPHIC GASTRITIS

Biology of Disease

■ Multifocal atrophic gastritis (MAG) is a biopsy finding, not a clinical disease entity.

■ There are several causes. Probably many cases arise as a long-term consequence of *Helicobacter pylori* infection; however, other environmental factors may also be involved in the causation of mucosal atrophy.

■ This type of gastritis is associated with intestinal adenocarcinoma of the stomach and is probably the precursor lesion.

Clinical Features

■ The prevalence of MAG increases with age.

■ It is most common in undeveloped countries and in the lower socioeconomic groups.

■ There are no specific endoscopic findings and no characteristic symptomatology.

■ Multifocal atrophic gastritis is common at the edge of gastric peptic ulcers and in stomachs with an intestinal adenocarcinoma.

Gross Pathology

■ No gross abnormalities are seen.

Microscopic Pathology

■ The disease involves fundic and antral mucosa in a patchy fashion but is maximal on the lesser curvature in the region of the incisura.

■ Atrophy of glands is present but may vary in extent and severity.

■ The lamina propria contains a mixed infiltrate of chronic inflammatory cells, which involves the full thickness of the mucosa.

■ Neutrophil infiltration of the epithelium is not present unless there is associated *Helicobacter* gastritis.

■ Intestinal metaplasia is very common, if not universal.

■ Reactive changes may be present in the pit-lining epithelium. These include cytoplasmic mucin loss, nuclear enlargement, and prominent nucleoli.

Differential Diagnosis

Helicobacter gastritis, autoimmune gastritis, Crohn's disease, and radiation gastritis may all be accompanied by MAG. Occasionally MAG is present with no other recognizable disease.

MAG is not a separate disease entity and likely can arise as a long-term consequence of a variety of causes. For this reason, it is unreasonable to present a strict differential diagnosis. However, the following points are offered to clarify use of the term MAG.

Helicobacter organisms are not present in foci of multifocal atrophic gastritis. However, both conditions are common and frequently coexist in the same stomach.

Autoimmune gastritis and radiation gastritis are generally diffuse, rather than focal, forms of gastric atrophy.

Multifocal atrophic gastritis does not have serum autoantibodies (to parietal cells and/or intrinsic factor) or hypergastrinemia.

Crohn's disease without granuloma formation may mimic multifocal atrophic gastritis but tends to have less prominent intestinal metaplasia. Almost all patients with Crohn's disease involving the stomach also have evidence of terminal ileal involvement.

MAG may be diagnosed in conjunction with other diseases or rarely as an isolated finding when other more specific forms of chronic inflammation have been excluded.

References

Correa P. Chronic gastritis—a clinico-pathological association. Am J Gastroenterol 1988;83:504–509.

Correa P, Yardley JH. Grading and classification of chronic gastritis. One American response to the Sydney system. Gastroenterology 1992;102:355–359.

Wyatt JI, Dixon MF. Chronic gastritis: a pathogenetic approach. J Pathol 1988;154:944–951.

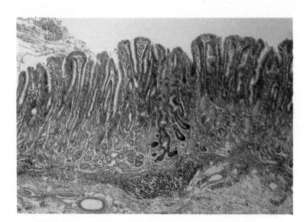

Figure 2–33. A single focus of atrophy and intestinal metaplasia.

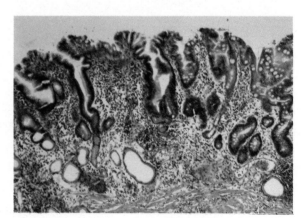

Figure 2–34. Extensive gland atrophy and metaplasia.

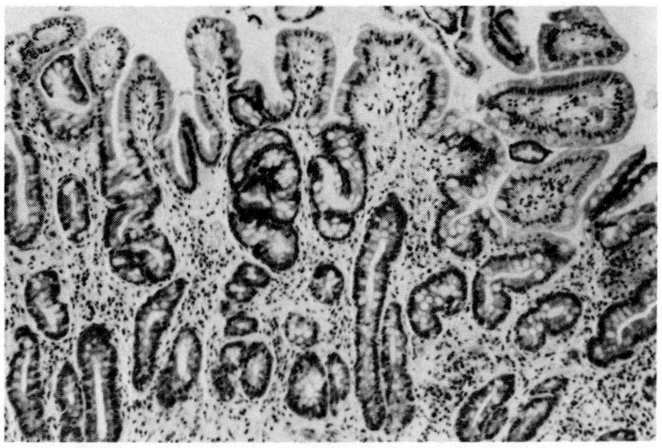

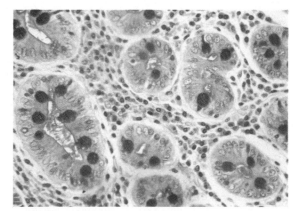

Figure 2–35. Extensive atrophy. Note the villiform surface mucosa.

Figure 2–37. Intestinal metaplasia (PAS).

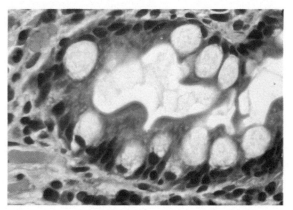

Figure 2–36. Intestinal metaplasia.

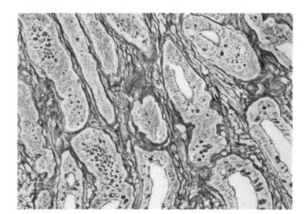

Figure 2–38. Reticulin stain showing condensed reticulin representing gland atrophy.

AUTOIMMUNE GASTRITIS

Biology of Disease

■ This condition accounts for fewer than 5% of all cases of chronic gastritis.

■ It results from autoimmune destruction of fundic acid– and enzyme-secreting glands with sparing of antral glands.

■ The mechanism of destruction is not fully elucidated. Evidence of cell-mediated immune reactions may be present, and autoantibodies may be detected in the serum.

Clinical Features

■ Some patients with this condition have established pernicious anemia (PA), but in others the hematologic abnormality is not fully manifest.

■ All patients have either hypochlorhydria or achlorhydria.

■ All patients have hypergastrinemia due to secondary antral G-cell hyperplasia.

■ Parietal cell antibodies are present in the serum of 80% to 90% of patients with established pernicious anemia and in 60% of patients who do not have PA.

■ Intrinsic factor antibodies are found less frequently but are virtually diagnostic of autoimmune gastritis.

■ Autoimmune gastritis is more common in elderly (> 60) female patients.

■ There are usually no symptoms referable to the stomach, and biopsies are usually obtained incidentally.

Gross Pathology

■ The fundic mucosa is thinner than normal and lacks the usual mucosal folds.

■ The antral mucosa is normal.

Microscopic Pathology

■ Atrophy is confined to the glands of the fundic mucosa, resulting in mucosa that is reduced to one quarter of its normal thickness.

■ A mild nonspecific chronic inflammatory infiltrate may be present in the lamina propria.

■ The pit-lining and surface epithelium shows extensive intestinal metaplasia. In addition to goblet cells, Paneth's cells and even rudimentary villi may be present.

32 ■ DISEASES OF THE STOMACH

- The changes are diffuse not focal, although minor variations in the extent of atrophy may be seen in different areas.
- Hyperplasia of G cells is present in biopsy tissue from the antral mucosa. This is almost universally present to a greater or lesser degree.
- In many cases, there is also a hyperplasia of enterochromaffin-like (ECL) cells of the fundic mucosa. This may be diffuse or nodular.

Differential Diagnosis

Multifocal atrophic gastritis, radiation gastritis.

Multifocal atrophic gastritis affects the antral and fundic mucosa. It is patchy with normal intervening mucosa. There are no serum autoantibodies and hypergastrinemia is not present.

Radiation may produce profound gastric atrophy. It is usually accompanied by obliterative lesions in submucosal vessels.

References

Borch K, Renvall H, Liedberg G. Gastric endocrine cell hyperplasia and carcinoid tumors in pernicious anemia. Gastroenterology 1985;88:638–648.

Flejou JF, Bahame P, Smith AC, et al. Pernicious anemia and *Campylobacter*-like organisms; is the gastric antrum resistant to colonization? Gut 1989;30:60–64.

Lewin KJ, Dowling F, Wright JP, Taylor KB. Gastric morphology and serum gastrin levels in pernicious anemia. Gut 1976;17:551–560.

Rode J, Dhillon AP, Papadaki L, et al. Pernicious anemia and mucosal endocrine cell proliferation of the non-antral stomach. Gut 1986;27:789–798.

Strickland RG, MacKay IR. A re-appraisal of the nature and significance of chronic gastritis. Am J Dig Dis 1973;18:426–440.

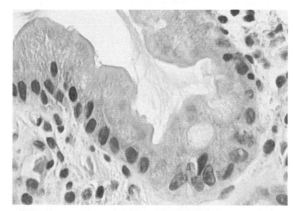

Figure 2–41. Intestinal metaplasia with brush border formation.

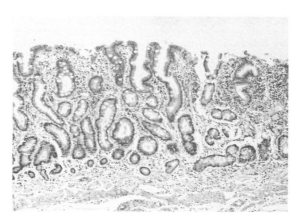

Figure 2–39. Complete mucosal atrophy.

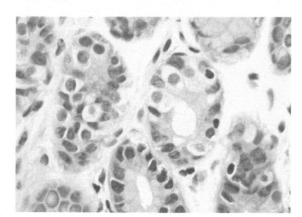

Figure 2–42. Endocrine cell hyperplasia in the gastric antrum.

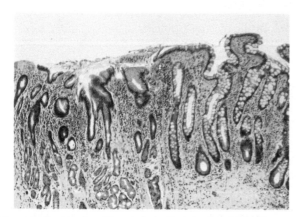

Figure 2–40. Atrophy with metaplasia. Occasional parietal cells are present.

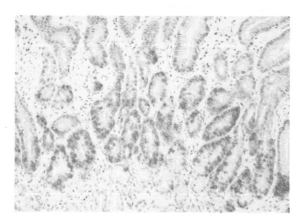

Figure 2–43. G-cell hyperplasia (immunostain for chromogranin).

INTESTINAL METAPLASIA

Biology of Disease

- Intestinal metaplasia (IM) is not a specific disease entity, but rather represents a common response of the gastric mucosa to a variety of injuries.
- It is encountered most commonly in autoimmune gastritis (usually in a diffuse pattern) and in multifocal atrophic gastritis (usually patchy).
- Intestinal metaplasia is common in persons over 60 years of age but typically is not extensive.
- Most intestinal-type gastric carcinomas of the distal stomach arise in foci of intestinal metaplasia.
- Because IM is so common, its presence is not useful in screening for the subsequent development of malignancy.

Clinical Features

- There are no specific clinical or endoscopic features that permit a diagnosis of IM.

Gross Pathology

- Grossly, IM is indistinguishable from normal mucosa.

Microscopic Pathology

- IM represents a change of mucosal pattern from gastric type to small bowel and/or colonic type.
- IM can affect any area of the stomach but is most common in the antrum.
- The normal gastric glands undergo progressive atrophy, and ultimately the mucosa may develop a villous pattern.
- Paneth's cells may be present in the base of the pits.
- Associated nonspecific chronic inflammation may be present in the lamina propria, but this is not an integral component of IM.
- The early stages of IM are termed *incomplete metaplasia*. There is no morphologic abnormality of the surface and pit-lining epithelium, but histochemically the normal neutral mucus of the surface epithelium changes to acidic mucins, either sulfomucin or sialomucin. This incomplete IM can only be detected histochemically.
- In the later stages of IM, there is complete metaplasia. As well as the histochemical change, there is a morphologic change whereby the normal columnar epithelial cells are converted to goblet cells and absorptive cells. The goblet cells also contain acidic mucin.

Special Techniques

- An Alcian blue stain performed at pH 2.5 will demonstrate all types of IM.
- An Alcian blue stain performed at pH 0.5 or a high iron diamine (HID) stain will selectively demonstrate sulfomucin.
- A combined Alcian blue (pH 2.5)–HID stain will simultaneously demonstrate sialomucin (light blue color) and sulfomucin (black or dark brown color).

Differential Diagnosis

Occasionally, degenerative changes will result in epithelial vacuolation. This is morphologically distinct from the regular goblet cell vacuole and is typically present in a subnuclear location.

References

Felipe MI, Potet F, Bogomoletz WV, et al. Incomplete sulphomucin-secreting intestinal metaplasia for gastric cancer. Preliminary data from a prospective study from three centers. Gut 1985;26:1319–1326.

Jass JR. Role of intestinal metaplasia in the histogenesis of gastric carcinoma. J Clin Pathol 1980;33:801–810.

Jass JR, Felipe MI. A variant of intestinal metaplasia associated with gastric carcinoma: a histochemical study. Histopathology 1979;3:191–199.

Rothery GA, Day DW. Intestinal metaplasia in endoscopic biopsy specimens of gastric mucosa. J Clin Pathol 1985;38:613–621.

Segura DI, Montero C. Histochemical characterization of different types of intestinal metaplasia in the gastric mucosa. Cancer 1983;52:498–503.

Teglbjaerg PS, Nielson HO. "Small intestinal type" and "Colonic type" intestinal metaplasia of the human stomach. Acta Pathol Microbiol Scand (A) 1978;86:351–355.

Thompson IW, Day DW, Wright NA. Subnuclear vacuolated cells: a novel abnormality of simple mucin-secreting cells of non-specialized gastric mucosa and Brunner's glands. Histopathology 1987;11:1067–1081.

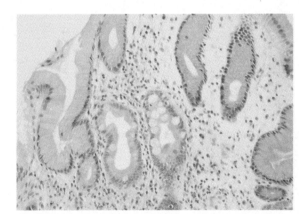

Figure 2–44. Focus of intestinal metaplasia characterized by goblet cells within gastric pits.

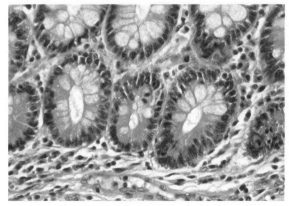

Figure 2–45. Paneth's cells at the base of gastric pits. No glands are present; they are completely atrophic.

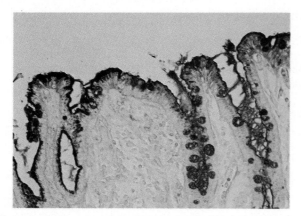

Figure 2–46. Focus of complete intestinal metaplasia (Alcian blue and PAS).

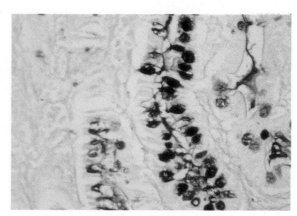

Figure 2–49. Complete intestinal metaplasia, large-bowel and small-bowel types (Alcian blue and High Iron Diamine).

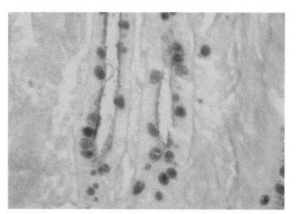

Figure 2–47. Pit showing complete intestinal metaplasia (PAS).

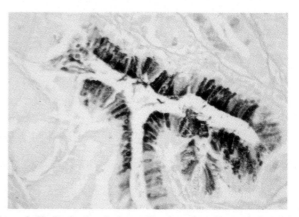

Figure 2–50. Predominantly incomplete large bowel metaplasia (Alcian blue and High Iron Diamine).

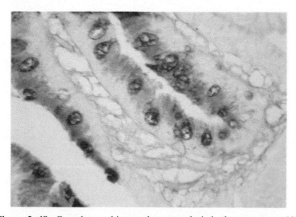

Figure 2–48. Complete and incomplete metaplasia in the same crypt (Alcian blue at pH 2.5).

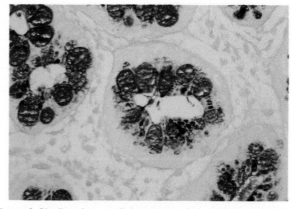

Figure 2–51. Complete small bowel metaplasia and incomplete large bowel metaplasia (Alcian blue and High Iron Diamine).

NONINFECTIOUS GRANULOMATOUS GASTRITIS

Biology of Disease

- Noninfectious granulomatous gastritis comprises three major entities: sarcoidosis, gastric Crohn's disease, and isolated granulomatous gastritis. Occasional examples of granulomas secondary to neoplasms may be seen.
- All of these diseases tend to affect the gastric antrum. In most cases, the disease is isolated to the mucosa and symptomatology is minimal.
- In a minority of cases, the inflammation spreads to involve deeper layers of the gastric wall, resulting in fibrosis and pyloric stenosis.

Clinical Features

- In the vast majority of cases, gastric granulomas are discovered incidentally in the investigation of dyspepsia.
- Sarcoidosis is more common in young black adults. Typically, granulomatous disease is also present at other sites (lungs, hilar nodes, salivary glands).
- Gastric Crohn's disease is almost invariably accompanied by Crohn's disease elsewhere in the bowel, usually the terminal ileum. It typically affects young, white patients.
- By definition, isolated granulomatous gastritis is not accompanied by disease at any other site. It is most common in the older white adult population.

Gross Pathology

- Granulomatous gastritis most commonly involves the antrum.
- In advanced cases, ulcers may occur that grossly resemble peptic ulcers or ulcers caused by nonsteroidal anti-inflammatory drugs (NSAIDs).
- Submucosal and muscle involvement may produce fibrosis and distortion of overlying mucosal folds.
- Rarely, the scarring may be severe and diffuse. The lesion may resemble a neoplasm, and there may be pyloric stenosis.

Microscopic Pathology

- In all three conditions, the granulomas are well circumscribed and noncaseating.
- In Crohn's disease, there is frequently an associated nonspecific chronic gastritis.
- Giant cells may or may not be found within the granulomas.
- Nonspecific ulcers may be present.
- Granulomas are most commonly encountered in the mucosa, but in advanced cases the submucosa and muscularis propria may be involved.

Special Techniques

- As with all granulomatous disease of unknown etiology, special stains for mycobacteria (Ziehl-Neelsen) and for fungi (Grocott and/or Diastase/PAS) should be performed.

Differential Diagnosis

Infectious granulomatous diseases (e.g., tuberculosis, fungal disease).

Caseation or necrosis of granulomas is not found in noninfectious diseases.

It is not always possible to detect organisms in infectious granulomas. A negative special stain, therefore, does not exclude these conditions, and culture of tissue fragments may be required to establish a definitive diagnosis.

In distinguishing among the various causes of noninfectious granulomas, the histologic features are not useful. Reliance has to be placed on clinical history and the patient's age.

References

Chinitz MA, Brandt LJ, Frank MS, et al. Symptomatic sarcoidosis of the stomach. Dig Dis Sci 1985;30:682–688.

Eras P, Goldstein MJ, Sherlock P. Candida infection of the gastrointestinal tract. Medicine 1972;51:367–379.

Fahimi HD, Deren JJ, Gottlieb MD, Zamcheck N. Isolated granulomatous gastritis: its relationship to disseminated sarcoidosis and regional enteritis. Gastroenterology 1963;45:161–175.

Subei I, Attar B, Schmitt G, Levendoglu H. Primary gastric tuberculosis: case report and literature review. Am J Gastroenterol 1987;82:769–772.

Van Spreeuwel JP, Lindeman J, Van der Wal AM, et al. Morphological and immunohistochemical findings in upper gastrointestinal biopsies of patients with Crohn's disease of the colon and ileum. J Clin Pathol 1982;35:934–940.

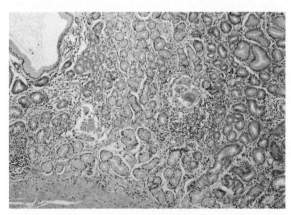

Figure 2–52. Isolated granulomatous gastritis. Granulomas are present with little background, nonspecific inflammation.

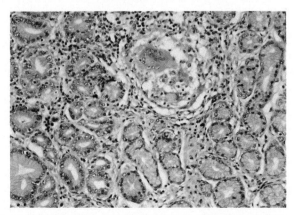

Figure 2–53. Granuloma with Langhans' giant cell. Case of isolated granulomatous gastritis.

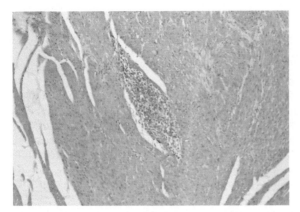

Figure 2–54. Isolated granulomatous gastritis with an intramuscular granuloma.

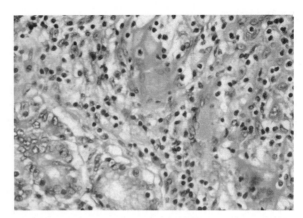

Figure 2–56. Crohn's granuloma in gastric antrum.

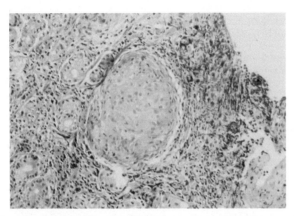

Figure 2–55. Gastric granuloma from a case of sarcoidosis. It is exceedingly well circumscribed, and the histiocytes have a well-developed epithelioid appearance.

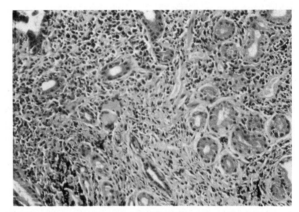

Figure 2–57. Crohn's disease of the stomach, showing a microgranuloma and extensive nonspecific chronic inflammation.

REFLUX GASTRITIS

Biology of Disease

■ Refluxed bile and pancreatic secretions are thought to be the agents injuring the gastric mucosa. Reflux changes are most commonly encountered in patients with a partial gastrectomy and gastroenterostomy.

■ The morphologic changes are considered to be the result of increased exfoliation of cells from the mucosal surface.

■ Similar changes have been described in cases in which the gastric mucosa is damaged by nonsteroidal anti-inflammatory drugs.

■ Polyps may occur immediately adjacent to a gastroenterostomy stoma. They may be multiple and form a ring around the stoma. They are the result of prolapse of mucosa through the stoma and are not primarily caused by reflux. They may, however, show changes similar to those encountered in flat mucosa damaged by reflux.

Clinical Features

■ The symptomatology is nonspecific, although many patients present with dyspepsia.

■ Bile may or may not be seen in the stomach at gastroscopy. There are no specific mucosal abnormalities, although erythema is commonly seen.

■ Changes are present in the antral mucosa in intact stomachs and in the prestomal region in patients with a gastroenterostomy.

■ Polyps, if present, are usually asymptomatic.

Gross Pathology

■ Erythema is commonly seen in flat mucosa.

■ Polypoid mucosal prolapse lesions are dome-shaped with a smooth surface and are seldom greater than 2 cm in diameter.

Microscopic Pathology

■ There is edema of the lamina propria with dilated congested capillaries present beneath the superficial epithelium.

■ Pit hyperplasia is present, usually manifested by increased pit depth, often with a corkscrew appearance. The lining cells show mucin depletion and nuclear hyperchromasia. There may be increased mitotic activity.

■ Pyloric glands are not involved in this process.

■ There is a minimal inflammatory cell infiltration.

■ Tongues of smooth muscle extend upward from the muscularis mucosae to the lamina propria in the subsurface epithelium.

■ Polyps resulting from mucosal prolapse resemble hyperplastic polyps. They consist of hyperplastic disorganized epithelium in which cysts are frequently present. Occasionally, these cysts extend into the gastric submucosa (gastritis cystica profunda). The epithelium of the polyps may show reactive changes similar to those encountered in flat mucosa.

Differential Diagnosis

Gastric antral vascular hyperplasia (GAVE).

The capillaries present in GAVE are larger than in reflux gastritis and may contain fibrin thrombi. GAVE does not show hyperplastic gastric pits.

References

Dixon MF, O'Connor HJ, Axon AT, et al. Reflux gastritis: a distinct histopathological entity? J Clin Pathol 1986;39:524–530.

Franzin G, Novelli P. Gastritis cystica profunda. Histopathology 1981;5:535–547.

Koga S, Watanabe H, Enjoji M. Stomal polypoid hypertrophic gastritis: a polypoid lesion at gastroenterostomy site. Cancer 1979;43:647–657.

Sobala GM, King RF, Axon AT, Dixon MF. Reflux gastritis in the intact stomach. J Clin Pathol 1990;43:303–306.

Stemmerman GN, Hayashi T. Hyperplastic polyps of the gastric mucosa adjacent to gastroenterostomy stomas. Am J Clin Pathol 1979;71:341–345.

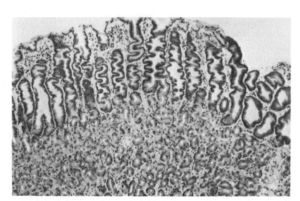

Figure 2–58. Tortuosity of gastric pits from a case of reflux gastritis.

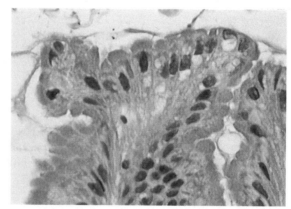

Figure 2–60. Reactive and degenerative changes in surface mucosa.

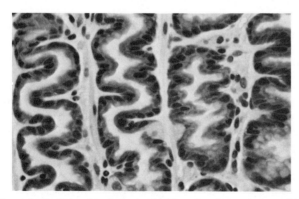

Figure 2–59. Tortuosity of gastric pits. Note the relative absence of inflammation.

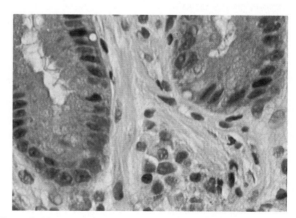

Figure 2–61. Muscle fibers in lamina propria.

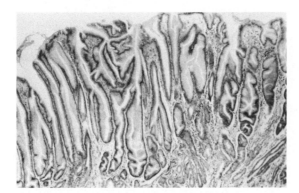

Figure 2–62. Mucosal prolapse showing hyperplastic tortuous gastric pits.

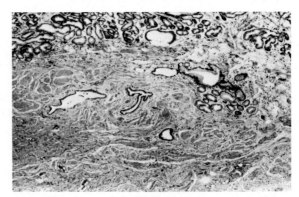

Figure 2–63. Gastritis cystica profunda. Note the epithelial proliferation between the layers of muscularis mucosae.

LYMPHOCYTIC GASTRITIS
(Varioliform Gastritis)

Biology of Disease

- The cause is unknown. Some cases are associated with *Helicobacter pylori* gastritis and some with celiac disease, which suggests a T-cell lymphocytic response to a variety of luminal antigens.
- The disease may be of variable severity. In the mildest cases, it is discovered incidentally at gastric biopsy; in more severe cases, it presents as a varioliform gastritis.
- Varioliform gastritis is an endoscopic description, rather than a specific pathologic entity. In many cases, it represents a late, florid phase of lymphocytic gastritis but may have other causes as well.

Clinical Features

- Most described cases have involved adults.
- There is no sex difference.
- No specific symptomatology has been described in early-stage disease. These cases may be discovered incidentally and have a normal endoscopic appearance.
- In more florid cases (varioliform gastritis), there are thickened mucosal folds, often with superficial chronic erosions at the tips.
- Patients with advanced disease can present with weight loss and anorexia. Occasionally, there may be protein loss sufficient to produce hypoproteinemia and edema.
- There is no specific treatment.

Gross Pathology

- Very little is known about the range of gross appearances, since gastrectomy is rarely performed.
- Early cases may have a normal appearing mucosa.
- Gastrectomy specimens (advanced cases) show rugal prominence and thickening, especially involving the fundic mucosa. This may mimic Menetrier's disease.
- Chronic erosions, 1 to 2 mm in diameter, are present on the tips of the mucosal folds.

Microscopic Pathology

- Variable numbers of chronic inflammatory cells, predominately lymphocytes, are present in the lamina propria.
- Large numbers of lymphocytes (50 or more per 100 epithelial cells) are present within the surface and pit-lining epithelium. In normal gastric surface epithelium, there are 2.5 lymphocytes per 100 epithelial cells, and in autoimmune gastritis, there are 3.5 lymphocytes per 100 epithelial cells.
- The intraepithelial lymphocytes are surrounded by a clear halo. This is considered to be a formalin fixation artifact.
- The lymphocytes are all small and regular, with rounded uniform nuclei.
- Lymphoepithelial lesions (clusters of three or more intraepithelial lymphocytes) are not seen or are exceedingly sparse.
- Chronic erosions may be present at the tips of mucosal folds.

Special Diagnostic Techniques

- Since the intraepithelial lymphocytes are all T cells, this may be confirmed using immunostains for CD8 markers.

Differential Diagnosis

Helicobacter gastritis, atrophic gastritis, malignant lymphoma (small cell lymphocytic types), Menetrier's disease.

Once the presence of large numbers of intraepithelial lymphocytes is recognized, all other forms of chronic atrophic gastritis can be eliminated from consideration.

The usual form of *H. pylori* gastritis is not characterized by an excess of intraepithelial lymphocytes. Therefore, if these features are found together, two diagnoses should be made. It is not yet clear whether this combination is a chance association or an unusual host reaction to the infection.

In most types of small cell lymphocytic lymphoma, the lymphocytic infiltrate in the lamina propria contains some medium-sized cleaved and noncleaved cells. Lymphocytic gastritis has only small round lymphocytes.

Lymphoepithelial lesions are typically found in lymphoma but rarely in lymphocytic gastritis.

Most gastric lymphomas are B-cell type. The intraepithelial lymphocytes of lymphocytic gastritis are T cells.

Lymphomas show clonal restriction (frozen tissue is needed to prove this).

The gross appearances of varioliform gastritis may be indistinguishable from Menetrier's disease. Indeed, some authors have suggested that these diseases frequently occur simultaneously; histologically, however, they are distinct. Menetrier's disease is accompanied by pit hyperplasia and gland atrophy. Lymphocytic gastritis is not.

References

Dixon MF, Wyatt JE, Burke DA, et al. Lymphocytic gastritis —relationship to *Campylobacter pylori* infection. J Pathol 1988;154:125–132.

Haot J, Bogomoletz WV, Jouret A, et al. Menetrier's disease with lymphocytic gastritis. An unusual association with possible pathogenetic associations. Hum Pathol 1991;22:379–386.

Haot J, Hamichi L, Wallez L, et al. Lymphocytic gastritis: a newly described entity. A retrospective endoscopic and histological study. Gut 1988;29:1258–1264.

Haot J, Jouret A, Willette E, et al. Lymphocytic gastritis: prospective study of its relationship with varioliform gastritis. Gut 1990;31:282–286.

Wolber R, Owen DA, DelBuono L, et al. Lymphocytic gastritis in patients with celiac sprue or sprue-like intestinal disease. Gastroenterology 1990;90:310–315.

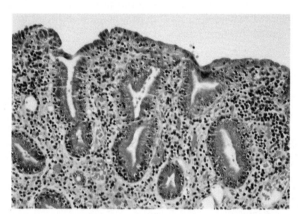

Figure 2–64. Low-power view showing extensive epithelial lymphocytosis, with moderate numbers of lymphocytes in the lamina propria.

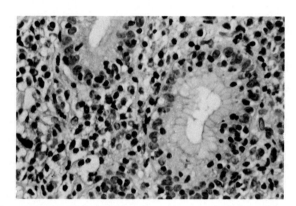

Figure 2–66. Epithelial lymphocytosis with a dense lymphocytic infiltrate in the lamina propria also. On cursory low-power examination, the epithelial lymphocytosis might be missed.

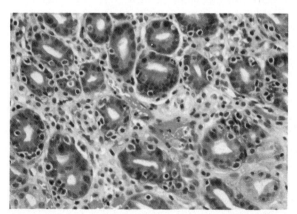

Figure 2–65. Epithelial lymphocytosis showing a clear halo (retraction artifact) surrounding the cells.

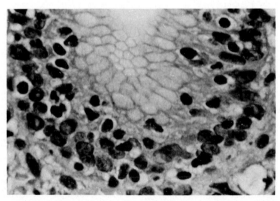

Figure 2–67. The lymphocytes are all fully mature with no atypical features.

GASTRIC ULCER

Biology of Disease

- Gastric ulcers can be acute or chronic.
- By definition, they must penetrate into the submucosal layer at least.
- Some gastric ulcers are due to chronic ingestions of non-steroidal anti-inflammatory drugs (NSAIDs). These are generally excluded from the general category of "peptic ulcer."
- For most gastric ulcers, no clear-cut cause exists, and they are considered to be the result of a combination of factors: hereditary predisposition, gastric acid and pepsin, environmental factors, such as smoking, and infection by *Helicobacter pylori*. These are generally termed peptic ulcers.
- Most gastric peptic ulcers probably arise in areas of multifocal atrophic gastritis.

Clinical Features

- Some gastric ulcers may be completely asymptomatic and discovered incidentally at endoscopy.
- The majority of gastric ulcers are symptomatic, and the most common complaint is epigastric pain, which may be relieved or exacerbated by food.
- The common complications of gastric ulcer include bleeding, which may be chronic or massive; perforation; penetration, usually into liver or pancreas; and scarring, with gastric stenosis.
- Ulcers occurring in the pyloric channel have the clinical and epidemiologic features of duodenal rather than gastric peptic ulcers.

Gross Pathology

- Most gastric ulcers occur at the antral-fundic junction along the lesser curvature.
- Most gastric ulcers are solitary and well circumscribed, usually measuring 0.5 to 2.5 cm in diameter.
- They have a sharp, punched-out edge.
- Developing fibrosis in chronic ulcers may be manifest by prominent mucosal folds radiating from the ulcer edge.
- The ulcer base is covered by a grayish-white exudate.

Microscopic Pathology

- A chronic ulcer has three histologic layers: the surface is covered by slough and inflammatory debris; beneath this is a layer of acute and chronically inflamed granulation tissue; the deep margin of the ulcer consists of stellate scar tissue.
- Vessels showing endarteritis obliterans may be present at the ulcer base.
- In acute ulcers, the layer of scar tissue is absent.
- At the edge of peptic ulcers, the mucosa shows multifocal atrophic gastritis. In addition, there is usually *H. pylori* gastritis with active inflammation. NSAID ulcers typically have little inflammation or atrophy at the edge, and *H. pylori* are not seen.
- In healing ulcers, the epithelium at the edge may show marked regeneration, which is sometimes difficult to distinguish from dysplasia.

Differential Diagnosis

Neoplastic ulcers, particularly superficial carcinomas and lymphomas.

Malignant ulcers may be multiple and irregular in contour with a rolled edge. They tend to be larger than benign ulcers.

Most benign ulcers have only a small amount of reactive lymphoid hyperplasia. Excess lymphoid tissue should raise the suspicion of a low-grade lymphoma (Maltoma) (see Chapter 8.)

Inflammatory epithelial atypia shows changes of varying severity with a gradual transition from normal to abnormal. True dysplasia has a more clearly defined edge.

Reactive nuclei tend to be vesicular with prominent nucleoli. They maintain their polarity. Dysplastic nuclei tend to have an overall hyperchromicity and are crowded and compressed with poor polarity.

References

Kurata JH, Haile BM. Epidemiology of peptic ulcer disease. Clin Gastroenterol 1984;13:289–307.

Soll AH, Kurata, J, McGuigan JE. Ulcers, non-steroidal anti-inflammatory drugs and related matters. Gastroenterology 1989;96:615–625.

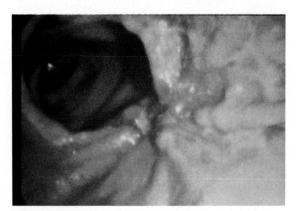

Figure 2–68. Endoscopic view of prepyloric ulcer. (Courtesy of Intellipath Inc., Santa Monica, CA.)

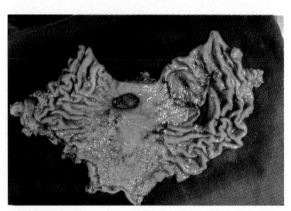

Figure 2–69. Typical gastric ulcer located on the lesser curvature. Note the sharply punched-out edges. (Courtesy of Intellipath Inc., Santa Monica, CA.)

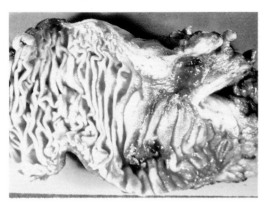

Figure 2–70. Recurrent peptic ulcer following gastroenterostomy. One ulcer is present at the anastomosis site and another in the small bowel opposite the anastomosis. (Courtesy of Intellipath Inc., Santa Monica, CA.)

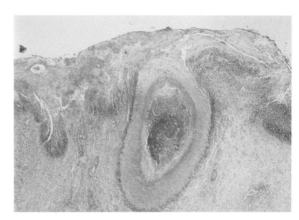

Figure 2–73. Large, partly eroded artery in ulcer bed.

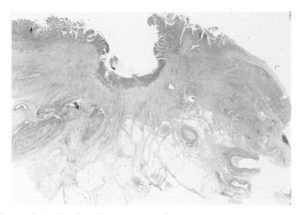

Figure 2–71. Peptic ulcer demonstrating submucosal, muscular, and serosal scarring.

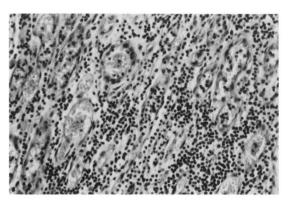

Figure 2–74. Granulation tissue from ulcer bed. Note the prominent endothelial cells.

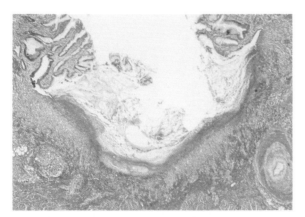

Figure 2–72. Scarring in ulcer bed (Trichrome). Fibrous tissue is staining blue.

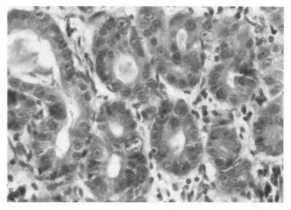

Figure 2–75. Reactive epithelium at the edge of ulcer.

HYPERPLASTIC POLYPS
(Regenerative or Hyperplaseogenic Polyps)

Biology of Disease

- This is the most common type of gastric polyp, comprising 70 to 85% of cases.
- Hyperplastic polyps occur predominately in stomachs involved by atrophic gastritis.
- They arise as a result of excessive regeneration in an inflamed mucosa.
- Morphologically and pathogenetically, they are comparable to inflammatory polyps (not hyperplastic polyps) of the large bowel.
- Malignancy develops in 2% of polyps, usually in those over 2 cm in diameter.

Clinical Features

- There is no family history, and polyps are not present elsewhere in the GI tract.
- The polyps arise mainly in older adults (>50 years of age).
- Most are discovered incidentally during gastroscopy or by radiologic examination.
- The location is mainly in the gastric antrum or at the antrofundic junction.
- There is no relation to sites of previous surgery.
- Most (80% of cases) are solitary.
- Multiplicity may occur (20% of cases), but generally fewer than 20 polyps are present.
- Occasionally, multiple polyps may coalesce, producing prominent mucosal folds. This condition has been called *hyperplastic gastropathy* and may be localized to inflamed mucosa surrounding peptic ulcers.
- Endoscopic removal is adequate treatment. Recurrence is rare.

Gross Pathology

- Size is in the range of 0.5 to 3.0 cm in diameter.
- Small polyps have a sessile configuration.
- Larger polyps (>1 cm diameter) may have a short broad stalk.
- The surface is coarsely lobulated. Some polyps have blunt papillae.
- The cut surface may show mucus-filled cysts 1 to 2 mm in diameter.
- Coalescent polyps may produce prominent antral folds.

Microscopic Pathology

- There is overgrowth and irregularity of gastric pits, which become branched, elongated, or cystic.
- Abundant edematous lamina propria is present.
- Acute and chronic inflammation are present to a variable extent but are usually mild and focal, except in larger polyps that may have undergone torsion.
- Foci of residual antral mucous glands may be present.
- Epithelial cells are mainly the normal columnar type found in the gastric pit mucosa. The cytoplasm may be hypertrophic.
- Intestinal metaplasia may be present to a variable degree, usually reflecting the degree of previous inflammation.
- Epithelial nuclei are bland, except for inflammatory changes consisting of nuclear enlargement and prominent nucleoli.
- Larger polyps may undergo torsion with congestion, bleeding into the stalk, and surface ulceration.

Differential Diagnosis

Juvenile polyps, Peutz-Jegher (PJ) polyps, polypoid mucosal prolapse, Canada-Cronkhite (CC) polyps, Menetrier's disease, gastric adenoma.

Clinical history is an extremely useful differential: Hyperplastic polyps occur in patients over 50 years old (compare with juvenile polyps, and PJ polyps). They are not associated with polyps at other sites in the GI tract (compare with juvenile polyps, PJ polyps, and CC polyps). They are not related to gastroenterostomy stoma sites (compare with polypoid mucosal prolapse).

Hyperplastic polyps do not generally have an overtly papillary appearance, and do not have an arborizing muscularis mucosae in the stalk (compare with PJ polyps).

Hyperplastic polyps may have focal epithelial crowding and atypia that are related to areas of inflammation. However, gastric adenomas consist uniformly of neoplastic epithelium and are similar to adenomas of the large bowel.

CC polyps are accompanied by abnormalities of skin and nails. Hyperplastic polyps have no systemic manifestations.

In Menetrier's disease, there are enlarged folds involving the fundus, and there is evidence of excessive mucosal protein loss.

References

Daibo M, Itabashi M, Hirota T. Malignant transformation of hyperplastic gastric polyps. Am J Gastroenterol 1987;82:1016–1025.

Dirschmid K, Walser J, Hugel H. Pseudomalignant erosions in hyperplastic polyps. Cancer 1982;54:2290–2293.

Komorowski RA, Caya JG. Hyperplastic gastropathy: clinico-pathologic correlation. Am J Surg Pathol 1991;15:577–585.

Laxen F, Sipponen P, Ihamaki T, et al. Gastric polyps, their morphological and endoscopical characteristics and relation to gastric carcinoma. Acta Pathol Microbiol Immunol Scand (A) 1982;90:221–228.

Ming SC. Classification and significance of gastric polyps. In: Yardley JH, Morson BC, Abell MR (eds). The Gastrointestinal Tract. International Academy of Pathology Monograph. Baltimore, Williams and Wilkins, 1977;149–175.

Stamp GWH, Palmer K, Misiewicz JJ. Antral hypertrophic gastritis. A rare cause of iron deficiency. J Clin Pathol 1985;38:390–392.

Tomasulo J. Gastric polyps: histologic types and their relationship to gastric cancer. Cancer 1971;27:1346–1355.

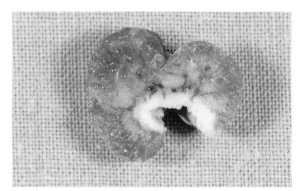

Figure 2–76. Hyperplastic polyp showing a fleshy appearance with mucus filled cysts. (Courtesy of Intellipath Inc., Santa Monica, CA.)

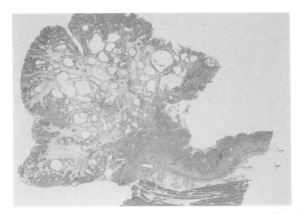

Figure 2–77. Lobulated surface with multiple cysts. (Courtesy of Intelli-path Inc., Santa Monica, CA.)

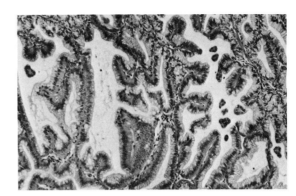

Figure 2–80. Branched pits from a hyperplastic polyp.

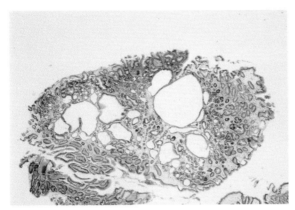

Figure 2–78. A mixture of cysts and complex branched pits.

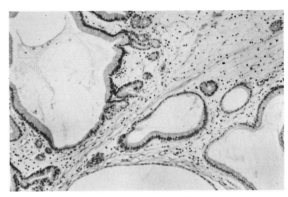

Figure 2–81. Cysts lined by attenuated epithelium.

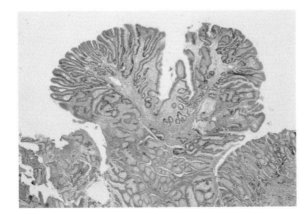

Figure 2–79. Hyperplastic polyp with multiply branched pits.

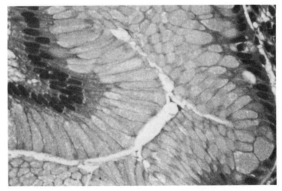

Figure 2–82. Hypertrophic mucus-secreting epithelium lining hyperplastic pits.

FUNDIC GLAND POLYPS

Biology of Disease

- The pathogenesis of these polyps is not clear, and they have variously been considered to be examples of focal hyperplasia or hamartomas.
- These lesions may occur as single polyps, small clusters of polyps, or many thousands of polyps (polyposis).
- Approximately 25% of patients with fundic gland polyposis have familial adenomatosis coli or Gardner's syndrome.
- The polyps have no malignant potential.

Clinical Features

- These polyps are asymptomatic and are always discovered incidentally. There are no clinical complications.
- Endoscopically, the polyps appear as small mucosal bumps. They are slightly paler than the surrounding mucosa.

Gross Pathology

- By definition, fundic gland polyps only involve areas of the gastric mucosa where the glands contain chief and parietal cells.
- The polyps are sessile with a smooth domed surface and measure 1 to 5 mm in diameter.

Microscopic Pathology

- The basic abnormality is a cystic dilatation of two to five adjacent fundic glands.

- The lining cells are attenuated, but otherwise are normal chief and parietal cells.
- Normally, there is no associated inflammation of either the epithelium or the lamina propria.
- The overlying gastric pits are normal.
- Solitary polyps and multiple polyps (polyposis) appear identical.

Differential Diagnosis

Cowden's disease.

The histology of fundic gland polyps is very specific and is not mimicked by any other condition. However, a related condition (i. e., antral gland polyps) may involve the antral mucosa in which small dilated glands are lined by mucus-secreting epithelium.

Cowden's disease is characterized by small polyps with cystic dilatation of pits and glands. However, these polyps also have an overgrowth of fibromuscular tissue in the lamina propria and excess nerves and ganglion cells.

References

Lee RS, Burt RW. The histopathology of fundic gland polyposis. Am J Clin Pathol 1986;86:498–503.

Sipponen P, Siurala M. Cystic "hamartomatous" gastric polyps: a disorder of oxyntic glands. Histopathology 1983;7:727–729.

Tatsuda M, Okuda S, Tamura H, et al. Gastric hamartomatous polyps in the absence of familial polyposis coli. Cancer 1980;45:818–823.

Watanabe H, Enjoji M, Yao T, Ohsato K. Gastric lesions in familial adenomatosis coli. Their incidence and histologic analysis. Hum Pathol 1978;9:269–283.

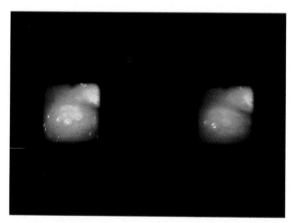

Figure 2–83. Endoscopic view of fundic gland polyps. (Courtesy of Intellipath Inc., Santa Monica, CA.)

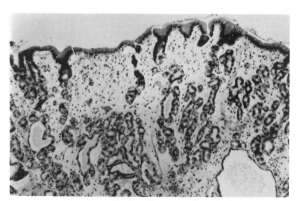

Figure 2–84. Occasional cystic glands lined by an attenuated epithelium.

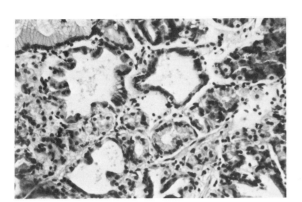

Figure 2–85. Attenuated fundic gland epithelium.

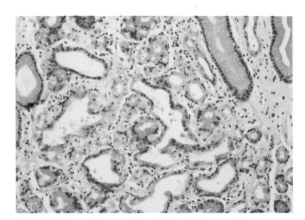

Figure 2–86. Minimally dilated fundic glands from a polyp.

GASTRIC ADENOMAS

Biology of Disease

- Adenomas comprise approximately 10% of all gastric polyps.
- The risk of malignancy developing in an adenoma is related to the size of the polyp. Overall, the risk is in the range of 5 to 10%. The risk is increased with polyps larger than 2 cm in diameter, but this has not been precisely quantified.
- When a gastric adenoma is present, there is a 5 to 10% increase in the likelihood of finding a malignancy elsewhere in the stomach.
- In contrast with the large bowel, the great majority of gastric cancers do not arise in preexistent adenomas.
- Most gastric adenomas occur in a sporadic fashion. However, small numbers of gastric adenomas are found in about two thirds of patients with familial adenomatosis coli and Gardner's syndrome.

Clinical Features

- Most gastric adenomas occur in patients older than 50 years of age. They are usually solitary.
- Most polyps are asymptomatic and are discovered incidentally. Occasionally, they may ulcerate at the tip and bleed. Massive hemorrhage is distinctly unusual, however. Large polyps, located in the antrum, may cause pyloric obstruction.
- Endoscopically, they are more darkly colored than the surrounding mucosa.

Gross Pathology

- Three separate types are recognized: tubular, villous, and flat.
- There are no gross features that reliably permit distinction from other types of gastric polyps; however, a prominent villous pattern is suggestive of an adenoma.
- Most adenomas are sessile and grow in a tubulovillous or pure villous pattern.

- Flat adenomas comprise 10% of all gastric adenomas. Grossly, they are recognized as shallow depressions measuring an average of 1.3 cm in diameter.

Microscopic Pathology

- Gastric adenomas are essentially similar histologically to adenomas occurring in the small and large bowel.
- The architecture may be tubular, villous, or a combination of both types.
- The apical portions of the cells have reduced quantities of cytoplasmic mucus.
- The nuclei are generally cigar shaped with an even distribution of chromatin, although small nucleoli may be present.
- There is nuclear crowding, loss of stratification, and increased mitotic activity.
- The degree of dysplasia (atypia) may vary from mild to severe.
- Inflammation is a variable feature, but it is usually not prominent.
- Surface ulceration and stromal congestion may be present, particularly if the polyp is large or has undergone torsion.

Differential Diagnosis

Polypoid adenocarcinoma, dysplasia, hyperplastic polyps, juvenile polyps, Peutz-Jegher (PJ) polyps, polypoid mucosal prolapse, Canada-Cronkhite (CC) polyps.

Distinguishing between an adenoma and an early carcinoma can be extremely difficult. Essentially, the difference is the presence or absence of invasion. When only intramucosal invasion is present, a low-power abnormality may be identified in one or more lobules of the polyp. This area of the epithelium looks hyperchromatic. At medium power, the gland pattern is abnormal with a back-to-back arrangement and an irregular outer contour. Invasion of tumor into the submucosa must be distinguished from pseudoinvasion. In true invasion, the glands are surrounded by a reactive fibrogenic stroma, rather than normal lamina propria. (See Chapter 5, Large Bowel Adenomas, for further discussion.) Generally, carcinomas are more severely dysplastic than adenomas, but this is not absolute and cannot always be relied on.

There is essentially no histologic difference between a gastric adenoma and gastric dysplasia. By convention, an adenoma is a localized nodule or plaquelike lesion, whereas dysplasia is a diffuse change involving mucosa that is not architecturally different from the surrounding areas. Since dysplasia is generally a widespread change, the risk of developing invasive malignancy is proportionately higher than for an adenoma.

Other differential diagnoses include all types of hyperplastic or hamartomatous polyps. The critical difference is in the nature of the constituent epithelium. Adenomas are composed exclusively of neoplastic epithelium. Non-neoplastic polyps may have focal atypical areas, but these are usually related to inflammation or ulceration.

Hamartomatous gastric polyps usually occur in young adults; polypoid mucosal hyperplasia is associated with gastroenterostomy stomas; and Canada-Cronkhite polyps are accompanied by ectodermal dysplasia.

References

Kamiya T, Morashita T, Asakura H, et al. Long term follow-up study on gastric adenoma and its relation to gastric protruded carcinoma. Cancer 1982;50:2496–2503.

Laxen P, Sipponen P, Ihamaki T, Dorschera Z. Gastric polyps; their morphologic characteristics and relation to gastric carcinoma. Acta Pathol Microbiol Immunol Scand (A) 1982;90:221–228.

Mark LK, Samter T. Villous adenomas of the stomach. Am J Gastroenterol 1975;64:137–139.

Nakamura K, Sakaguchi H, Enjoji M. Depressed adenoma of the stomach. Cancer 1988;62:2197–2202.

Tomasulo J. Gastric polyps: histologic types and their relationship to gastric cancer. Cancer 1971;27:1346–1355.

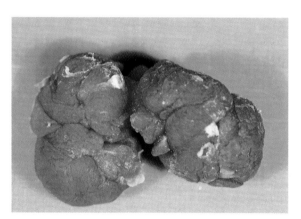

Figure 2–87. Gastric adenoma with lobulated surface. (Courtesy of Intellipath Inc., Santa Monica, CA.)

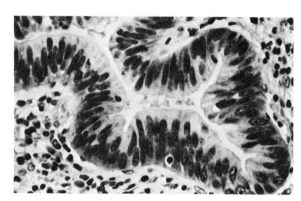

Figure 2–89. Low-grade dysplasia in an adenoma.

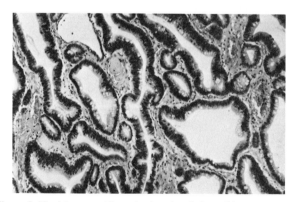

Figure 2–88. Adenoma with predominantly tubular architecture.

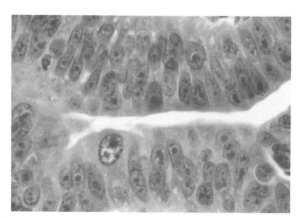

Figure 2–90. High-grade dysplasia in an adenoma.

ZOLLINGER-ELLISON SYNDROME

Biology of Disease

■ Zollinger-Ellison (ZE) syndrome is caused by a massive oversecretion of gastrin.

■ This oversecretion is usually secondary to a neoplasm, most commonly in the head of the pancreas, but occasionally in the duodenum. In about 20% of cases, the excess gastrin is produced by a primary G-cell hyperplasia of the gastric antrum.

■ In about 20% of cases, the pancreatic neoplasm is part of multiple endocrine neoplasia (MEN) syndrome type I. Tumors in these patients are frequently multifocal.

■ The excess gastrin causes proliferation and hyperplasia of gastric parietal cells. Their mass has been estimated to be three to six times greater than in normal individuals. The result is increased secretion of acid.

Clinical Features

■ Peptic ulceration occurs in 95% of patients with ZE syndrome. Most ulcers (75%) occur in the first part of the duodenum, but they can also affect more distal duodenum and jejunum (11%). When compared with the usual isolated peptic ulcer, ZE ulcers tend to be larger, multiple, and more difficult to heal.

■ The secretory diarrhea that affects one third of patients is the result of concentrated acid entering the small bowel.

■ Smaller numbers of patients may have steatorrhea due to inactivation of pancreatic enzymes by excess acid.

■ There are usually no symptoms referable to the enlarged gastric folds.

Gross Pathology

■ Only the acid-secreting fundic zone of the stomach is involved.

■ The mucosal folds are enlarged and thrown into a cerebriform pattern.

■ Gastric ulceration is unusual, but if present is typically prepyloric.

Microscopic Pathology

■ The fundic mucosa is up to two times thicker than normal.

■ The parietal cells crowd out chief cells and mucus neck cells from the glands.

■ Parietal cells may be larger in size than normal.

■ Inflammation and cyst formation is not a feature.

■ Hyperplastic endocrine cells may be present within the fundic glands. These are enterochromaffin-like (ECL) cells that also proliferate due to the trophic action of gastrin. They produce histamine, which may further stimulate acid production by parietal cells.

Differential Diagnosis

Exaggerated normal gastric folds, Menetrier's disease, hypertrophic hypersecretory gastropathy, lymphocytic gastritis, diffuse carcinoma (linitis plastica), lymphoma.

In exaggerated normal gastric folds, the mucosa is normal and the folds are due to excessively long cores of submucosa.

In Menetrier's disease, there is hyperplasia of the pit portion of the gastric mucosa with microcyst formation. The glands are atrophic.

One form of hypertrophic hypersecretory gastropathy closely resembles the ZE syndrome, but the patients do not have hypergastrinemia. Fundic gland hyperplasia and acid hypersecretion appear to result from an abnormal sensitivity of the parietal cells to normal gastrin levels. The other type of hypertrophic hypersecretory gastropathy is accompanied by mucosal protein loss and is similar to Menetrier's disease.

Mucosal inflammation is prominent in lymphocytic gastritis, which is not a feature of ZE syndrome.

Malignant infiltration of the stomach mucosa may produce prominent folds that grossly simulate ZE syndrome. Microscopically, the presence of malignant cells allows easy distinction from ZE syndrome.

References

Deveney CW, Deveney KE. Zollinger-Ellison syndrome (gastrinoma): current diagnosis and treatment. Surg Clin North Am 1987;67:411–422.

Komorowski RA, Caya JG. Hyperplastic gastropathy: clinico-pathologic correlation. Am J Surg Pathol 1991;15:577–585.

Wolfe MM, Jensen RT. Zollinger-Ellison syndrome: current concepts in diagnosis and management. N Engl J Med 1987;317:1200–1209.

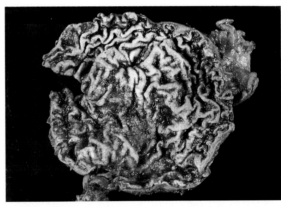

Figure 2–91. Zollinger-Ellison syndrome showing prominent enlarged mucosal folds. (Courtesy of Intellipath Inc., Santa Monica, CA.)

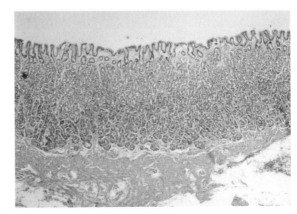

Figure 2–92. Low-power view of mucosa showing fundic gland hyperplasia.

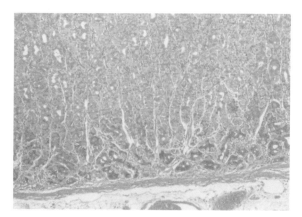

Figure 2–93. Tightly packed fundic glands.

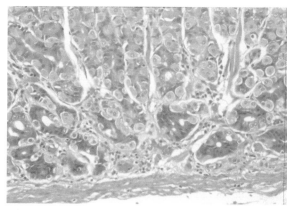

Figure 2–94. Parietal cells extending to the base of the fundic glands and crowding out the chief cells.

MENETRIER'S DISEASE

Biology of Disease

■ For many years, there was no agreement as to exactly what constituted Menetrier's disease. The literature on the subject was confusing and consisted largely of single case reports, so that it was difficult to make definite statements about the disease biology. Formerly, all gastric diseases characterized by giant folds and mucosal protein loss were labeled Menetrier's disease, provided that other causes of giant folds (e.g., carcinoma or lymphoma) had been excluded.

■ Recently, a more precise clinicopathologic definition has been proposed and is gaining acceptance. Menetrier's disease, therefore, is characterized by (1) giant gastric folds, especially in the gastric fundus; (2) low acid production, even after stimulation; (3) mucosal protein loss; and (4) histologic findings of pit hyperplasia and glandular atrophy.

■ The cause of Menetrier's disease is unknown. Recently, it has been postulated that in some cases there is a relationship with lymphocytic gastritis, but as yet this is unconfirmed.

■ A condition resembling Menetrier's disease has been described in children. The majority of these cases resolve spontaneously and are likely the result of a variety of viral infections.

■ In adults, Menetrier's disease, as defined above, is usually a progressive condition.

Clinical Features

■ Menetrier's disease is most common in men over the age of 50.

■ Symptoms are variable and include pain, weight loss, diarrhea, and sometimes peripheral edema.

■ Laboratory findings include anemia and hypoproteinemia secondary to mucosal blood and serum loss from superficial erosions.

■ Usually, some form of partial gastrectomy is needed to control symptoms and hypoproteinemia.

■ The association of carcinoma with Menetrier's disease is controversial. Probably, there is a slight increase in risk, but this is likely the same as for patients who have received a partial gastrectomy for other reasons.

Gross Pathology

■ Large folds are present in the gastric fundus and may also involve the antrum. In fully developed cases, a cerebriform appearance is seen.

■ Ulcers may be visible on the tips of the folds.

Microscopic Pathology

■ This disease involves the gastric mucosal pits, which are elongated and sometimes cystically dilated.

■ The cysts extend downward, involving the glandular portion of the mucosa, which is atrophic due to compression and replacement.

■ Cysts may extend through the muscularis mucosae into the submucosa (gastritis cystica profunda).

■ The superficial lamina propria is often edematous and variably inflamed.

■ Superficial ulcers (erosions) may be present.

Differential Diagnosis

Exaggerated normal gastric folds, hyperplastic polyps and hyperplastic folds secondary to chronic inflammation (hyperplastic gastropathy), Zollinger-Ellison syndrome, hypertrophic hypersecretory gastropathy, lymphocytic gastritis, Canada-Cronkhite syndrome, carcinoma (linitis plastica), lymphoma.

In exaggerated normal gastric folds, the abnormality is excessively long cores of submucosa. These are covered by unremarkable gastric mucosa.

Hyperplastic polyps and hyperplastic folds are usually localized to the antrum. Menetrier's disease primarily involves the fundus.

In Zollinger-Ellison syndrome, there is hyperplasia of the glandular portion of the mucosa. Cysts are not a feature.

Hypertrophic hypersecretory gastropathy is exceedingly rare. The protein-losing variant of this condition resembles Menetrier's disease but also has features of the Zollinger-Ellison syndrome, including hypergastrinemia.

In lymphocytic gastritis, there is infiltration of the pit-lining epithelium by mature T lymphocytes. Recently, an association between Menetrier's disease and lymphocytic gastritis has been described.

The Canada-Cronkhite syndrome may be morphologically indistinguishable from Menetrier's disease but is characterized by polyps elsewhere in the gastrointestinal tract and epidermal dysplasia.

Gastric neoplasms may infiltrate and expand the lamina propria in a single-cell growth pattern but are not associated with epithelial hyperplasia.

References

Appelman HD. Localized and extensive expansions of the gastric mucosa: mucosal polyps and giant folds. In: Appelman HD (ed). Pathology of the Esophagus, Stomach and Duodenum. Contemporary Issues in Surgical Pathology. New York, Churchill Livingstone, 1984:79–119.

Burke AP, Sobin LH. The pathology of Cronkhite-Canada polyps. A comparison to juvenile polyposis. Am J Surg Pathol 1989;13:940–946.

Chouraqui JP, Roy CC, Brochu P, et al. Menetrier's disease in children: report of a patient and review of 16 other cases. Gastroenterology 1981;80:1042.

Fieber SS, Rickert RR. Hyperplastic gastropathy. Analysis of 50 selected cases from 1955–1980. Am J Gastroenterol 1981;76:321–329.

Haot J, Bogomoletz WV, Jouret A, Mainguet P. Menetrier's disease with lymphocytic gastritis: an unusual association with possible pathologic implications. Hum Pathol 1991;22:379–386.

Komorowski RA, Caya JG. Hyperplastic gastropathy: Clinicopathologic-correlation. Am J Surg Pathol 1991;15:577–585.

Overholt BG, Jeffries GH. Hypertrophic, hyposecretory protein-losing gastropathy. Gastroenterology 1970;58:80–87.

Stamp GWH, Palmer K, Misiewicz JJ. Antral hypertrophic gastritis. A rare cause of iron deficiency. J Clin Pathol 1985;38:390–392.

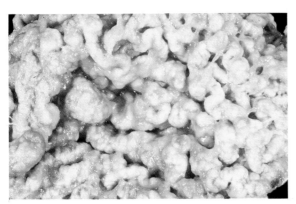

Figure 2–95. Hyperplastic enlarged mucosal folds from a case of Menetrier's disease. (Courtesy of Intellipath Inc., Santa Monica, CA.)

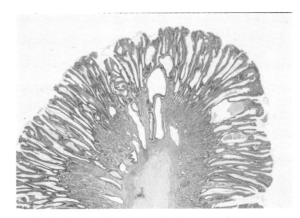

Figure 2–97. Hyperplastic mucosa at tip of mucosal fold.

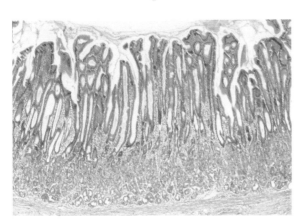

Figure 2–96. Hyperplastic pits occupying two thirds of the mucosal thickness.

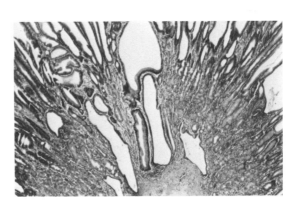

Figure 2–98. Hyperplastic pits with cyst formation.

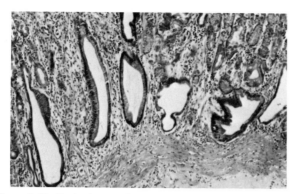

Figure 2–99. Cystic pits crowding out glands at the base of the mucosa.

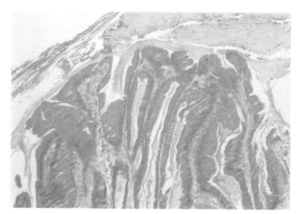

Figure 2–100. Excess mucus production on the surface of the mucosa.

INTESTINAL GASTRIC ADENOCARCINOMA

Biology of Disease

- Intestinal carcinomas may be located in the distal stomach or in the esophagocardiac region. Although histologically similar, cancers at these two locations are epidemiologically distinct.
- Esophagocardiac cancer is similar to carcinoma arising in Barrett's esophagus (see Chapter 1). The cause is unknown, but there is no relation to multifocal atrophic gastritis or *Helicobacter pylori* infection. Its incidence in North America is increasing.
- Distal gastric cancer is becoming less prevalent in North America, although it is still common in some undeveloped countries. It is thought to arise in areas of multifocal atrophic gastritis.
- Intestinal adenocarcinoma of the distal stomach is primarily a disease of the elderly (60+).

Clinical Features

- Intestinal carcinomas can present in a variety of ways. Local symptoms include obstruction, loss of appetite, early satiety, and foul-smelling breath. Sudden massive hematemesis and melena are uncommon.
- General symptoms include weight loss and anemia.
- Lymphatic spread is initially to local lymph nodes, then to nodes in the para-aortic, mediastinal, and cervical regions.
- Hematogenous spread to the liver and lungs is common.
- Transserosal spread, with production of ascites, is not common, although an enlarging mass may become adherent to other abdominal organs.

Gross Pathology

- Intestinal tumors tend to be large, usually over 2 cm in diameter and frequently in excess of 10 cm.
- Tumors may have a nodular, polypoid, or ulcerated appearance.

- Nodular or polypoid tumors are very commonly ulcerated on the surface, particularly when the tumor is large.
- Ulcerated tumors typically have a rolled edge with a distinct lip.
- Grossly, the tumors tend to be moderately well circumscribed, although they can have an irregular border as they infiltrate omental fat. The circumscription is most apparent on the cut surface.

Microscopic Pathology

- Most intestinal carcinomas have a well-defined glandular or papillary pattern.
- In poorly differentiated tumors, there may be only poorly formed glands, and the neoplasm may have a sheetlike growth pattern.
- Individual cells are columnar or cuboidal with a basally located nucleus.
- Mucin may be present within glands but is usually not found within the cytoplasm.
- There is usually an identifiable growing edge of the tumor. This may be irregular and not precisely defined.
- Multifocal atrophic gastritis and intestinal metaplasia are almost universally present in non-neoplastic mucosa adjacent to the tumor.
- About 10% of gastric carcinomas cannot be satisfactorily classified as either intestinal or diffuse.

Differential Diagnosis

Adenoma, early gastric cancer, peptic ulcer, diffuse carcinoma.

Adenomas are by definition noninvasive. It is recommended that the term *carcinoma in situ* not be used with respect to gastrointestinal malignancy. Severely dysplastic adenomas should be called high-grade adenomas and a comment made as to whether or not intramucosal invasion (early gastric cancer) is present.

By definition, early gastric cancer involves invasion extending no deeper than the submucosa.

Peptic ulcers may be indistinguishable from ulcerated carcinomas by gross inspection. Peptic ulcers typically have a punched-out edge to which adjacent mucosal folds extend. Carcinomas have a rolled edge, and the adjacent mucosal folds flatten out before they reach the edge.

References

Antonioli DA, Goldman H. Changes in location and type of gastric carcinoma. Cancer 1982;50:775–781.

Correa P, Cuello C, Duque E. Carcinoma and metaplasia of the stomach in Colombian migrants. J Natl Cancer Inst 1970;44:207–306.

Lauren P. The two histological main types of gastric carcinoma: diffuse and so-called intestinal type. Acta Pathol Microbiol Scand (A) 1965;64:31–49.

MacDonald WC, MacDonald JB. Adenocarcinoma of the esophagus and/or gastric cardia. Cancer 1982;60:1094–1098.

Morson BC. Carcinoma arising from areas of intestinal metaplasia in the gastric mucosa. Br J Cancer 1955;9:377–385.

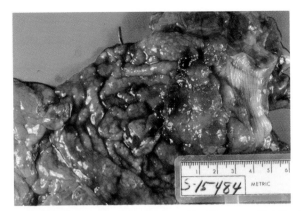

Figure 2–103. Carcinoma of the gastric cardia. (Courtesy of Intellipath Inc., Santa Monica, CA.)

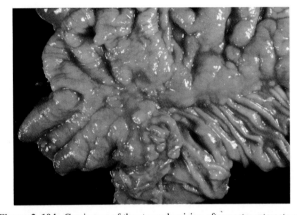

Figure 2–104. Carcinoma of the stomach arising after gastroenterostomy. (Courtesy of Intellipath Inc., Santa Monica, CA.)

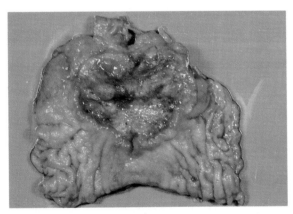

Figure 2–101. Large ulcerated carcinoma with rolled edge. (Courtesy of Intellipath Inc., Santa Monica, CA.)

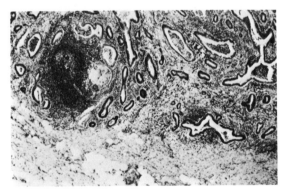

Figure 2–105. Sharply circumscribed edge of tumor.

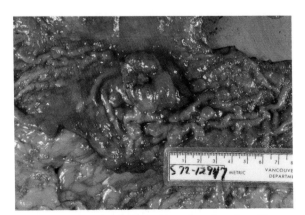

Figure 2–102. Polypoid carcinoma with surface ulceration. (Courtesy of Intellipath Inc., Santa Monica, CA.)

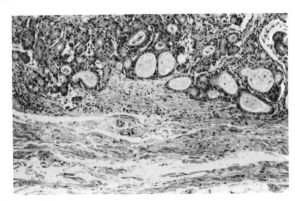

Figure 2–106. Edge of tumor.

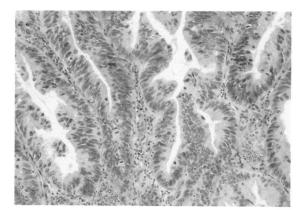

Figure 2–107. Well-differentiated intestinal-type carcinoma.

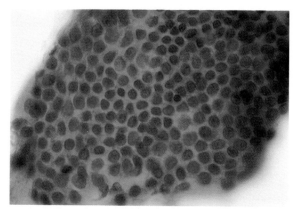

Figure 2–109. Brush cytology of gastric mucosa showing normal epithelial cells.

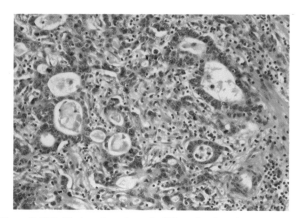

Figure 2–108. Moderately and poorly differentiated carcinoma.

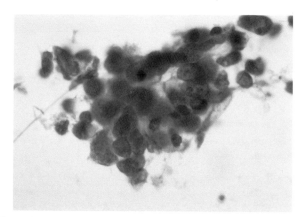

Figure 2–110. Brush cytology of intestinal adenocarcinoma.

DIFFUSE GASTRIC CARCINOMA

Biology of Disease

- Diffuse carcinomas may involve the antrum, the fundus, or both. Frequently, they are very extensive.
- Diffuse cancers account for fewer than 20% of gastric neoplasms.
- These neoplasms occur in a wider age group than intestinal carcinomas (age 25+).
- The worldwide incidence is similar.
- There is no association with intestinal metaplasia and multifocal atrophic gastritis. The precursor lesion has not been identified.

Clinical Features

- The presentation is similar to that of intestinal-type gastric carcinoma, but diffuse carcinoma tends to be diagnosed at a later stage.
- Transserosal spread to the ovaries may occur, producing Krukenberg's tumor.
- Stage for stage, the prognosis is similar to that of intestinal-type carcinoma.

Gross Pathology

- The surface component is frequently inconspicuous. There may be a plaquelike appearance or only a small area of ulceration accompanied by extensive submucosal spread.
- In advanced cases, the mucosal folds are flattened and the stomach shrunken (linitis plastica).
- The wall of the stomach, especially the submucosa, is thickened.
- By gross inspection, the edge of the tumor is poorly delineated.

Microscopic Pathology

- The growth pattern is one of single cells or small clumps and clusters. Glands are usually not present.
- The tumor margin is exceedingly ill defined.
- There is frequently a strong host fibroblastic response (scirrhous carcinoma).
- Individual cells may contain intracytoplasmic mucus, often in the form of a vacuole, producing a "signet ring" appearance.
- Extracytoplasmic mucin is usually absent.

- The nuclei are large but otherwise may appear deceptively bland.
- The intramucosal component of the tumor is often quite small.
- Intestinal metaplasia and multifocal atrophic gastritis are either absent or found only in small foci.

Differential Diagnosis

Gastric lymphoma.

Large cell lymphomas may have a growth pattern identical to that of diffuse carcinomas, and the differential diagnosis can be exceedingly difficult on endoscopic biopsy.

Special stains may be quite useful. Carcinomas may contain cytoplasmic mucin, which is PAS/Diastase posi-tive. Carcinoma cells may also be cytokeratin and carcinoembryonic antigen (CEA) positive by immunostaining. Lymphomas may be leukocyte common antigen (LCA) and L26 positive.

References

Grabiec J, Owen DA. Carcinoma of the stomach in young persons. Cancer 1985;56:388–396.

Kubo T. Histologic appearance of gastric carcinoma in high and low mortality countries. Comparison between Kyushu, Japan and Minnesota, U.S.A. Cancer 1971;28:726–734.

Lauren P. The two histological main types of gastric carcinoma: diffuse and so-called intestinal type. Acta Pathol Microbiol Scand (A) 1965;64:31–49.

Munoz N, Correa P, Cuello C, et al. Histologic types of gastric cancer in high- and low-risk areas. Int J Cancer 1968;3:809–818.

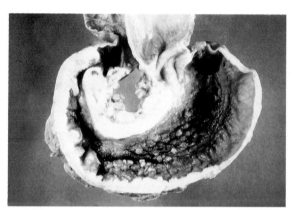

Figure 2–111. Linitis plastica. Note thickening of gastric wall. (Courtesy of Intellipath Inc., Santa Monica, CA.)

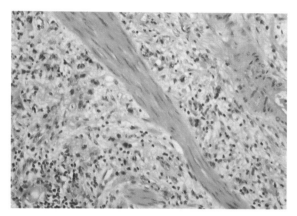

Figure 2–114. Tumor cells infiltrating the muscularis propria. The nuclei are deceptively bland.

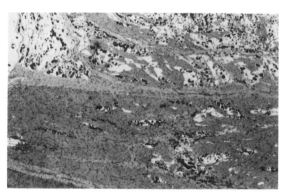

Figure 2–112. Poorly delineated edge of tumor.

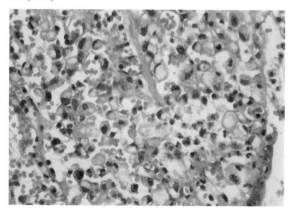

Figure 2–115. Signet ring cells.

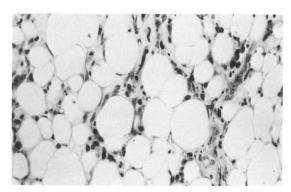

Figure 2–113. Tumor diffusely infiltrating omental fat.

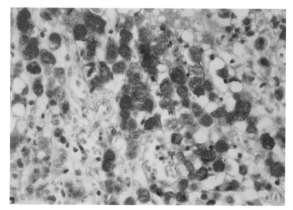

Figure 2–116. Signet ring cells (PAS).

EARLY GASTRIC CANCER

Biology of Disease

■ Early gastric cancer is an invasive tumor that is confined to the mucosa and submucosa of the stomach.

■ Gastric carcinoma in situ and gastric dysplasia, in contrast, are noninvasive lesions.

■ Early gastric cancer has a high cure rate when treated surgically (>80% 5-year survival).

Clinical Features

■ At endoscopic examination, these tumors may be flat, elevated, protruded, depressed, excavated, or a combination of these (Japanese Gastroenterological Endoscopic Society Classification).

■ These tumors are predominately asymptomatic and are discovered incidentally or on screening gastroscopy (used in some centers in Japan).

Gross Pathology

■ Early gastric cancer is most commonly encountered in the distal stomach.

■ In 10% of cases, multicentric neoplasms are present.

■ Most tumors are 2 cm in diameter or less.

■ Lesions may be flat, elevated, or ulcerated.

■ The gross findings are similar to those for larger, more deeply infiltrating tumors.

Microscopic Pathology

■ Most tumors are intestinal in type, but occasionally early diffuse cancer is encountered.

■ By definition, infiltration extends no deeper than the submucosa.

■ The presence of lymph node or even hepatic metastases is possible. Only the extent of the primary tumor is considered when determining whether a cancer is "early." Metastases reduce the prognosis, but only slightly.

References

Bogomoletz WV. Early gastric cancer. Am J Surg Pathol 1984;8:381–391.

Green PH, O'Toole KM, Weinberg LM, Goldfarb JP. Early gastric cancer. Gastroenterology 1981;81:247–256.

Ohta H, Noguchi Y, Takagi K, et al. Early gastric carcinoma with special reference to macroscopic classification. Cancer 1987;60:1099–1106.

Qizilbash AH, Stevenson GW. Early gastric cancer. Pathol Annu 1979;14:317–351.

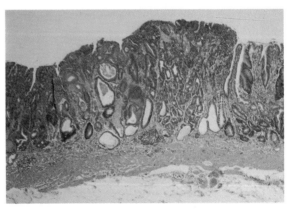

Figure 2–117. Early gastric cancer. Note that tumor does not infiltrate the muscularis propria.

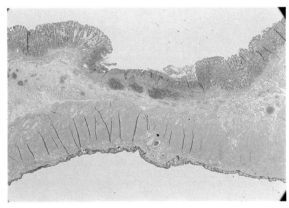

Figure 2–119. Ulcerated type of early gastric cancer. Some solid tumor is present at the left side of the crater.

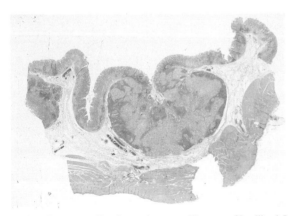

Figure 2–118. Very small early gastric cancer. (Courtesy of Intellipath Inc., Santa Monica, CA.)

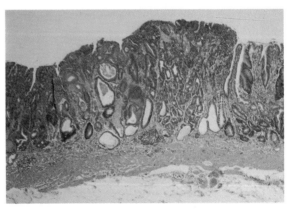

Figure 2–120. Early gastric cancer confined to the mucosa.

GASTRIC DYSPLASIA

Biology of Disease

- *Dysplasia* is defined as a morphologic or cytologic alteration that is (1) distinct from reactive or regenerative change, and (2) distinct from infiltrating carcinoma.
- The morphologic appearance and clinical significance of dysplasia and adenomas of the stomach are similar. By convention, however, adenomas are polypoid and dysplasia is a flat lesion.
- Dysplasia carries an increased risk of evolving into infiltrating carcinoma.
- Dysplasia may be high or low grade, depending on the severity of the morphologic abnormality.
- The term *carcinoma in situ* is not used with respect to gastric mucosa. High-grade dysplasia incorporates this morphologic abnormality.

Clinical Features

- In most cases, dysplasia cannot be identified endoscopically and is a chance finding.
- Mild dysplasia is a relatively innocuous lesion that generally does not progress and may even regress. It should receive routine follow-up.
- Up to 60% of patients diagnosed with severe dysplasia will have coincidental carcinoma and a further 25% will develop cancer within 15 months.

Gross Pathology

- The mucosa usually appears normal.
- If a gross lesion is identified in a patient with biopsy-proven gastric dysplasia, suspicion should be aroused that malignancy has already developed.

Microscopic Pathology

- Considerable interobserver variation is encountered in the diagnosis of dysplasia. This may be on the order of up to 50%, depending on the type of biopsy and the experience of the observer.
- Reactive changes are extremely difficult to distinguish from dysplasia and early carcinoma. Both architectural and cytologic criteria may be applied. Architectural features suggestive of dysplasia include glandular proliferation and crowding with budding and branching producing a back-to-back or cribriform pattern. The cytologic criteria are listed below.
- There are two types of dysplasia: type I, or adenomatous dysplasia, and type II, or hyperplastic dysplasia.
- Type I dysplasia histologically resembles an adenoma with pseudostratified crowded cigar-shaped nuclei and abundant amphophilic cytoplasm. Cytoplasmic mucin is present in scanty amounts.

- In type II dysplasia, the nuclei are round and vesicular with prominent nucleoli and an irregular chromatin pattern. The cytoplasm is pale and inconspicuous.
- The distinction between high- and low-grade dysplasia is one of degree of morphologic abnormality. In low-grade dysplasia (type I), the nuclei are more or less confined to the basal portion of the cell, whereas in high-grade dysplasia, they fill up most of the cell with loss of superficial cytoplasm. High-grade dysplasia of both types is characterized by an increasingly complex architecture.
- In biopsy material, the distinction of high-grade dysplasia from early infiltrating carcinoma can be extremely difficult. However, it is not critical as treatment for both lesions is similar.
- The criteria for the diagnosis of dysplasia are basically similar for all sites in the gastrointestinal tract.

Differential Diagnosis

Reactive atypia, adenoma, carcinoma.

In reactive atypia, the nuclear abnormalities are mild and generally will be confused only with low-grade dysplasia.

Reactive changes are usually accompanied by active inflammation. Diagnostic problems may be resolved by repeating the biopsies after treating the gastritis.

By convention, an adenoma is a tumorlike mass and dysplasia is a completely flat lesion. Otherwise the cytologic abnormalities are similar.

Carcinoma can be distinguished from severe dysplasia by the presence of invasion. Sometimes this can be difficult, but irregularly shaped or budding glandular structures suggest that invasion has occurred.

References

Cuello C, Correa P, Zarama G, et al. Histopathology of gastric dysplasias: correlations with gastric juice chemistry. Am J Surg Pathol 1979;3:491–500.

De Dombal FT, Price AB, Thompson H, et al. The British Society of Gastroenterology early gastric cancer/dysplasia survey: an interim report. Gut 1990;31:115–120.

Falck VG, Novelli MR, Wright NA, Alexander N. Gastric dysplasia: interobserver variation, sulphomucin staining and nucleolar organizer region counting. Histopathology 1990;16:141–149.

Ghandur-Mnaymneh L, Paz J, Roldau E, Cassady J. Dysplasia of non-metaplastic gastric mucosa: a proposal for its classification and its possible relationship to diffuse-type gastric carcinoma. Am J Surg Pathol 1988;12:96–114.

Jass JR. A classification of gastric dysplasia. Histopathology 1983;7:181–193.

Lansdown M, Quirke P, Dixon MF, Johnston D. High grade dysplasia of the gastric mucosa: a marker for gastric carcinoma. Gut 1990;31:977–983.

Ming SC, Bajtai A, Correa P, et al. Gastric dysplasia: significance and pathologic criteria. Cancer 1984;54:1794–1801.

Saraga E-P, Gardiol D, Costa J. Gastric dysplasia: significance and pathologic criteria. Am J Surg Pathol 1987;11:788–796.

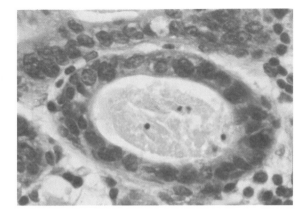

Figure 2–121. Type II dysplasia, low grade.

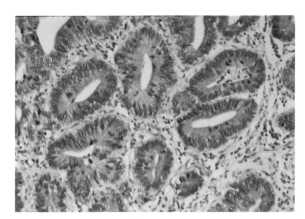

Figure 2–125. Type I dysplasia, low grade.

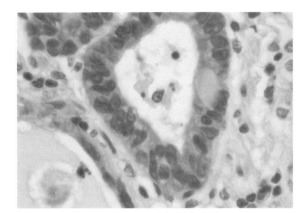

Figure 2–122. Type II dysplasia, high grade.

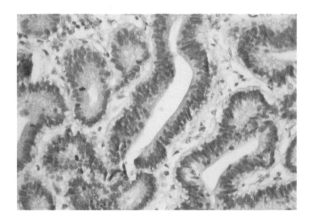

Figure 2–126. Type I dysplasia, low grade.

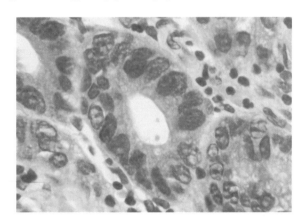

Figure 2–123. Type II dysplasia, high grade.

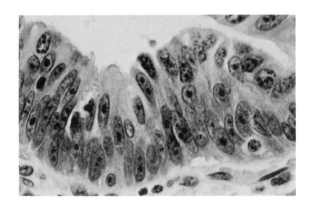

Figure 2–127. Type I dysplasia, high grade.

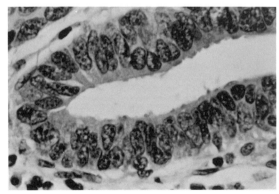

Figure ■ 2–124. Type II dysplasia. Note vesicular nuclei.

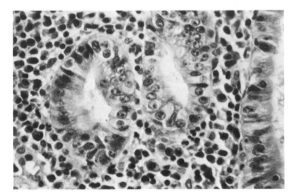

Figure 2–128. Reactive changes in epithelium for comparison.

RARE TYPES OF GASTRIC CARCINOMA

Biology of Disease

- This category includes squamous carcinoma, adenosquamous carcinoma, carcinosarcoma, carcinoma with lymphoid stroma, parietal cell carcinoma, hepatoid carcinoma, and composite carcinoma.
- In most instances, these neoplasms are variants of intestinal adenocarcinoma of the distal stomach.
- These variants account for fewer than 5% of all gastric carcinomas.
- The prognosis for carcinomas with lymphoid stroma and for parietal cell carcinomas is better than for the usual type of gastric cancer. The prognosis for the other variants is generally poorer.
- The term *composite carcinoma* refers to a combination of adenocarcinoma and carcinoid tumor.

Clinical Features

- The presence of a rare type of carcinoma is usually apparent only by histologic examination of biopsy or resection specimens.
- Hepatoid carcinomas have grossly elevated alpha-fetoprotein levels.

Gross Pathology

- The gross features of these tumors are usually nonspecific and closely resemble those of intestinal adenocarcinoma of the distal stomach. They have well-circumscribed edges.
- Parietal cell carcinomas may be bulky and friable.
- Carcinomas with lymphoid stroma may be extremely soft with a white-grey cut surface (medullary carcinoma).

Microscopic Pathology

- To diagnose squamous and adenosquamous carcinomas, it is necessary that squamous pearls or unequivocal prickles (desmosomes) be present. A sheetlike growth pattern is, on its own, not sufficient for a diagnosis.
- The squamous and glandular elements of adenosquamous carcinomas are intimately mixed. In *collision tumors*, one part of the tumor is purely squamous and the other part purely glandular.
- Carcinosarcomas consist of adenocarcinoma and a stromal component. In most cases, the stroma is composed of undifferentiated spindle cells, although rarely, osseous, cartilaginous muscle, or fatty differentiation is present. The stromal areas are generally positive with immunostains for cytokeratin and are considered to be foci of spindle cell differentiation in a carcinoma.
- In carcinomas with lymphoid stroma, the epithelial cells take the form of single cells, small clumps, or acini widely separated by the lymphoplasmacytic stroma.

- Parietal cell carcinomas are composed of solid sheets of boxlike or polygonal cells with large quantities of eosinophilic cytoplasm.
- Hepatoid carcinomas closely resemble true liver carcinomas even to the extent of having bile plugs in the canaliculi. There may be trabecular, pseudoacinar, papillary, or clear cell areas of differentiation.
- Composite carcinomas consist of adenocarcinomas with areas of carcinoid differentiation. The neuroendocrine cells may be variably differentiated.

Special Diagnostic Techniques

- Electron microscopy will help to distinguish a true carcinosarcoma from a carcinoma with spindle cell components. Evidence of smooth muscle differentiation may be identified.
- Ultrastructural examination will also identify neurosecretory granules in a composite carcinoma and intracellular canaliculi in a parietal cell tumor.
- Immunohistochemical examination will identify areas of carcinoid differentiation (chromogranin) and hepatoid differentiation (alpha-fetoprotein, alpha$_1$-antitrypsin).

References

Ali MH, Davidson A, Azzopardi JG. Composite gastric carcinoid and adenocarcinoma. Histopathology 1984;8:529–536.

Bansal M, Mamoru K, Gordon RE. Carcinosarcoma and separate carcinoid tumor of the stomach. A case report with light and electron microscopic studies. Cancer 1982;50:1876–1881.

Burke AP, Yen TS, Shekitkak M, Sobin LH. Lymphoepithelial carcinoma of the stomach with Epstein-Barr virus demonstrated by polymerase chain reaction. Mod Pathol 1990;3:277–380.

Copella G, Frigerio B, Cornaggia M, et al. Gastric parietal cell carcinoma—a newly recognised entity: light microscopic and ultrastructural features. Histopathology 1984;8:813–824.

Ishikura H, Kirimoto K, Shamoto M, et al. Hepatoid adenocarcinoma of the stomach. Cancer 1986;58:119–126.

Mori M, Fukada T, Enjoji M. Adenosquamous carcinoma of the stomach. Histogenetic and ultrastructural features. Gastroenterology 1987; 92:1078–1082.

Mori M, Iwashita A, Enjoji M. Squamous carcinoma of the stomach: report of three cases. Am J Gastroenterol 1986;81:339–342.

Mori M, Iwashita A, Enjoji M. Adenosquamous carcinoma of the stomach. Cancer 1986;57:330–339.

Robey-Cafferty SS, Grignon DJ, Ro JY, et al. Sarcomatoid carcinoma of the stomach. Report of three cases with immunohistochemical and ultrastructural observations. Cancer 1990;65:1601–1606.

Ruck P, Wehrman M, Campbell M, et al. Squamous carcinoma of the gastric stump. Case report and review of the literature. Am J Surg Pathol 1989;13:317–324.

Siegal A, Freund U, Gal R. Carcinosarcoma of the stomach. Histopathology 1988;13:350–353.

Ulich TR, Kollin M, Lewin KH. Composite gastric carcinoma. Report of a tumor of the carcinoma—carcinoid spectrum. Arch Pathol Lab Med 1988;112:91–93.

Watanabe H, Enjoji M, Imai T. Gastric carcinoma with lymphoid stroma. Its morphologic characteristics and prognostic correlations. Cancer 1976;38:232–243.

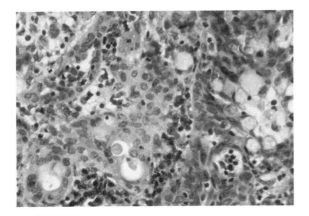

Figure 2–129. Adenosquamous carcinoma.

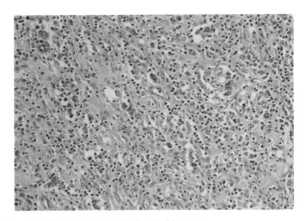

Figure 2–132. Carcinoma with lymphoid stroma.

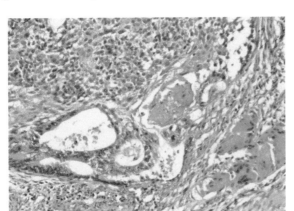

Figure 2–130. "Carcinosarcoma" epithelial area.

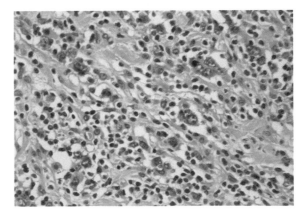

Figure 2–133. Carcinoma with lymphoid stroma.

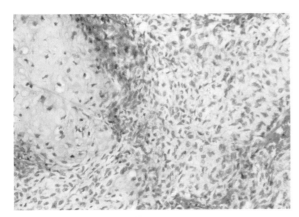

Figure 2–131. "Carcinosarcoma" sarcomatous area.

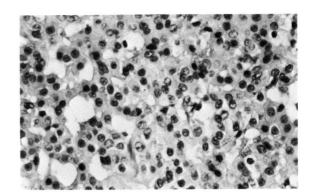

Figure 2–134. Hepatoid carcinoma of stomach.

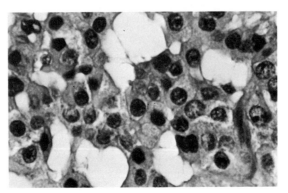

Figure 2–135. Hepatoid carcinoma. The spaces represent canalicular structures.

CARCINOID TUMORS

Biology of Disease

- Gastric tumors account for 5% of all gastrointestinal carcinoids.
- Most gastric carcinoids occur in association with autoimmune gastritis. These patients have secondary antral G-cell hyperplasia and nodular hyperplasia of fundic enterochromaffin-like (ECL) cells. The ECL hyperplasia may give rise to multiple microcarcinoids and one or more grossly identifiable carcinoid tumors. Although ECL cells secrete histamine, there is no syndrome of histamine overproduction associated with autoimmune gastritis.
- Sporadic gastric carcinoids unassociated with autoimmune gastritis may occur. These may produce 5-hydroxytryptophan, gastrin, or ACTH.
- Most carcinoids (70%) have not metastasized at the time of presentation. Factors associated with metastases include size (>2 cm) and atypical histology (features intermediate between those of typical carcinoid and oat cell carcinoma).

Clinical Features

- Many cases are discovered incidentally.
- Larger tumors may present with nonspecific symptoms, such as abdominal pain or dyspepsia.
- The carcinoid syndrome is rare, and if present is usually atypical (red flush rather than cyanotic flush). This is the result of 5-hydroxytryptophan overproduction.

Gross Pathology

- Most tumors are located in the gastric fundus, since this is the site of hyperplastic ECL cells.
- Most tumors are polypoid and superficially ulcerated.

Microscopic Pathology

- A typical foregut carcinoid appearance is seen, with a predominately ribbonlike arrangement of cells. Occasionally trabecular and rosette formations are present.
- Microcarcinoids are characterized by endocrine cells budding off the base of fundal pits.
- The nuclei are bland with an even distribution of chromatin. The cytoplasm is amphophilic.
- Mitoses are present but not abundant.

Special Techniques

- Gastric carcinoids are generally argentaffin negative and argyrophil positive. They will therefore stain with Grimelius but not with Fontana-Masson.
- Immunostains with chromogranin are positive.

Differential Diagnosis

Glomus tumor.
Glomus tumors have a distinctive vascular pattern, with tumor cells closely related to the walls of venules.
Glomus tumors are negative for chromogranin but positive for smooth muscle immunostains (smooth muscle actin).

References

Borch K, Renvall H, Kullman E, Willander E. Gastric carcinoid tumor associated with a syndrome of hypergastrinemic atrophic gastritis: a prospective analysis of 11 cases. Am J Surg Pathol 1987;11:435–444.

Borch K, Renvall H, Liedberg G. Gastric endocrine cell hyperplasia and carcinoid tumors in pernicious anemia. Gastroenterology 1985;88:638–648.

Chejfec G, Gould VE. Malignant gastric neuroendocrinomas. Ultrastructural and biochemical characterization of their secretory activity. Hum Pathol 1977;8:433–434.

Muller J, Kirchner T, Muller-Hermelink HK. Gastric endocrine cell hyperplasia and carcinoid tumors in atrophic gastritis type A. Am J Surg Pathol 1987;11:909–917.

Sandler M, Snow PJ. An atypical carcinoid tumor secreting 5-hydroxytryptophan. Lancet 1958;1:137–139.

Wilander E, El-Salhy M, Pitkanen P. Histopathology of gastric carcinoids: a survey of 42 cases. Histopathology 1984;8:183–193.

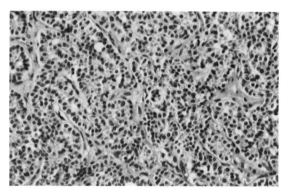
Figure 2–136. Carcinoid tumor showing a trabecular pattern.

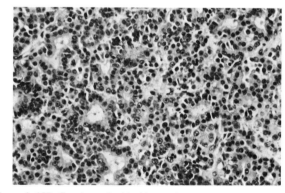
Figure 2–137. Gastric carcinoid with an acinar pattern.

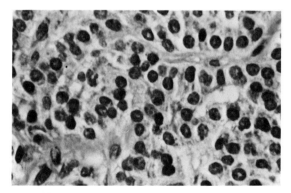
Figure 2–138. Carcinoid tumor. Note the nuclear regularity.

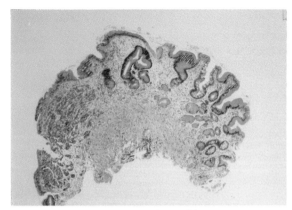

Figure 2–139. Microcarcinoid tumor in atrophic mucosa.

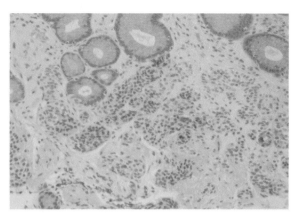

Figure 2–140. Microcarcinoid tumor. Note the clumps of cells present in the muscularis mucosae.

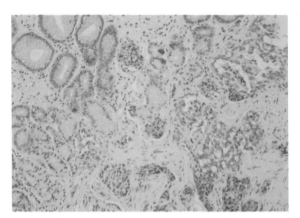

Figure 2–141. Microcarcinoid tumor (chromogranin).

CHAPTER ■ 3

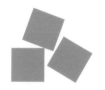

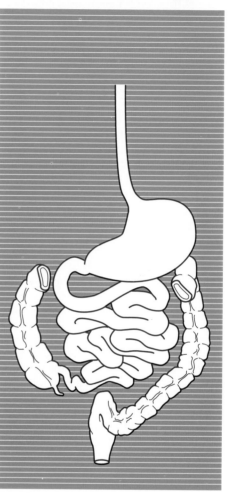

DISEASES OF THE
SMALL BOWEL

THE NORMAL SMALL BOWEL

Gross Anatomy

■ The small bowel comprises the duodenum, jejunum, and ileum. The duodenum is approximately 25 cm long, extends from the pylorus to the ligament of Treitz, and forms a loop around the head of the pancreas. It is composed of four parts. The *first part* is the duodenal cap or bulb; the *second part* is the descending portion, which includes the ampulla of Vater; the *third part* is the horizontal portion, and the *fourth part* ascends left of the second lumbar vertebra to the ligament of Treitz. The duodenum is entirely retroperitoneal.

■ The jejunum consists of the proximal two fifths of the intraperitoneal small bowel, and the ileum the distal three fifths. Characteristically, the lumen of the jejunum is wider than that of the ileum, and its mucosal folds (valvulae conniventes) are higher. There is no fixed anatomical landmark at the jejunoileal junction.

■ The jejunum, ileum, and fourth part of the duodenum are supplied by the superior mesenteric artery through a series of branching arcades. The duodenum is supplied by the superior pancreaticoduodenal branches of the gastroduodenal artery, which is derived from the celiac axis, and by the inferior pancreaticoduodenal branches of the superior mesenteric artery. The veins drain to the superior mesenteric vein, which joins the splenic vein to form the portal vein. The veins, lymphatics, and autonomic nerves accompany the arteries. The lymph drains to mesenteric nodes and thence to para-aortic nodes.

■ The mucosa of the small bowel forms concentric folds (called valvulae conniventes, plicae circulares, or mucosal folds), which considerably increase the surface area of the mucosa. The muscularis mucosae is part of the mucosa and forms the structural basis of the folds.

■ The muscle coat (muscularis propria or muscularis externa) is composed of an inner circular layer and an outer longitudinal layer. The myenteric plexus (Auerbach's plexus) lies between the layers of muscle.

■ The coils of intraperitoneal small bowel are anchored to the posterior abdominal wall by the mesentery, a loose mesenchymal tissue that is rich in fat cells and is strengthened by the vascular (including lymphatic) arcades and nerves that run through it. The mesenteric attachment polarizes the bowel in its longitudinal axis. Arterial blood flows from the mesenteric to the antimesenteric border, whereas venous blood and lymph flow the opposite way. The antimesenteric border may be more susceptible to hypotensive ischemia. The mesenteric anchor influences disease processes on the mesenteric border; for example, the sinuses of Crohn's disease usually penetrate into the mesentery.

Microscopic Appearances

■ The mucosa has three components: the *epithelium*, with its crypts and villi, a loose connective tissue called the *lamina propria*, and a muscular layer, the *muscularis mucosae*. The villi are 300 to 500 μm in height and are four to five times the height of the crypts. Villi are tallest in the jejunum and shortest in the duodenal bulb and terminal ileum.

■ The epithelium is a single cell layer that turns over every 5 to 6 days in the jejunum and every 3 days in the ileum. The stem cell zone is located a short distance above the base of the crypt. Paneth's cells and endocrine cells migrate downwards from the stem cell zone. Absorptive cells, goblet cells, and endocrine cells migrate upwards. Endocrine cells display fine eosinophilic, subnuclear granules that take up silver stains and show chromogranin immunoreactivity.

■ The villi are covered by columnar absorptive cells with basally located nuclei and a brush border of microvilli on the luminal surface. Mucin-secreting goblet cells are interspersed among the absorptive cells. Goblet cells store their secretory granules as a compact apical mass limited by a dense, cup-shaped layer of cytoplasm called the *theca*, which contains an orderly arrangement of microtubules and intermediate filaments.

■ The lamina propria of the villus displays a capillary network immediately beneath the epithelium. A central lymphatic channel, occasional smooth muscle cells, lymphocytes, macrophages, eosinophils, and mast cells are also present. Mucosal mast cells can be identified by using special stains such as toluidine blue and sulfated alcian blue. The villi are supplied by a central arteriole that opens into a network of capillaries at the villus tip. The arrangement is suitable for countercurrent exchange of gases and solutes.

■ The *submucosa* is a loose connective tissue that links the mucosa and muscle coat, allowing both independent play. Blood vessels, lymphatics, and nerves course through it and it contains the nerve plexus of Meissner.

■ The muscle coat is separated from the peritoneum by a thin connective tissue layer except at the attachment of the mesentery. The *myenteric plexus of Auerbach* consists of a meshwork of nerve cells and fibers that, on conventional sections, appear as clusters of ganglion cells, perineurial cells, and nerve fibers.

■ The peritoneal surface consists of a single row of cuboidal mesothelial cells. These overlie an elastic lamina and a loose connective tissue layer, the *serosa*, which separates the peritoneum from the muscle coat.

■ The duodenum contains *Brunner's glands*, which are mainly located below the muscularis mucosae but are also present above it in the duodenal bulb. They form lobules of pale-staining cells that secrete mucin, pepsinogen type II, and (possibly) bicarbonate into the crypts. Small numbers of endocrine cells are also present in Brunner's glands.

■ The normal duodenal bulb mucosa shows foci of gastric surface metaplasia, blunt villi, and a mixed cell population in the lamina propria, including plasma cells, eosinophils, macrophages, and lymphocytes.

■ Solitary lymphoid follicles are present throughout the small bowel but are abortive in the normal duodenum and jejunum. They may be visible grossly in children or adolescents as randomly scattered, 2- to 3-mm elevations of the terminal ileal mucosa. There are specialized *membranous enterocytes*, cells adapted for antigen sampling, on the dome of each follicle. Antigen is passed to lymphocytes and to dendritic cells in the underlying lymphoid follicle. There, it is processed and lymphocytes are instructed. The *Peyer's patches* along the antimesenteric border of the ileum are aggregates of these lymphoid follicles. Nefarious bacteria and viruses (such as *Salmonella typhi, Yersinia enterocolitica*, and reoviruses) exploit the membranous enterocytes to invade the gut. Peyer's patches may have a dusky or black appearance because they take in and retain swallowed atmospheric dust.

References

Antonioli DA, Madara JL. Functional anatomy of the gastrointestinal tract. In: Ming S-C, Goldman H (eds). Pathology of the Gastrointestinal Tract. Philadelphia: WB Saunders, 1992;24–32.

Deschner EE, Lehnert T. Cell renewal in health and disease. In: Ming S-C, Goldman H (eds). Pathology of the Gastrointestinal Tract. Philadelphia: WB Saunders, 1992;98–110.

Phillips AD. The small intestinal mucosa. In: Whitehead R (ed). Gastrointestinal and Esophageal Pathology. New York: Churchill Livingstone, 1989;29–39.

Segal GH, Petras RE. Small intestine. In: Sternberg SS (ed). Histology for Pathologists. New York: Raven Press, 1992;547–571.

Specian RD, Neutra MR. Cytoskeleton of intestinal goblet cells in rabbit and monkey. The theca. Gastroenterology 1984;87:1313-1325.

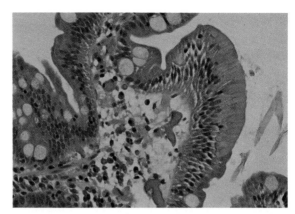

Figure 3–3. Normal duodenal bulb mucosa showing focal gastric metaplasia (*right*).

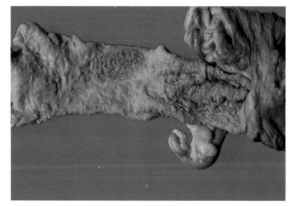

Figure 3–4. Normal Peyer's patches in the terminal ileum of an 18-year-old man. Solitary lymphoid follicles are the tiny mucosal bumps.

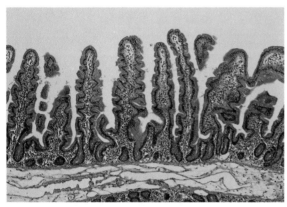

Figure 3–1. Normal duodenal mucosa (second part) displays tall villi and short crypts.

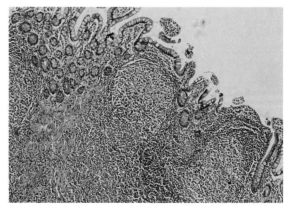

Figure 3–5. A portion of a Peyer's patch displays two mucosal lymphoid follicles (*right*).

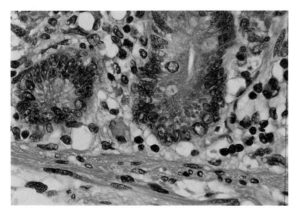

Figure 3–2. The base of the crypt shows Paneth's cells with large supranuclear granules. An enterochromaffin cell on the lateral wall of the crypt shows fine subnuclear granules.

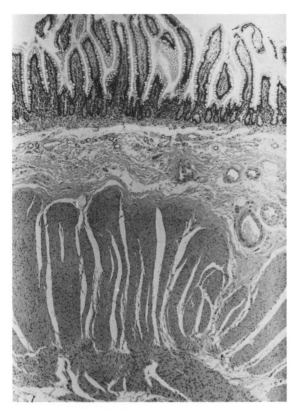

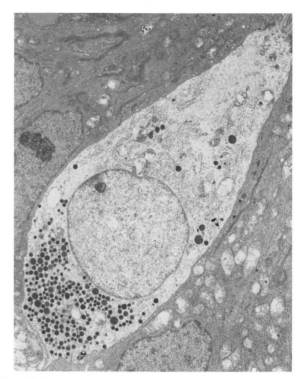

Figure 3–8. Normal endocrine cell containing dense-core granules.

Figure 3–6. Normal ileum showing mucosa, submucosa, inner circular, and outer longitudinal muscle coats.

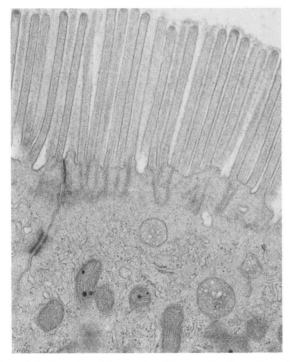

Figure 3–7. Normal small bowel microvilli covered by fuzzy glycocalyx and anchored by actin rootlets.

CONGENITAL ATRESIA OR STENOSIS

Biology of Disease

- *Stenosis*, which means narrowing of the lumen, may be due to intrinsic disease of the bowel or to external pressure such as from an annular pancreas or peritoneal band. Congenital stenoses are more common in the duodenum than elsewhere in the small bowel.
- *Atresia* is a congenital absence of the lumen of a portion of bowel. It is thought to be due to intrauterine failure of lumen formation or ischemia. Atresias are randomly distributed in the small bowel. Forty percent occur in duodenum, and 60% in jejunum or ileum. Atresias are more common than stenoses.

Clinical Findings

- Maternal hydramnios or a single umbilical artery may be a harbinger of duodenal atresia.
- About 25% of cases of duodenal stenosis or atresia are associated with Down's syndrome.
- Congenital malformations such as malrotation, annular pancreas, and congenital heart disease are associated with duodenal atresia but not with jejunoileal atresia.

Gross Pathology

- Atresias may be single (80%) or multiple (20%). The normal bowel may be dilated between multiple atretic lesions.
- Three types of atresia are recognized:
  Type 1 atresia is an imperforate septum in an otherwise continuous bowel.
  Type 2 atresia is replacement of a length of bowel by a thin cord of fibromuscular tissue.
  Type 3 atresia is complete absence of a segment of bowel between two blind ends.
- The bowel proximal to an atresia is dilated and may become gangrenous, whereas the distal bowel is empty and narrowed.
- Stenoses are of two types: (1) an incomplete septum and (2) narrowing of bowel, which retains more or less normal structure.

Microscopic Pathology

- Septa in type 1 atresia are covered on both surfaces by mucosa with underlying submucosa and muscularis mucosae.
- In a stenotic or type 2 atretic segment, mucosa may be absent, having been replaced by granulation tissue.
- At the margin of the lesion, the mucosa may consist of a single layer of epithelium or simple crypts without villi.
- The muscularis mucosae may be absent, fibrosed, thickened, or fused with the muscularis propria. Hemosiderin-laden macrophages may be found within the scar tissue or granulation tissue.
- Some atresias consist of thin fibrous cords with little residual bowel structure.

References

Bodian M, White LLR, Carter CO, Louw JH. Congenital duodenal obstruction and mongolism. Br Med J 1952;1:77–78.

De Sa DJ. Congenital stenosis and atresia of the jejunum and ileum. J Clin Pathol 1972;25:1063–1070.

Lynn HB, Espinas EE. Intestinal atresia: an attempt to relate location to embryologic processes. Arch Surg 1959;79:357–361.

O'Neill JF, Anderson K, Bradshaw HH, et al. Congenital atresia of small intestine in newborn. Am J Dis Child 1948;75:214–237.

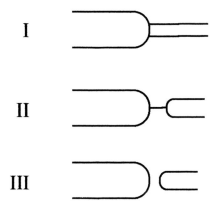

Figure 3–9. Types of atresia. Type 1, an imperforate septum; type 2, a fibrous cord; type 3, a complete separation.

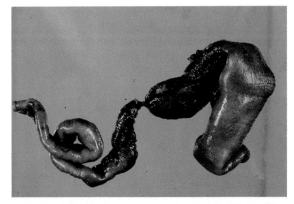

Figure 3–10. Small bowel atresia (type 2) in a 2-day-old infant. Note the enormous dilatation of the proximal bowel (*right*), the cordlike stricture, and the narrowed distal bowel. (Courtesy of Dr. Geoffrey Machin.)

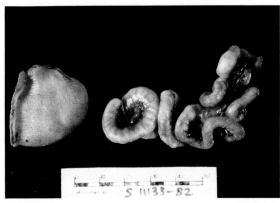

Figure 3–11. Type 3 atresia with discontinuity between the dilated proximal bowel (*left*) and the narrowed distal bowel (*right*). (Courtesy of Dr. Geoffrey Machin.)

MECKEL'S DIVERTICULUM

Biology of Disease

- *Meckel's diverticulum* is a congenital diverticulum of the ileum derived from a remnant of the embryonic vitellointestinal duct. It may be tethered to the umbilicus by a fibrous remnant of the duct. Its wall includes all the layers of the normal small bowel.
- The mucosal lining may contain ectopic gastric fundic mucosa or pancreas.

Clinical Findings

- Meckel's diverticulum is usually a symptomless finding at autopsy or surgery. Symptomatic cases may manifest in infancy or childhood but often do not arise until adult life. Symptoms include blood loss, perforation, and bowel obstruction.
- Ectopic gastric mucosa may cause peptic ulceration and give rise to anemia, fecal occult blood, and, rarely, perforation.
- Meckel's diverticulum may undergo inversion and become the lead point of an intussusception.
- A foreign body may lodge in Meckel's diverticulum and perforate it.
- Acute diverticulitis may manifest as appendicitis and may be associated with the presence of an enterolith.
- A vitellointestinal band may act as the apex of a volvulus or ensnare a segment of bowel, producing obstruction.

Gross Pathology

- The Rule of 2's is a useful mnemonic: Meckel's diverticulum occurs in about 2% of the population, is located 2 feet from the cecum, averages 2 inches in length, and is symptomatic in 2% of cases.
- Meckel's diverticulum is located on the antimesenteric border, about 30 cm proximal to the cecum in the infant and about 60 cm proximal to the cecum in the adult.
- Ectopic gastric mucosa may have a whitish color clearly distinguishing it from the remainder of the mucosa or it may be grossly invisible.
- Meckel's diverticulum may be contained in hernias. It may be complicated by ulceration and perforation, enterolith formation, endometriosis, secondary diverticula, diverticulitis, pancreatic heterotopia, carcinoids, leiomyomas, or other tumors.
- Intussusception, ulceration, perforation, or foreign body impaction may be the presenting pathology. Peptic ulceration may be located in the bowel distal to the diverticulum or in the diverticulum itself. Scarring may give the diverticulum an hourglass appearance.

Microscopic Pathology

- Most diverticula are lined by normal small bowel mucosa alone.
- Ectopic gastric fundic mucosa comprises pits and glands, including chief and parietal cells.
- Intussusception may be associated with ischemic intestinal necrosis and acute peritonitis.

References

Berman EJ, Schneider A, Potts WJ. Importance of gastric mucosa in Meckel's diverticulum. JAMA 1954;156:6–7.

Soltero MJ, Bill AH. The natural history of Meckel's diverticulum and its relation to incidental removal: a study of 202 cases of diseased Meckel's diverticulum found in King County, Washington, over a fifteen year period. Am J Surg 1976;132:168–173.

Vico JJ, Nosanchuk JS. Calculi in Meckel's diverticulum. Arch Pathol Lab Med 1982;106:206–207.

Weinstein EC, Cain JC, ReMine WH. Meckel's diverticulum: 55 years of clinical and surgical experience. JAMA 1962;182:251–253.

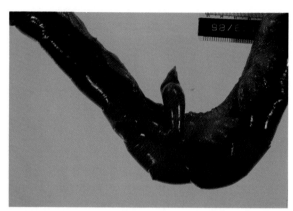

Figure 3–12. Meckel's diverticulum found incidentally at autopsy.

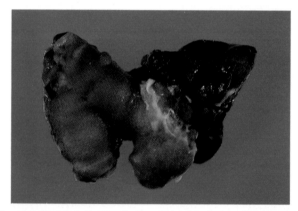

Figure 3–13. Meckel's diverticulum. This diverticulum shows extreme congestion and purulent exudate on the surface secondary to a perforated peptic ulcer.

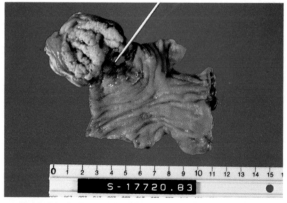

Figure 3–14. Meckel's diverticulum. Heterotopic gastric fundus–type mucosa appears whiter than the small bowel mucosa. Near the ectopic mucosa there is a peptic ulcer, and the probe is in a perforation.

DUODENAL DIVERTICULA

Biology of Disease

■ Duodenal diverticula may be intraluminal or extraluminal. Extraluminal diverticula are commonly seen on barium swallow or at autopsy, with a reported prevalence varying from 1% to 8.6%. Most are acquired, single, and located on the medial wall of the second part of the duodenum. One third of cases are located in the third or fourth part of the duodenum. Congenital duodenal diverticula are rare.

■ Intraluminal diverticula are not true diverticula, but rather congenital mucosal webs or diaphragms that become distended by food. They have been likened to a windsock within the duodenum. They are always postbulbar and usually near the ampulla.

Clinical Findings

■ Extraluminal diverticula are rarely symptomatic. Complications such as diverticulitis, biliary obstruction, pancreatitis, hemorrhage, and perforation are described rarely.

■ Intraluminal diverticula are rare. They are asymptomatic in childhood but ultimately produce symptoms in adulthood. The symptoms are abdominal pain, vomiting, and, sometimes, blood loss. Pancreatitis may occur.

Gross Pathology

■ Extraluminal diverticula are outpouchings of the bowel wall that generally contain all the layers of the bowel wall. Most are found incidentally at autopsy or radiologically as solitary lesions on the medial wall of the duodenum.

Microscopic Pathology

■ Diverticula are lined predominantly by small bowel–type mucosa. Heterotopic gastric fundic mucosa may be abundant proximal to intraluminal diverticula.

■ Intraluminal diverticula are thin sheets of tissue lined on both sides by mucosa.

References

Critchlow JF, Shapiro ME, Silen W. Duodenojejunostomy for the pancreaticobiliary complications of duodenal diverticulum. Ann Surg 1985;202:56–58.

Juler GL, List JW, Stemmer EA, Connolly JE. Perforating duodenal diverticulitis. Arch Surg 1969;99:572–578.

Kennedy RH, Thompson MH. Are duodenal diverticula associated with choledocholithiasis? Gut 1988;29:1003–1006.

Sreide JA, Seime S, Sreide O. Intraluminal duodenal diverticulum: case report and update of the literature 1975–1986. Am J Gastroenterol 1988;83:988–991.

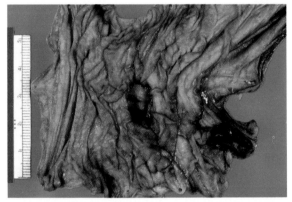

Figure 3–15. Duodenal diverticulum. The central depression is a diverticulum of the second part of the duodenum that was discovered incidentally at autopsy. The pylorus is at *left*.

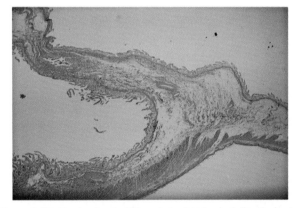

Figure 3–16. Duodenal web. This web (or intraluminal diverticulum) is covered on both surfaces by mucosa and contains a submucosal core. The lack of mucosal histologic detail is due to autolysis; the specimen was obtained at autopsy.

JEJUNAL DIVERTICULA

Biology of Disease

■ *Jejunal diverticula* are acquired outpouchings of mucosa passing through the muscle coat into the mesentery. They are pseudodiverticula (they do not include all layers of the bowel wall) and are seen on 1% of barium studies.

■ Jejunal diverticulosis may arise from primary pseudo-obstruction due to visceral neuropathy or myopathy.

■ Most patients with jejunal diverticula are over 50 years of age.

Clinical Findings

■ The majority of jejunal diverticula are asymptomatic and are often discovered incidentally at surgery or autopsy, or on radiologic studies.

■ Complications such as diverticulitis with perforation or peritonitis, massive hemorrhage, and enterolith formation can occur.

■ Less common complications are steatorrhea, malabsorption, and vitamin B_{12} deficiency. These are secondary to bacterial overgrowth within the diverticula. Bacteria consume ingested vitamin B_{12} and deconjugate bile acids, resulting in steatorrhea. Vitamin B_{12} deficiency may occur independently of steatorrhea.

Gross Pathology

■ Multiple diverticula are present on the mesenteric border of the gut. They vary in diameter from 1 to 4 cm. They have thin walls consisting of mucosa and serosa, which is typical of pulsion diverticula. Localized peridiverticular inflammation or peritonitis may be visible grossly.

Microscopic Pathology

■ Diverticula are lined by normal mucosa and longitudinal muscle coat. They penetrate the muscle coat where the blood vessels enter the bowel wall.
■ Foamy macrophages may accumulate in the submucosa of diverticula as a response to local lymphatic obstruction.
■ The jejunal muscle coat may appear normal or may show changes similar to those seen with familial visceral myopathy or progressive systemic sclerosis.
■ Fabry's disease, in which there is neuronal degeneration, neuronal intranuclear inclusions, or accumulation of glycolipid in the myenteric plexus, may be complicated by diverticulosis.
■ Diverticulitis consists of ulceration of the mucosa in the diverticulum with peridiverticular inflammation or abscess. Inflammatory rupture of the wall of an artery may be found occasionally.

References

Butler RW. Multiple intramesenteric diverticula of the small intestine. Br J Surg 1933;21:329–346.
Cooke WT, Cox EV, Fone DJ, et al. The clinical and metabolic significance of jejunal diverticula. Gut 1963;4:115–131.
Fraser I. The diverticula of the jejunoileum. Br J Surg 1933;21:183–211.
Krishnamurthy S, Kelly MM, Rohrman CA, Schuffler MD. Jejunal diverticulosis: a heterogenous disorder caused by a variety of abnormalities of smooth muscle or myenteric plexus. Gastroenterology 1983;65:538–547.
Lee FD. Submucosal lipophages in diverticula of the small intestine. J Pathol Bacteriol 1966;92:29–33.
Palder SB, Frey CB. Jejunal diverticulosis. Arch Surg 1988;123:889–894.
Sheppe WM. False diverticula of the jejunum. JAMA 1924;82:1118–1119.

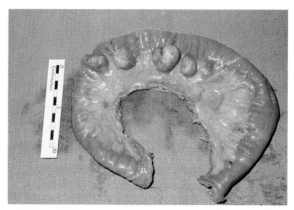

Figure 3–17. Jejunal diverticulosis. Several diverticula are present in the mesenteric attachment of the jejunum.

PANCREATIC HETEROTOPIA

Biology of Disease

■ *Pancreatic heterotopia* is pancreatic tissue located distant from the normal pancreas.
■ Heterotopias are submucosal, tumorlike masses usually 3 to 20 mm in diameter.
■ Sixty percent of cases involve the stomach or duodenum. The remainder are found in the small bowel or in a Meckel's diverticulum.

Clinical Findings

■ Pancreatic heterotopia is most often an incidental finding at surgery or autopsy. The incidence is approximately 1 per 380 upper GI operations.
■ It may manifest as an intussusception or a cause of occult blood loss.

■ The male-to-female ratio is 3:1.
■ Rarely, cystic change and inflammation in heterotopic pancreas of the duodenal wall result in duodenal or biliary stenosis, causing abdominal pain, nausea, and vomiting. On ultrasonography, and computed tomography, the lesions may mimic carcinoma. Whipple's procedure (which may carry significant mortality) was carried out in several cases of heterotopia because they were suspected to be malignancies.

Gross Pathology

■ Heterotopic pancreas is a submucosal tumorlike nodule. The overlying mucosa is intact. Ducts may empty into the bowel through a central punctum.
■ The cut surface resembles normal pancreas. The nodule often extends into the muscle coat.
■ Cystic change may be present. Rarely, the cysts measure

up to 3 cm in diameter and bulge as nodules into the gastric antral or duodenal lumen.

Microscopic Pathology

■ Exocrine pancreatic glands, excretory ducts, and islets of Langerhans may all be present. Relative excess of dilated ductal elements and atrophy of exocrine glands may make identification of the lesion difficult.

■ The ectopic pancreas may display the full spectrum of pancreatic pathology, including pancreatitis, tumors, and islet cell lesions.

Differential Diagnosis

Heterotopic gastric fundic mucosa, adenomyoma.

Heterotopic gastric fundic mucosa is distinguished by the presence of chief cells, parietal cells, and gastric pits.

Adenomyoma is a condition similar to pancreatic heterotopia but consisting of exocrine ducts alone, without exocrine acini.

References

De Castro Barbosa JJ, Dockerty MB, Waugh JM. Pancreatic heterotopia. Review of the literature and report of 41 authenticated surgical cases of which 25 were clinically significant. Surg Gynecol Obstet 1946; 82:527–542.

Fléjou J-F, Potet F, Molas G, et al. Cystic dystrophy of the gastric and duodenal wall developing in heterotopic pancreas: an unrecognized entity. Gut 1993;34:343–347.

Nickels J, Laasonen EM. Pancreatic heterotopia: review. Scand J Gastrointerol 1970;5:639–640.

Stewart MJ, Taylor AL. Adenomyoma of the stomach. J Pathol Bacteriol 1925;28:195–202.

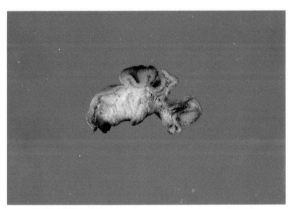

Figure 3–18. Heterotopic pancreas. A nodule in the wall of the jejunum found coincidentally at surgery has yellowish lobular appearance resembling that of normal pancreas.

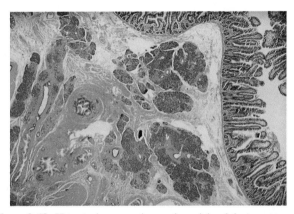

Figure 3–19. Heterotopic pancreatic exocrine acini and ducts are present in the submucosa and muscle coat of the jejunum. The overlying jejunal mucosa is normal.

GASTRIC HETEROTOPIA

Biology of Disease

■ Heterotopic gastric fundic mucosa forms small pink nodules in the duodenal bulb and is found in 2% of endoscopic examinations.

■ Rarely, gastric heterotopia is found at other sites, including upper esophagus, rectum, Meckel's diverticulum, gallbladder, and enteric duplications.

Clinical Findings

■ Gastric heterotopia in the duodenal bulb is usually asymptomatic. In other locations, it may lead to peptic ulceration or, rarely, an obstructing mass.

Gross Pathology

■ Endoscopically, one or multiple pink nodules, less than 1 cm in diameter, are seen in the duodenal bulb, especially on the anterior wall.

Microscopic Pathology

■ Gastric body mucosa complete with chief cells, parietal cells, and overlying foveolar mucosa is present. *Helicobacter pylori* may colonize this mucosa and induce active chronic inflammation.

Differential Diagnosis

Gastric pit metaplasia, pancreatic heterotopia.

In gastric pit metaplasia, foci of gastric pit epithelium are admixed with duodenal epithelium on the surfaces of villi. Gastric body glands are not present.

Pancreatic heterotopia is distinguished by the lobules of exocrine acini and the ducts that drain them.

References

Haglund U, Rehnberg O, Elander B, et al. Acid secreting gastric heterotopia in the duodenum. Acta Chir Scand 1982;148:693–696.

Hoedemaeker J. Heterotopic gastric mucosa in the duodenum. Digestion 1970;3:165–173.

Lessells AM, Martin DF. Heterotopic gastric mucosa in the duodenum. J Clin Pathol 1982;35:591–595.

Remmele W, Hartmann W, Von der Laden U, et al. Three other types of duodenal polyps: mucosal cysts, focal foveolar hyperplasia, and hyperplastic polyps originating from islands of gastric mucosa. Dig Dis Sci 1989;34:1468–1472.

Soule EH, Hallenbeck GA. Polypoid gastric heterotopia of the jejunum and ileum causing subacute intestinal obstruction. Surg Gynecol Obstet 1959;108:282–288.

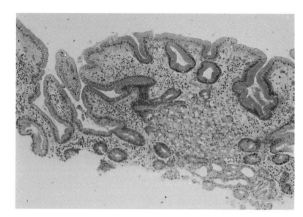

Figure 3–20. Heterotopic gastric mucosa. This duodenal biopsy displays gastric pits and gastric fundus–type glands.

BRUNNER'S GLAND POLYPS AND HYPERPLASIA

Biology of Disease and Gross Appearances

■ Brunner's gland polyps are located in the first or second portion of the duodenum. They form either single or multiple, smooth-surfaced nodules or polyps.

■ Single lesions have been called adenomas, hamartomas, hyperplasias, and polyps. In fact, all are hyperplasias of Brunner's glands and not adenomas (dysplastic lesions).

■ The majority are idiopathic; however, uremia or peptic ulceration may predispose to Brunner's gland hyperplasia.

Clinical Findings

■ The majority of Brunner's gland polyps are asymptomatic and are discovered incidentally at endoscopy or autopsy. A minority manifest as ulceration, hemorrhage, or obstruction.

Microscopic Pathology

■ Lobules of Brunner's glands are surrounded by bands of muscularis mucosae and appear structurally normal.

■ Cystically dilated glands are often present. There may be focal lymphoid infiltration.

■ Endocrine cells may be numerous, and microcarcinoids have been reported.

■ Mucoceles or cysts of Brunner's glands may alone cause duodenal nodules.

References

Buchanan EB. Nodular hyperplasia of Brunner's glands of the duodenum. Am J Surg 1961;101:253–257.

Franzin G, Musola R, Ghidini O, et al. Nodular hyperplasia of Brunner's glands. Gastrointest Endosc 1985;31:374–378.

Goldman RL. Hamartomatous polyp of Brunner's glands. Gastroenterology 1963;44:57–62.

Matsui T, Lida I, Fujischima M, et al. Brunner's gland hamartoma associated with microcarcinoids. Endoscopy 1989;21:37–38.

Miyawaki EH, Straehley CJ. Mucoceles of Brunner's glands. Am J Surg 1973;126:688–690.

Re Mine WH, Brown PW, Gomes MMR, Harrison EG. Polypoid hamartomas of Brunner's glands. Arch Surg 1970;100:313–316.

Robertson HE. The pathology of Brunner's glands. Arch Pathol 1941;31:112–130.

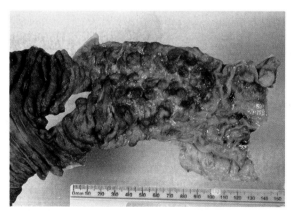

Figure 3–21. Brunner's gland hyperplasia. Multiple nodules of Brunner's gland hyperplasia are present in the duodenum, which was removed at autopsy from a patient with renal failure.

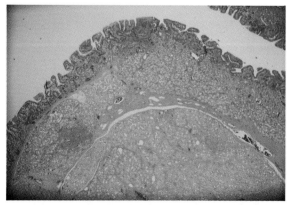

Figure 3–22. Brunner's gland polyp. This duodenal polyp removed endoscopically is composed of hyperplastic Brunner's glands. (Courtesy of Dr. Patrick Dean.)

INTUSSUSCEPTION

Biology of Disease

- *Intussusception* is bowel telescoped into bowel.
- The most common intussusception involves telescoping of the terminal ileum into the ascending colon.
- Intussusception is usually the result of a lesion in the wall of the ileum that acts as a lead point. The lead point may be a polyp, hypertrophied Peyer's patch, carcinoid, lipoma, leiomyoma, lymphoma, adenoma, adenocarcinoma, hemangioma, endometrioma, cyst, hematoma, or helminthoma. Henoch-Schönlein purpura may manifest as intussusception.

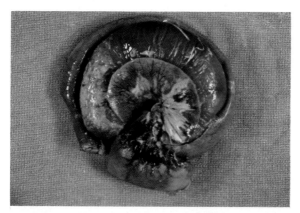

Figure 3–23. Ileoileal intussusception. The sausage-shaped portion of telescoped bowel (intussusceptum) lies within an opened portion of bowel (the intussuscepiens). The intussusceptum has the plum color of congestion and ischemia. There is a purulent exudate on the left side.

Clinical Findings

- Intussusception occurs most often in infants. The lead point is usually a hypertrophied Peyer's patch.
- The classic presentation is severe, colicky abdominal pain, vomiting (and occasionally hematemesis), and hematochezia in the form of "red-currant jelly" stools. Peritonitis and complete obstruction may be late presenting signs.

Gross Pathology

- Venous obstruction of the involved bowel produces extreme congestion and ischemia, which may result in partial- or full-thickness infarction.
- A specific lesion at the lead point may not be identifiable in all cases.

Microscopic Pathology

- The spectrum of changes includes congestion, edema, infarction, perforation, and peritonitis.
- The lead-point lesion may undergo infarction.

References

Bell TM, Steyn JH. Viruses in lymph nodes of children with mesenteric adenitis and intussusception. Br Med J 1962;2:700–702.

Goodall P. Intussusception in adults complicating specific inflammatory diseases of the intestine. Gut 1963;4:132–135.

Newman J, Schuh S. Intussusception in babies under 4 months of age. Can Med Assoc J 1987;136:266–272.

Perrin WS, Lindsay EC. Intussusception: a monograph based on 400 cases. Br J Surg 1921;9:46–71.

Sarason EL, Prior JT, Prowda RL. Recurrent intussusception associated with hypertrophy of Peyer's patches. N Engl J Med 1955; 253:905–908.

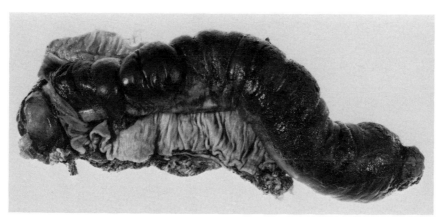

Figure 3–24. Ileocolic intussusception in Peutz-Jeghers syndrome. The telescoped bowel is ischemic. There is a Peutz-Jeghers polyp at the apex of the intussusceptum (*right*).

GALLSTONE ILEUS

Biology of Disease

■ *Gallstone ileus* is acute bowel obstruction due to impaction of a gallstone.

■ The gallstone ulcerates through the gallbladder into the duodenum or jejunum. It then travels within the bowel lumen until it is passed in the feces or causes obstruction.

■ Most often the gallstone impacts in the terminal ileum or sigmoid colon, because these are the narrowest parts of the bowel.

Clinical Findings

■ Gallstone ileus accounts for 1% to 2% of acute mechanical intestinal obstructions.

■ Patients are usually elderly women. The male-to-female ratio is 1:4. The mean duration of symptoms prior to admission is 3 to 4 days. The symptoms are those of intermittent acute obstruction.

■ Plain films of the abdomen may show air in the biliary tree and dilated loops of small bowel with air-fluid levels. If the gallstone is calcified, it may be visible on radiography. All three of these signs are present in only 10% of cases.

■ There is a high rate of death from perforation and peritonitis if diagnosis is delayed. The overall 30-day postoperative mortality in one recent study was 13.5%. Because the patients are elderly, many have concomitant cardiovascular disease or diabetes mellitus, and the principal cause of death is intra-abdominal sepsis.

Gross Pathology

■ Grossly, there is obstruction of the bowel by one or more gallstones. The gallstone is usually 2.5 cm in diameter or larger. Ulceration is often seen at the point of impaction.

■ The proximal bowel is dilated. The mucosa of the proximal bowel demonstrates flattening, granularity, and small, ill-defined ulcers. The serosa may show local peritonitis.

Microscopic Pathology

■ The crests of mucosal folds may show blunted villi or ulcers.

■ The ulcers are nonspecific. They may contain clefts that penetrate into the muscle coat and are surrounded by granulation tissue with widely dilated capillaries.

■ Perforations may arise from fissures or thinned, ulcerated areas.

References

Day EA, Marks C. Gallstone ileus: review of the literature and presentation of thirty-four new cases. Am J Surg 1975;129:552–558.

Kurtz RJ, Heimann TM, Kurtz AB. Gallstone ileus: a diagnostic problem. Am J Surg 1983;146:314–317.

Safaie-Shirazi S, Zike WL, Printen KJ. Spontaneous entero-biliary fistulas. Surg Gynecol Obstet 1973;137:769–772.

Schutte H, Bastias J, Csendes A et al. Gallstone ileus. Hepatogastroenterology 1992;39:562–565.

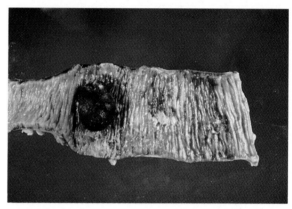

Figure 3–25. Gallstone ileus. The specimen displays a gallstone impacted in the ileum. There are dilatation of the bowel and mucosal ulceration proximal to the obstruction.

PEPTIC BULBITIS (DUODENITIS)

Biology of Disease

■ *Nonspecific duodenitis* refers specifically to inflammation of the mucosa of the duodenal bulb (referred to hereafter as *bulbitis*). Bulbitis is the minimal form of peptic ulcer disease of the duodenal bulb. Follow-up studies have shown that 80% of patients with bulbitis develop peptic ulceration within 2 years. Conversely, bulbitis is present is all patients with duodenal ulcers.

Clinical Findings

■ Patients may suffer from non-ulcer dyspepsia. (They have the typical symptoms of duodenal ulcer, but no ulcer is detected by barium meal or endoscopy.)

■ The incidence of bulbitis increases with age.

Gross Pathology

■ Endoscopic features include erythema, congestion, and erosions.

Microscopic Pathology

■ Normally, the villi of the duodenal bulb are much shorter than those in the third part of the duodenum, and the normal bulbar lamina propria contains a moderate number of plasma cells and eosinophils.

■ In bulbitis, the capillaries are congested, and the lamina propria displays edema, increased numbers of lymphocytes and plasma cells, and a neutrophil infiltrate of variable severity. Neutrophils may also infiltrate the crypt epithelium.

■ Gastric pit metaplasia is a normal finding in the duodenal bulb. It may be colonized by *Helicobacter pylori*, which elicits a neutrophil infiltrate and larger numbers of plasma cells. The surface epithelium may show reactive hyperchromatism. Epithelial lymphocytes are not increased. The mucosa may appear even flatter than normal.

■ Duodenal erosions show partial-thickness necrosis of the mucosa. A neutrophil infiltrate is present at the junction of viable and necrotic tissue.

Differential Diagnosis

Celiac disease, Crohn's disease, infections.

The duodenal bulb should not be sampled for biopsy if there is a suspicion of celiac disease; rather, specimens should be taken from the second or third part of the duodenum, distal to the ampulla of Vater, so that bulbitis does not enter into the differential diagnosis. Nevertheless, duodenal bulb biopsies do show the characteristic flat mucosa, increased epithelial lymphocytes, and increased plasma cells of celiac disease.

Crohn's disease is suggested by focal inflammation and granulomas at any level of the GI tract; however, Crohn's disease of the duodenal bulb is extremely uncommon in the absence of terminal ileal disease.

Infection by *Strongyloides*, hookworm, cytomegalovirus, or *Cryptosporidium* may be associated with bulbitis or distal duodenitis.

References

Corachan M, Oomen HAPC, Sutorius FJM. Parasitic duodenitis. Trans R Soc Trop Med Hyg 1981;75:385–387.

Greenlaw R, Sheahan DG, DeLuca V, et al. Gastroduodenitis. A broader concept of peptic ulcer disease. Dig Dis Sci 1980;25:600–672.

Johnston BJ, Reed PI, Ali MH. Campylobacter-like organisms in duodenal and gastric endoscopic biopsies: relationship to inflammation. Gut 1986;27:1132–1137.

Kreuning J, Bosman FT, Kuiper G, et al. Gastric and duodenal mucosa in healthy individuals. An endoscopic and histopathologic study of 50 volunteers. J Clin Pathol 1978;31:69–77.

Kreuning J, Wal AM, Kuiper G, Lindeman J. Chronic nonspecific duodenitis. A multiple biopsy study of the duodenal bulb in health and disease. Scand J Gastroenterol 1989;24 (suppl 167):16–20.

Shousha S, Spiller RC, Parkins RA. The endoscopically abnormal duodenum in patients with dyspepsia: biopsy findings in 60 cases. Histopathology 1983;7:23–34.

Sircus W. Duodenitis: a clinical endoscopic and histopathological study. Q J Med 1985;45:593–600.

Wyatt JI, Rathbone BJ, Dixon MF, Heatley RV. *Campylobacter pyloridis* and acid induced gastric metaplasia in the pathogenesis of duodenitis. J Clin Pathol 1987;40:841–848.

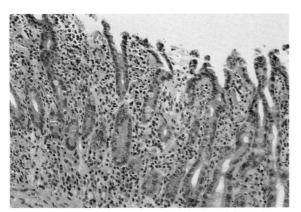

Figure 3–26. Nonspecific duodenitis. Biopsy of the duodenal bulb displays a flat mucosa with crypt hyperplasia and increased numbers of inflammatory cells. The epithelial cells are hyperchromatic, and there is tufting of epithelial cells at the surface.

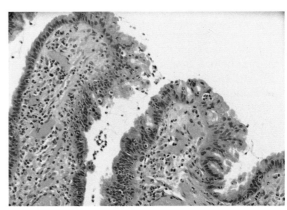

Figure 3–27. Nonspecific duodenitis. The villi are blunted; there is gastric metaplasia and neutrophil infiltration. *Helicobacter pylori* was present but is not visible at this magnification.

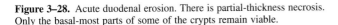

Figure 3–28. Acute duodenal erosion. There is partial-thickness necrosis. Only the basal-most parts of some of the crypts remain viable.

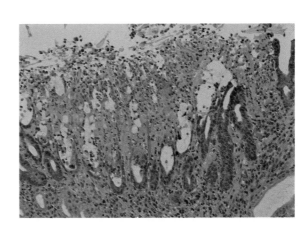

DUODENAL ULCER

Biology of Disease

- *Duodenal ulcer* is a full-thickness ulceration of the duodenal mucosa. Bulbitis is the main predisposing lesion. A chronic ulcer persists for years if untreated.
- The point prevalence rate is about 1.4% of the population. The lifetime prevalence is estimated at 10% for men and 4% for women.
- Yearly incidence (of new cases), about 1.5 per 1,000 in men and 0.3 per 1,000 in women, is decreasing. Age-specific incidence increases linearly with age. Incidence is declining in western countries.
- Active chronic gastritis with *Helicobacter pylori* is present in 95% of patients with duodenal ulcer and is the major causative factor. If *H. pylori* is eliminated by antibiotic treatment, the rate of relapse is much lower than if colonization persists. Chronic *H. pylori* infection elicits hyperchlorhydria by a variety of mechanisms.
- Cirrhosis, pulmonary emphysema, hypercalcemia, and renal failure are associated with duodenal ulcers. Syndromes that may cause duodenal ulcer include Zollinger-Ellison syndrome and multiple endocrine neoplasia type 1 (MEN I). Ulcer healing is adversely affected by smoking, nonsteroidal anti-inflammatory drugs (NSAIDs), and corticosteroids.

Clinical Findings

- Symptoms include burning or hunger-type epigastric pain occurring 1 to 3 hours after meals, nausea, vomiting, heartburn, and loss or gain of appetite. Epigastric pain may wake the patient at night or early in the morning. Epigastric tenderness is found on physical examination.
- Perforation and hemorrhage are major complications.
- Low-grade blood loss may cause iron deficiency anemia and positive stool occult blood test result.

Gross Pathology

- Duodenal ulcers are located in the first part of the duodenum on the anterior wall, the posterior wall, or both.
- The ulcer forms a rounded crater with flat margins. If the ulcer has been bleeding, an artery may be visible. The ulcer may perforate or penetrate into the pancreas or liver.

Microscopic Pathology

- Biopsy specimens from ulcer craters show necrotic debris, inflammatory exudate, and granulation tissue.

- The mucosa at the margin of the ulcer shows neutrophil infiltration and epithelial hyperchromatism. Gastric metaplasia and colonization by *Helicobacter pylori* may be seen.

Special Diagnostic Techniques

- Barium double-contrast radiography is about 90% sensitive and is used in uncomplicated cases.
- Upper GI endoscopy is performed in cases resistant to treatment or complicated by bleeding or gastric outlet obstruction.

Differential Diagnosis

Acute erosions.

Acute erosions are often multiple and show only partial-thickness ulceration and necrosis of the mucosa.

References

Bonnevie O. The incidence of duodenal ulcer in Copenhagen County. Scand J Gastroenterol 1975;10:385–393.

Dragstedt LR. Cause of peptic ulcer. JAMA 1959;169:203–209.

Graham DY. Treatment of peptic ulcers caused by *Helicobacter pylori*. N Engl J Med 1993;328:349–350.

Magnus HA. The pathology of peptic ulceration. Postgrad Med J 1954; 30:131.

Marshall BJ, McGechie DB, Rogers PA, Glancy RJ. Pyloric campylobacter infection and gastroduodenal disease. Med J Austr 1985;142: 439–444.

Marshall BJ, Warren JR. Unidentified curved bacilli in the stomach of patients with gastritis and peptic ulceration. Lancet 1984;1:1311–1315.

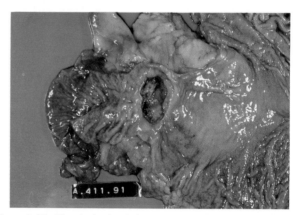

Figure 3–29. Chronic duodenal ulcer at autopsy. The tissue was fixed before photography.

CELIAC DISEASE AND GLUTEN SENSITIVITY

Biology of Disease

- *Celiac disease* is a condition in which the small bowel mucosa is immunologically sensitive to the gliadin subfraction of gluten and related prolamins of wheat, rye, barley, and oats in genetically predisposed individuals. Ingestion of these proteins causes enterocyte damage, resulting in a threefold increase in cell loss, an expanded proliferative zone in the crypts, higher mitotic index, reduced cell cycle time, and more rapid epithelial migration. The result is a flat mucosa with greater crypt depth and malabsorption. There is a great increase in epithelial lymphocytes.
- The estimated prevalence of celiac disease is 0.03% of the population. Celiac disease, which occurs mainly in people of Northern European ancestry, is the most common primary malabsorptive disorder of the small bowel.
- Celiac disease is strongly associated (>90%) with the HLA haplotype DQw2, which is in strong linkage disequilibrium with DR3 and B8. Between 10% and 20% of first-degree relatives of a proband have the disorder.
- Celiac disease, frank or latent, may be associated with dermatitis herpetiformis.
- Rare but major complications of celiac disease include T-cell lymphoma of the jejunum, carcinoma of the upper GI tract, and idiopathic ulcerative nongranulomatous jejunoileitis.
- Adenovirus type 12 contains a protein that shares homology with alpha-gliadin, and many celiac patients have antibodies to the virus. These facts support the speculation that the virus might trigger celiac disease by immunologic cross-reactivity.

Clinical Findings

- Celiac disease in childhood may manifest as steatorrhea, malabsorption, failure to thrive, and failure to grow. Adults with celiac disease may present with anemia due to iron or folate deficiency, steatorrhea, weight loss, osteomalacia, vague ill health, psychological disturbances, abdominal pain, or arthropathy. Other DQw2-linked autoimmune diseases may be present, too: chronic hepatitis, pernicious anemia, diabetes mellitus, or thyroiditis.
- A wider spectrum of gluten sensitivity has been defined. In 50% to 60% of patients, gluten sensitivity may be asymptomatic or latent. Such patients display a range of intestinal mucosal involvement, from increases in epithelial lymphocytes alone to flat mucosa.

Gross Pathology

- Two endoscopic signs of celiac disease are flattening and scalloping of the mucosal folds.

Microscopic Pathology

- The wider spectrum of mucosal abnormality in gluten sensitivity includes four mucosal lesions that form a spectrum of increasing severity: (1) mucosa displaying normal villus-to-crypt ratio and increased epithelial lymphocytes ("infiltrative lesion"), (2) increased lymphocytes with mucosal hyperplasia ("infiltrative-hyperplastic"), (3) classic flat lesion ("flat-destructive"), and (4) "irreversible hypoplastic-atrophic" — the unresponsive end-stage disease with progressive intestinal failure, ulceration, and lymphoma. The first two are minimal or latent lesions that may be converted to the flat lesion by gluten challenge.
- Classic celiac disease displays severe shortening or loss of villi (flat mucosa) with crypt hyperplasia (greater crypt depth and higher numbers of mitotic figures). The mucosal height remains near normal.
- Surface epithelial cells are reduced in height, show basophilic cytoplasm, and may show lipid vacuolization.
- Greater numbers of plasma cells are present in the lamina propria.
- Intraepithelial lymphocytes are greatly increased from a normal of one lymphocyte per six epithelial cell nuclei to approximately one lymphocyte per epithelial cell nucleus.
- Endocrine cells are increased in number. Paneth's cell numbers may be normal or decreased.

Special Diagnostic Techniques

- To firmly establish the diagnosis, mucosal biopsy specimens from the second or third part of the duodenum should show a flat mucosa with increased epithelial lymphocytes and laminal plasma cells. Withdrawal of gluten should be followed by full clinical remission. A second biopsy showing recovery of villi after elimination of gluten from the diet and a third biopsy showing deterioration after gluten challenge are no longer considered necessary. Biopsy of the jejunum is also unnecessary.
- Serum antigliadin antibody has approximately 90% sensitivity and specificity for gluten sensitivity and gives positive and negative predictive values of 45% and 98%, respectively.

Differential Diagnosis

Protein sensitivity, drug-induced enteropathy, immunodeficiency syndromes, bacterial overgrowth, Crohn's disease, viral enteritis, AIDS enteropathy, infections, idiopathic nongranulomatous jejunoileitis, microvillus inclusion disease.

Conditions that flatten the mucosa include cow's milk, beef and soya protein sensitivities. These disorders are diagnosed by selective withdrawal of specific foods, confirmed by challenge testing, and treated by withdrawal of the offending agent.

Drugs that may cause a flat mucosa include triparanol and neomycin. A variety of other drugs may cause malabsorption by various mechanisms. Withdrawal of the drug gives prompt relief.

Immunodeficiency syndromes, particularly hypogammaglobulinemia, may be associated with celiac disease. Plasma cells are absent in hypogammaglobulinemia.

Bacterial overgrowth, due to chronic pseudo-obstruction (either primary or secondary to scleroderma, drugs, or diabetes mellitus) may be associated with flat mucosa.

The focal inflammatory lesions of Crohn's disease may be associated with local villous flattening, but adjacent mucosa is normal. Granulomas may be present.

Other causes of villous shortening are viral enteritis, AIDS enteropathy, AIDS-related infections (such as cytomegalovirus, cryptosporidiosis, isosporiasis, and microsporidiosis), tropical sprue, kwashiorkor, and idiopathic nongranulomatous ulcerative jejunoileitis. Infectious causes are recognized by identifying the relevant pathogen. The other conditions are diagnosed by exclusion, clinical features, or response to treatment.

Microvillus inclusion disease is an inherited disorder of the brush border of the enterocyte. Inclusion cysts of brush border form within the cytoplasm of enterocytes. Affected infants evince severe congenital diarrhea. On light microscopy, the small bowel mucosa is flat. Immunostains or cytochemistry for surface antigens or enzymes demonstrate the inclusion cysts on light microscopy.

References

Brocchi E, Corazza G, Caletti G, et al. Endoscopic demonstration of loss of duodenal folds in the diagnosis of celiac disease. N Engl J Med 1988;319:741–744.

Cutz E, Rhoads JM, Drumm B, et al. Microvillus inclusion disease: an inherited defect of brush-border assembly and differentiation. N Engl J Med 1989;320:646–651.

Marsh MN. Gluten, major histocompatibility complex, and the small intestine: a molecular and immunobiologic approach to the spectrum of gluten sensitivity. Gastroenterology 1992;102:330–354.

Marsh MN. Gluten sensitivity and latency: can patterns of intestinal antibody secretion define the great 'silent majority'? Gastroenterology 1993;104:1550–1562.

Mee AS, Burke M, Vallon AG, et al. Small bowel biopsy for malabsorption: comparison of the diagnostic adequacy of endoscopic forceps and capsule biopsy specimens. Br Med J 1985;291:769–772.

Sjolund K, Alumets J, Berg N-O, et al. Enteropathy of celiac disease in adults: increased number of enterochromaffin cells in the duodenal mucosa. Gut 1982;23:42–48.

Variend S, Placzek M, Raafat F, Walker-Smith JA. Small intestinal mucosal fat in childhood enteropathies. J Clin Pathol 1984;37:373–377.

Walker-Smith JA, Guandalini S, Schmitz J, et al. Revised criteria for diagnoses of celiac disease. Arch Dis Child 1990;65:909–911.

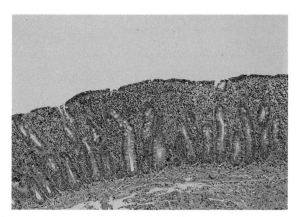

Figure 3–30. Celiac disease. Biopsy from the second part of the duodenum shows a flat mucosa, crypt hyperplasia, and increased number of lymphocytes in the lamina propria. The inflammatory cells are predominantly in the upper half of the mucosa.

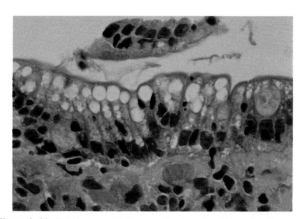

Figure 3–32. Focal areas of fatty vacuolization of surface epithelium may be seen in celiac disease. This appearance is not specific to celiac disease.

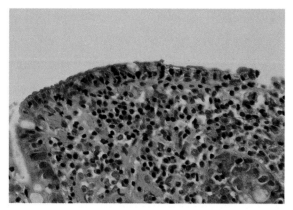

Figure 3–31. Celiac disease. There are increased numbers of plasma cells in the lamina propria. The surface epithelial height is diminished, and epithelial lymphocytes are more numerous.

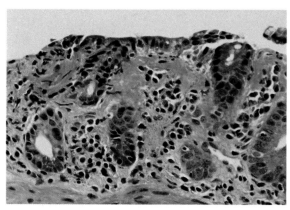

Figure 3–33. Collagenous sprue. This trichrome stain demonstrates considerable collagenization of the superficial part of the lamina propria. This patient's mucosa reverted to normal after the patient was started on a gluten-free diet.

INTESTINAL ULCERATION WITH MALABSORPTION (ULCERATIVE DUODENOJEJUNOILEITIS)

Biology of Disease

- *Idiopathic nongranulomatous ulcerative duodenojejunoileitis* is an uncommon condition in which middle-aged or elderly individuals manifest steatorrhea, intestinal hemorrhage, multiple ulcers of the small intestine, and/or perforation. The ulcers are benign and nonspecific histologically.
- Half of these patients have had celiac disease for many years. They present with relapse of symptoms despite a gluten-free diet. Other cases present de novo.
- Multifocal primary intestinal T-cell lymphoma complicating celiac disease also manifests as multiple small bowel ulcers, and some authors believe that all cases of ulcerative duodenojejunoileitis are examples of lymphoma. There do appear to be two distinct entities, however both with poor prognosis and sometimes one leading into the other. Benign ulcers may antedate lymphoma by years or may coexist with lymphoma.
- Treatments employed include resection of bowel, corticosteroids, and nutritional support. The prognosis is poor. The average survival is 3 years.

Clinical Findings

- Patients present with abdominal pain, distention, weight loss, diarrhea, intestinal hemorrhage, perforation, or steatorrhea. The diarrhea or steatorrhea may be present for years before presentation to a physician. Fever, anemia, hypocalcemia, hypoproteinemia, and clubbing of the fingers may all be found.

Gross Pathology

- Multiple shallow ulcers in the jejunum and ileum with little or no thickening of the bowel wall. The ulcers often cause a mild degree of stricturing.
- Healed ulcers are slightly depressed scars interrupting the mucosal folds.
- Mesenteric lymph nodes may be greatly enlarged and cavitated. The spleen is generally atrophied.

Microscopic Pathology

- Duodenal or jejunal biopsy specimens show a flat mucosa, and sometimes the lesion is patchy in distribution. Epithelial lymphocytes may not be increased in number as they are in celiac disease. Neutrophil infiltration may be present, including crypt abscesses.
- The ulcer floors show necrotic debris, granulation tissue, and a chronic inflammatory infiltrate. The ulcers may penetrate into the muscle coat or may even perforate.

- Pyloric metaplasia and disruption of the muscularis mucosae indicate healed ulcers.
- The mucosa in between ulcers shows villous flattening and crypt hyperplasia in most patients but a minority of patients show normal mucosa.

Special Diagnostic Techniques

- Barium follow-through studies may show dilatation of small bowel loops, strictures, and coarse mucosal folds.
- Immunostaining with B-cell and T-cell markers may help to characterize the lymphoma.
- Gene rearrangement studies may demonstrate T-cell gene rearrangement confirming lymphoma.

Differential Diagnosis

Lymphoma, NSAID-induced ulcers, Crohn's disease, other ulcerative disorders.

Lymphomas display an atypical infiltrate of large cells in the ulcer floor that extend into the muscle coat. There may be an associated infiltrate of small lymphocytes and eosinophils that initially suggests inflammation. Immunostaining and gene rearrangement studies confirm the diagnosis.

Ulcers induced by nonsteroidal anti-inflammatory drugs (NSAIDs) should be considered when the ileum is more involved than jejunum. Mucosal diaphragms suggest NSAID-induced ulcers.

Crohn's disease usually shows distinct signs of chronicity, including stenosis and mucosal scarring. The terminal ileum is involved in most cases. Granulomas are present in about 60% of cases.

Rarer ulcerative disorders, such as tuberculosis, syphilis, vascular disorders, potassium chloride–induced ulcer, and Zollinger-Ellison syndrome, may also need to be excluded.

References

Baer AN, Bayless TM, Yardley JH. Intestinal ulceration and malabsorption syndromes. Gastroenterology 1980;79:754–765.

Barry RE, Morris JS, Read EA. A case of small-intestinal mucosal atrophy. Gut 1970;11:743–747.

Goulston KJ, Skyring AP, McGovern VJ. Ulcerative jejunitis associated with malabsorption. Australas Ann Med 1965;14:57–64.

Lance P, Gazzard BG. Ulcerative enteritis and liver disease and a patient with coeliac disease. Gut 1983;24:433–437.

Mills PR, Brown IL, Watkinson G. Idiopathic chronic ulcerative enteritis: report of five cases and review of the literature. Q J Med 1980;194:133–149.

Modigliani R, Poitras P, Galian A, et al. Chronic non-specific ulcerative duodenojejunoileitis: Report of four cases. Gut 1979;20:318–328.

Robertson DAF, Dixon MF, Scott BB, et al. Small intestinal ulceration: diagnostic difficulties in relation to coeliac disease. Gut 1983;24:565–574.

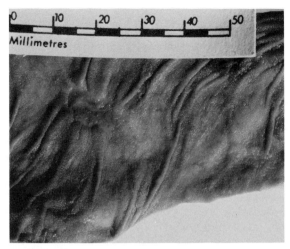

Figure 3–34. Idiopathic ulcerative, nongranulomatous jejunoileitis. Shallow ulcer in the jejunum.

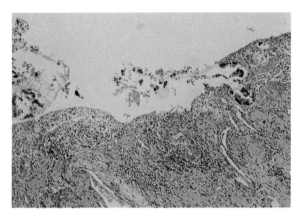

Figure 3–36. The ulcer shows nonspecific inflammation and granulation tissue.

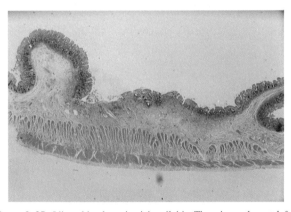

Figure 3–35. Idiopathic ulcerative jejunoileitis. There is an ulcer at *left of center.*

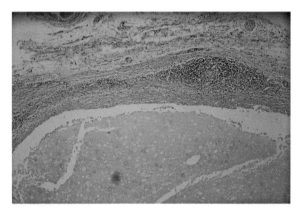

Figure 3–37. A cavitated mesenteric lymph node in idiopathic ulcerative, nongranulomatous jejunoileitis. The cystic cavity may enlarge the lymph node up to a diameter of 5 cm. The spleen may be atrophied.

GIARDIASIS

Biology of Disease

■ *Giardia lamblia* is a cosmopolitan protozoan parasite and the most common cause of epidemic water-borne diarrhea. It is especially prevalent in children in developing countries, and although the majority of such infections are asymptomatic, some are associated with chronic diarrhea and weight loss. Re-infection after spontaneous or treatment cure is common.

■ Cysts of *Giardia* are highly infectious for humans, and ingestion of as few as ten viable cysts can result in patent infection. Cysts resist chlorination but are removed by filtration. Direct fecal-oral transmission occurs particularly in child daycare centers and among homosexual men. Food-borne transmission is recognized but less common.

■ Hypochlorhydria and immunodeficiency predispose to giardiasis. In atrophic gastritis the gastric mucosa may also be colonized.

■ Severe giardiasis with chronic diarrhea and malabsorption may complicate hypogammaglobulinemia, selective IgA deficiency, or AIDS.

Clinical Findings

■ The clinical presentation consists of vomiting and diarrhea, often a traveler's diarrhea, and sometimes steatorrhea. Steatorrhea is mainly seen in immunocompromised patients who have a heavy parasite burden; they may develop a flat mucosa and lymphoid hyperplasia.

■ Giardiasis is treated with either quinacrine hydrochloride or metronidazole.

Microscopic Pathology

- *Giardia* trophozoites measure 10 to 14 μm long and 5 to 7 μm wide. They are seen on the luminal surface and between the villi as curved or sickle-shaped hematoxyphilic organisms. When cut en face, they appear pear-shaped, and display two symmetric nuclei with single central nucleoli like a pair of eyes. Cysts are not seen in duodenal biopsy specimens.
- Changes in the villous morphology are usually minimal. In immunodeficient patients, giardiasis may be associated with nodular lymphoid hyperplasia, villous atrophy, neutrophil cryptitis, and crypt abscesses. Villous morphology returns to normal after the parasite is eliminated.

Special Diagnostic Techniques

- Microscopic examination of duodenal fluid aspirates and stool microscopy may be used to detect *Giardia*.

Differential Diagnosis

No other gut pathogen looks like *Giardia*.

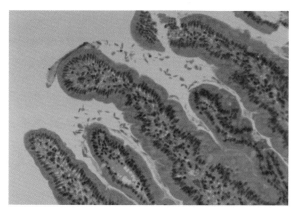

Figure 3–38. Giardiasis. Numerous semilunar organisms are present between normal villi.

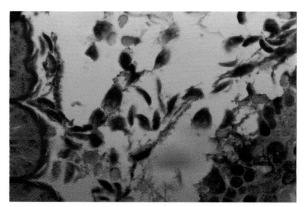

Figure 3–39. Giardiasis. The paired nuclei remain unstained in this alcian blue–PAS stain.

References

Adam RD. The biology of *Giardia* spp. Microbiol Rev 1991;55:706–732.

Doglioni C, DeBoni M, Cielo R, et al. Gastric giardiasis. J Clin Pathol 1992;45:964–967.

Hartvong WA, Gourley WK, Arvanitakis C. Giardiasis: clinical spectrum and functional-structural abnormalities of the small intestinal mucosa. Gastroenterology 1979;77:61–69.

Raizman RE. Giardiasis. Am J Dig Dis 1976;21:1070–1074.

Yardley JH, Takano J, Hendrix TR. Epithelial and other mucosal lesions of the jejunum in giardiasis. Jejunal biopsy studies. Bull Johns Hopkins Hosp 1964;115:389–406.

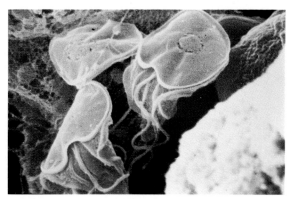

Figure 3–40. Scanning electron micrograph of three giardia from a human duodenal biopsy. The organisms resemble jellyfish. The flagellae emerge from the caudal end, but they actually arise anterior to the midline on the ventral surface. (Courtesy of Drs. Michael J. O'Brien and Peter Dervan.)

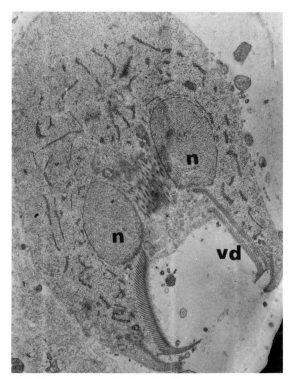

Figure 3–41. Transmission electron micrograph of *Giardia lamblia* cut en face. The paired nuclei (*n*) and a portion of the ventral striated sucking disc (*vd*) are evident. The ends of the disc curve inwards, giving a clawlike appearance.

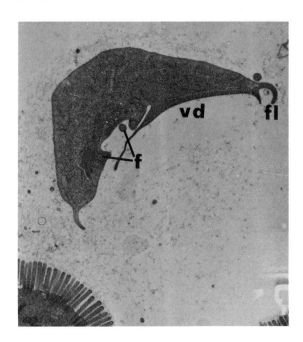

Figure 3–42. *Giardia lamblia.* Flagellae (*f*), ventral sucking disc (*vd*), and ventrolateral flange (*fl*) are evident.

CRYPTOSPORIDIOSIS

Biology of Disease

■ *Cryptosporidium* is a protozoan parasite that colonizes the brush border of columnar epithelia and causes a diarrheal illness. Outbreaks in children in daycare centers are an important public health problem and usually involve person-to-person spread.

■ The infectious forms—sporozoites, merozoites and microgametes—are motile by body flexion, gliding, or undulation.

■ *Cryptosporidium* commonly infects wild and domestic animals and is transmitted by the fecal-oral route.

Life Cycle. Ingested oocysts excyst in the duodenum and release banana-shaped sporozoites that invade epithelial cells. Each sporozoite differentiates into a spherical trophozoite with a prominent nucleus. The trophozoite nucleus divides asexually, in the process known as merogony or schizogony, into six or eight nuclei. Each nucleus becomes incorporated into a merozoite, a form closely resembling the sporozoite. On release, each merozoite is capable of invading another epithelial cell and developing into either a type I schizont, which forms eight merozoites, or a type II schizont, which produces four merozoites. Merozoites from type II schizonts initiate sexual reproduction when they parasitize new host cells and develop into either microgamonts or macrogamonts, the sperm (male) and ovum (female) equivalents, respectively. In microgamonts, the nucleus divides, and each nucleus becomes incorporated into a microgamete, which will fertilize the equivalent of an ovum, the macrogamont. The fertilized macrogamont develops into an oocyst containing four sporozoites. Thick-walled oocysts leave the body in the feces. Thin-walled oocysts may remain in the host and release sporozoites that can repeat the cycle of schizogony, gametogeny, and sporogony.

■ Oocysts may survive chlorination, so that treated water may be a vehicle for transmission of infection.

■ In immunocompetent individuals, the infection is self limited, but immunosuppressed patients may fail to clear *Cryptosporidium* and may develop a debilitating chronic watery diarrhea. Paromomycin and sinefungin are promising new therapeutic agents.

■ The jejunum is most heavily colonized, but any columnar mucosa, including the biliary and respiratory mucosa, may be involved in immunosuppressed individuals.

Clinical Findings

■ Infection in nonimmunosuppressed individuals produces a self-limited diarrhea of variable severity lasting up to 14 days that sometimes requires hospitalization. Children under 5 years are most often affected.

■ Immunosuppressed patients, especially patients with AIDS who have CD4 lymphocyte counts below 200×10^6/L may develop persisting infection and may present with profuse watery diarrhea with malabsorption.

■ Biliary tract involvement may cause sclerosing cholangitis and acalculous cholecystitis in some AIDS patients.

Microscopic Pathology

■ In tissue sections, cryptosporidia are round, 2 to 4 μm, PAS-positive organisms that are incorporated into the microvillous border of the mucosa of the stomach, small bowel, large bowel, or biliary tract. They line both surface epithelium and crypts. In semithin sections, various stages in the life cycle of the organism may be identified.

- Ultrastructurally, trophozoites, meronts, microgamonts, macrogamonts, and oocysts may be identified. The parasites develop in parasitophorous vacuoles, which replace the microvillous border of the gut, and are covered by host cell membrane (therefore they are intracellular).
- The tissue reaction is active chronic inflammation, including increased numbers of mononuclear cells in the lamina propria, neutrophil infiltration of the epithelium, and variable epithelial damage, villous blunting, crypt elongation, and crypt dilatation.

Special Diagnostic Techniques

- Diagnosis usually rests on demonstration of oocysts in stool concentrates stained by the Ziehl-Neelsen or trichrome methods.
- Organisms can also be recognized in gastrointestinal biopsy specimens because of their distinctive location and morphology.

Differential Diagnosis

No other human pathogen gives the pattern of small organisms on the brush border.

References

Dubey JP, Speer CA, Fayer R (eds). Cryptosporidiosis of Man and Animals. Boca Raton, FL: CRC Press, 1991.

Fayer R, Ungar BLP. Cryptosporidium spp. and cryptosporidiosis. Microbiol Rev 1986;50:458–483.

Flanigan T, Whalen C, Turner J, et al. *Cryptosporidium* infection and CD4 lymphocyte counts. Ann Intern Med 1992;116:840–842.

Guarda LA, Stein SA, Cleary KA, Ordonez NG. Human cryptosporidiosis in the acquired immunodeficiency syndrome. Arch Pathol Lab Med 1983;107:562–566.

Lefkowitch JH, Krumholtz S, Feng-Chen K-C, et al. Cryptosporidiosis of the human small intestine: a light and electron microscopic study. Hum Pathol 1984;15:746–752.

Marcial MM, Madara JL. Cryptosporidium: cellular localisation, structural analysis of absorptive cell-parasite membrane-membrane interactions in guinea pigs, and suggestions of protozoan transport by M cells. Gastroenterology 1986;90:583–594.

Meisel JL, Perera DR, Meligro C, Rubin CE. Overwhelming watery diarrhea associated with a cryptosporidium in an immunosuppressed patient. Gastroenterology 1976;70:1156–1160.

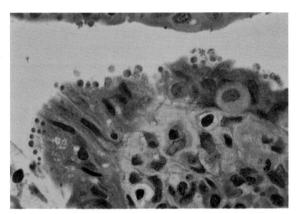

Figure 3–43. Cryptosporidiosis. The surface epithelium is lined by small, round hematoxiphilic organisms measuring 2 to 4 μm in diameter.

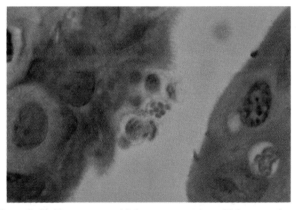

Figure 3–45. Two cryptosporidial meronts contain multiple merozoites.

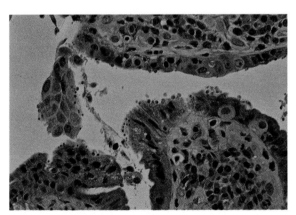

Figure 3–44. Cryptosporidia implanted on the microvillous border of the duodenum.

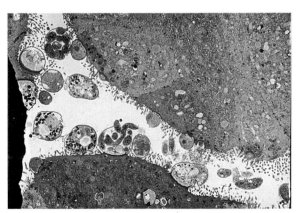

Figure 3–46. Cryptosporidiosis. Several phases of the life cycle are evident in this picture, including meronts and macrogamonts. (Courtesy of Dr. Jan Marc Orenstein.)

MICROSPORIDIOSIS

Biology of Disease

■ Microspora is a phylum of ubiquitous spore-forming, intracellular, protozoan parasites that cause disease in all five classes of vertebrates. Three genera of microspora have been reported in humans—*Nosema, Encephalitozoon*, and *Enterocytozoon*. Only *Enterocytozoon* has been found in the small gut.

■ A new genus and species of Microspora, *Enterocytozoon bieneusi*, was first identified in small bowel biopsy specimens from AIDS patients with unexplained chronic diarrhea. A second new genus identified in the small bowel epithelium is named *Septata intestinalis*. Neither of these organisms has been found outside small bowel mucosa.

■ The defining feature of Microspora is the presence in each spore of a coiled polar filament.

■ A spore attaches to an enterocyte, uncoils its polar tube, inserts the tube into the enterocyte, and injects its nucleus. The spore then enters the (plasmodial) proliferative phase, becoming first a meront and later a sporont.

■ Jejunal biopsies give a higher yield of positive results than duodenal biopsies.

Clinical Findings

■ Microsporidia are a major cause of chronic diarrhea in patients with AIDS who have no other demonstrable pathogen.

■ Patients are generally in the late stages of AIDS, with CD4-positive lymphocyte counts less than 100×10^6/L. They suffer from chronic watery diarrhea or steatorrhea. Albendazole is the treatment of choice.

Microscopic Pathology

■ Light microscopy usually shows partial villous atrophy and mild inflammation of the lamina propria. Only the oldest enterocytes near the villous tip are infected.

■ By light microscopy, plasmodia may occasionally be visible on the luminal side of the enterocyte nuclei. They may indent the nucleus and lie in a vacuole, which is thought to be an artifact of fixation. Definite identification requires demonstration of spores in silver (Warthin-Starry), Gram, or Ziehl-Neelsen stains, in 1- μm plastic–embedded, toluidine blue–stained sections, or on ultrastructural study. Diagnosis from hematoxylin-eosin sections is possible in some cases but is not reliable.

■ Microsporidial spores stained by the Ziehl-Neelsen, Warthin-Starry, or Gram stain form clusters in the supranuclear cytoplasm of enterocytes at the tops of villi.

■ In semithin sections stained with toluidine blue, the spores are also recognizable as multiple intracytoplasmic bodies, 1 to 1.5 μm in diameter. No stain identifies meronts; consequently, cases can be missed by light microscopic studies.

■ Organisms may be identified, both intracellularly and liberated from cells, in touch preparations of biopsy specimens that are air dried, methanol fixed, and Giemsa stained. They appear as hyaline, pale blue bodies ranging from 2 to 9 μm in diameter, with from one to many reddish purple nuclei.

Special Diagnostic Techniques

■ The spores may be demonstrated by Gram, Ziehl-Neelsen, or Warthin-Starry stain.

■ On transmission electron microscopy, *E. bieneusi* is seen within the supranuclear cytoplasm of enterocytes but not in a parasitophorous vacuole. The organisms are rimmed by host mitochondria from which they are presumed to derive energy.

■ Various stages in the life cycle can be identified, including meronts and sporonts. Meronts measure about 5 μm in diameter and are more electron-lucent than the cytoplasm of the host cell. Meronts display one to six nuclei and a highly characteristic feature is the presence of empty clefts. When the spore-forming phase begins, stacks of electron-dense discs are formed. Later, the discs aggregate to form polar tubes, which surround the nucleus of each spore. There may be up to 12 spores per cell. Mature spores are electron dense and contain a single nucleus, a coiled polar tube, an anchoring disc, and a polarplast.

■ The organisms display absence of mitochondria, various stages of sporogenesis, and electron-dense, disclike, coiled polar filaments. Sporoblasts measure up to 5 μm in diameter and mature spores measure 0.5 μm x 1.5 μm.

■ *Septata intestinalis* forms spores within septate parasitophorous vacuoles and lacks polar discs and clear clefts. It also infects laminal macrophages.

■ Examination of fecal smears stained with a modified trichrome stain may be a more sensitive diagnostic tool than electron microscopy.

Differential Diagnosis

Isosporiasis.

Isospora belli also colonizes the supranuclear cytoplasm of enterocytes but is larger than *Microsporidium*; also, its merozoites are banana-shaped and have a central nucleus with a perinuclear halo.

References

Cali A, Kotler DP, Orenstein JM. *Septata intestinalis* N. G., N. Sp., an intestinal microsporidian associated with chronic diarrhea and dissemination in AIDS patients. J Euk Microbiol 1993;40:101–112.

Cali A, Owen RL. Intracellular development of Enterocytozoon, a unique microsporidian found in the intestine of AIDS patients. J Protozool 1990;37:145–155.

Curry A, McWilliam LJ, Haboubi NY, Mandal BK. Microsporidiosis in a British patient with AIDS. J Clin Pathol 1988;41:477–478.

Desportes I, Le Charpentier Y, Gallan A, et al. Occurrence of a new microsporidian: *Enterocytozoon bieneusi* n. g., n. sp., in the enterocytes of a human patient with AIDS. J Protozool 1985;32:250–254.

Gourley WK, Swedo JL. Intestinal infection by microsporidia *Enterocytozoon bieneusi* of patients with AIDS: an ultra-structural study of the use of human mitochondria by a protozoan. Mod Pathol 1988;1:35A.

Ledford DK, Overman MD, Gonzalvo A, et al. Microsporidiosis myositis in a patient with the acquired immunodeficiency syndrome. Ann Intern Med 1985;102:628–630.

Modigliani R, Bories C, LeCharpentier Y, et al. Diarrhoea and malabsorption in acquired immune deficiency syndrome: a study of four cases with special emphasis on opportunistic protozoan infestations. Gut 1985;26:179–187.

Orenstein JM, Chiang J, Steinberg W, et al. Intestinal microsporidiosis as a cause of diarrhea in human immunodeficiency virus-infected patients: A report of 20 cases. Hum Pathol 1990;21:475–481.

Orenstein JM, Tenner M, Coli A, Kotler DP. A microsporidian previously undescribed in humans, infecting enterocytes and macrophages, and associated with diarrhea in an acquired immunodeficiency syndrome patient. Hum Pathol 1992;23:722–728.

Weber R, Bryan RT, Owen RL, et al. Improved light-microscopical detection of Microsporidia spores in stool and duodenal aspirates. N Engl J Med 1992;326:161–166.

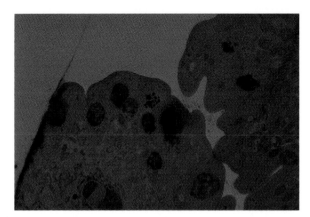

Figure 3–49. Microsporidiosis. Toluidine blue stain showing microsporidial spores within enterocytes in a 1-μm plastic-embedded section.

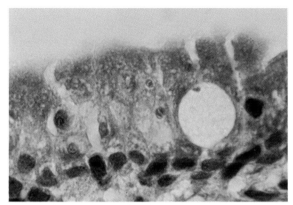

Figure 3–47. Microsporidiosis. High magnification of oblique cut surface epithelium displays small intracytoplasmic inclusions in the supernuclear cytoplasm that may represent microsporidial meronts.

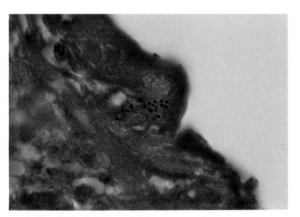

Figure 3–48. Microsporidiosis. Ziehl-Neelsen stain displays microsporidial spores within enterocytes.

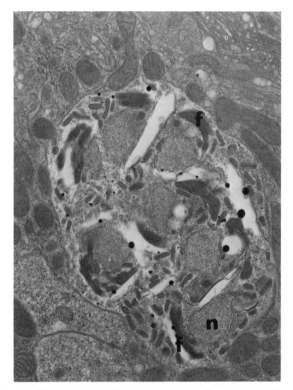

Figure 3–50. A microsporidial meront shows the characteristic clefts and portions of seven spores with their micronuclei (*n*) and coiled filaments (*f*). Note the rim of host cell mitochondria, which fuel the parasite.

ISOSPORIASIS

Biology of Disease

■ *Isospora belli* and *Isospora hominis* are morphologically similar protozoans that proliferate within the cytoplasm of small bowel absorptive cells.

Life Cycle. Infection begins with ingestion of oocysts. These excyst in the proximal small bowel, releasing sporozoites that invade epithelial cells. There they become round trophozoites and enter the asexual stage, schizogony, in which they divide into variable numbers of merozoites. On release, the merozoites invade other epithelial cells, where they may undergo further schizogony or may enter the sexual stage, becoming gametocytes. When the macrogametocyte (female) is fertilized by a microgamete (male), it becomes an unsporulated oocyst, which is extruded into the intestinal lumen and passed in the feces.

■ Treatment with sulfamethoxazole-trimethoprim or sulfadoxine-pyrimethamine is successful, and recurrence is prevented by ongoing prophylaxis.

Clinical Findings

■ Affected patients are usually immunosuppressed or have AIDS and present with persistent unexplained diarrhea or steatorrhea.

Microscopic Pathology

■ There is mild to moderate villous atrophy and crypt hyperplasia with clubbed villi.
■ Numbers of lymphocytes and plasma cells in the lamina propria are increased, and eosinophil numbers may be.
■ Isospora reside within the surface epithelium of villi. They are seen within vacuoles, which displace the nucleus toward the luminal surface. The appearance of the vacuolar contents depends on the stage of the life cycle. All stages of the life cycle may be seen in the small bowel mucosa. Merozoites are most often identified. They are banana-shaped, about the same size as epithelial nuclei, and have central nuclei with perinuclear halos.

Special Diagnostic Techniques

■ Acid-fast oocysts are concentrated from stool by flotation techniques and diagnosed by microscopic examination.

Differential Diagnosis

Microsporidiosis.

Microsporidia, when visible in paraffin sections, do not have the distinctive morphology of isospora, but rather a distinctive morphology of their own. Their spores are gram positive and acid fast.

References

Brandborg LL, Goldberg SB, Breidenbach WC. Human coccidiosis—a possible cause of malabsorption: the life cycle in small bowel mucosal biopsies as a diagnostic feature. N Engl J Med 1970;283:1306–1313.
DeHovitz JA, Pape JW, Boncy M, Johnson WD. Clinical manifestations and therapy of *Isospora belli* infection in patients with the acquired immunodeficiency syndrome. N Engl J Med 1986;315:87–90.
Henry K, Bird RG, Doe WF. Intestinal coccidiosis in a patient with alpha-chain disease. Br Med J 1974;1:542–543.
Tanowitz HB, Weiss LM, Wittner M. Diagnosis and treatment of protozoan diarrheas. Am J Gastroenterol 1988;83:339–350.
Trier JS, Moxey PC, Schimmel EM, Robles E. Chronic intestinal coccidiosis in man: intestinal morphology and response to treatment. Gastroenterology 1974;66:923–935.
Westerman EL, Christensen RP. Chronic *Isospora belli* infection treated with co-trimoxazole. Ann Intern Med 1979;91:413–414.

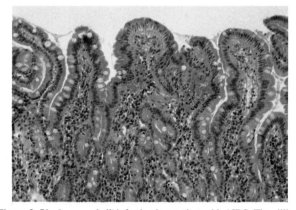

Figure 3–51. *Isospora belli* infection in a patient with AIDS. The villi are blunt, and there is a minimal increase in inflammatory cells in the lamina propria. (Microscope slide courtesy of Dr. Audrey Lazenby.)

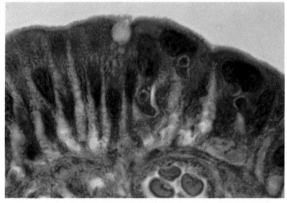

Figure 3–52. *Isospora belli.* Banana-shaped organisms are present within the infranuclear cytoplasm of the enterocytes. Note the characteristic nuclei with perinuclear clear areas.

STRONGYLOIDIASIS

Biology of Disease

■ Strongyloidiasis is caused by *Strongyloides stercoralis* and is common in warm climates where soil is contaminated by human feces owing to lack of sewage systems. Larvae excreted in feces mature in the soil. The filariform

larvae penetrate the skin of people who walk barefoot in the soil.

Life Cycle. In warm soil, rhabditiform larvae excreted in stool develop into infective filariform larvae. The latter penetrate the skin, enter veins, and are carried in the blood stream to the lungs. There they enter alveoli, migrate up the trachea, are swallowed, and finally reach their breeding ground in the proximal small bowel. Female worms lay eggs in the duodenal crypts. Eggs hatch into rhabditiform larvae, which are excreted in the stool. Adult male worms have not been reliably identified; they are believed to exist, but this belief currently rests more on emotional aversion to parthogenesis than on evidence!

- An estimated half of all infections are asymptomatic. Symptoms may include fleeting skin rashes, cutaneous larval tracts of migrating larvae, chronic diarrhea, malabsorption, and even protein-losing enteropathy. Pulmonary symptoms include cough, dyspnea, hemoptysis, and pleural effusions.
- Sexual transmission by penile invasion of larvae during anal intercourse or by oral-anal contact is possible.
- Infection is life long and may only become clinically manifest 30 years or more after primary infection.
- *Hyperinfection* is a severe disseminated form of infection, with a huge parasitic burden, that occurs in immunosuppressed or debilitated patients. Hyperinfection results from autoinfection, with completion of the life cycle within the host and diminished host resistance. Filariform larvae develop in the gut, invade the colon, rectum, and perineum, and migrate to the lungs. Pneumonic symptoms often predominate, and filariform larvae are present in bronchial lavage fluid. Granulomas may form around dead larvae in the wall of the large bowel. Ultimately, small ulcers may form owing to parasitic penetration, and secondary bacterial infection may lead to a severe colitis.

Clinical Findings

- Patients include immigrants from endemic areas, residents in psychiatric institutions, and former soldiers who served in Southeast Asia. Typical patients spent time in endemic areas many years earlier and subsequently became immunosuppressed from malignancy, corticosteroid therapy, or cytotoxic chemotherapy.
- Chronic asymptomatic infection may precede hyperinfection by years. Signs of infection include fever, migratory macular erythema over the distal extremities (larva currens rash), and cough. Abdominal pain, weight loss, and diarrhea may occur.
- Hyperinfection may manifest as enterocolitis, pneumonitis, intestinal obstruction, perforation, sepsis, gastritis, or esophagitis.
- Laboratory findings include eosinophil leukocytosis, iron deficiency anemia, positive stool occult blood test result, and hypoalbuminemia.
- Thiabendazole, the drug of choice until now, may be replaced by albendazole, which has fewer side-effects. All cases should be treated.

Gross Pathology

- Three forms of enteritis are described—catarrhal with excess mucus secretion, edematous with severe edema of the bowel wall, and ulcerative with mucosal ulceration and hypotonia. Ulcers are usually small (2 to 8 mm), with elevated swollen edges surrounded by a smooth, bright red mucosa.
- Rarely, invasion of the bowel wall produces an helminthic pseudotumor. This happens most often at the ileocecal junction.

Microscopic Pathology

- In duodenal biopsy specimens, cross-sections of coiled adult female worms, rhabditiform larvae, or ova are seen in mucosal crypts.
- The adult worm measures 30 to 60 μm in diameter, has a cuticle 1 to 2 μm in thickness, and is usually wedged between crypt epithelial cells, not in the lumen. The anterior third of the worm contains a long cylindrical esophagus, whereas the posterior two thirds contain the intestine and paired reproductive organs.
- Eggs are ovoid, measuring 50 to 58 μm long by 30 to 34 μm in diameter. They are deposited by females between crypt epithelial cells. They have a dense hematoxyphilic staining and a lobated structure.
- Rhabditiform larvae measure 10 to 12 μm in diameter and do not have a cuticle. They are most often seen within thin-walled cysts formed from crypt epithelium. Cysts develop from the intercellular spaces, where eggs are laid. As cysts enlarge, they bulge into the lumen of the crypt.
- The infestation may elicit little reaction or may provoke an intense mixed inflammatory infiltrate, including lymphocytes, plasma cells, macrophages, and neutrophils with or without eosinophils.
- Mucosa may appear flattened, with loss of villi and crypt hyperplasia, or may be reasonably well preserved.
- In autopsy or resection specimens, larvae producing autoinfection may be seen within the deeper layers of the wall of either the colon or small bowel. They may elicit no inflammation, a lymphocytic or eosinophil response, or granulomas. In severe infections, there are marked edema of the bowel wall, inflammation, villous atrophy, crypt hyperplasia, and many ulcers.

Special Diagnostic Techniques

- Microscopic examination of stool or duodenal fluid for larvae is the usual means of diagnosis.
- In duodenal biopsy specimens, female worms, ova, and larvae are seen in mucosal crypts. Less often, they may be seen in gastric or colonic biopsy specimens. Mucosal biopsy is not an efficient way of making the diagnosis in the majority of cases with low parasite loads.
- Pulmonary lavage fluid or sputum may contain larvae in cases of hyperinfection. Affected patients may have pneumonic symptoms and radiologic pulmonary infiltrates.

References

Archibald LK, Beeching NJ, Gill GV, et al. Albendazole is effective treatment for chronic strongyloidiasis. Q J Med 1993;86:191–195.

Genta RM. Predictive value of an enzyme-linked immunosorbent assay (ELISA) for the serodiagnosis of strongyloidiasis. Am J Clin Pathol 1988;89:391–394.

Genta RM, Caymmi Gomes M. Pathology. In: Grove DI (ed). Strongyloidiasis, a Major Roundworm Infection of Man. London: Taylor and Francis, 1989;105–132.

Milner PF, Irvine RA, Barton CJ, et al. Intestinal malabsorption in *Strongyloides stercoralis* infestation. Gut 1965;6:574–781.

Purtilo DT, Meyers WM, Connor DH. Fatal strongyloidiasis in immunosuppressed patients. Am J Med 1974;56:468–493.

Schad GA. Morphology and life history of *Strongyloides stercoralis*. In: Grove DI (ed). Strongyloidiasis, a Major Roundworm Infection of Man. London: Taylor and Francis, 1989;85–104.

Stemmerman GN. Strongyloidiasis in migrants. Pathological and clinical considerations. Gastroenterology 1967;53:59–70.

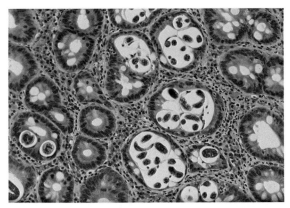

Figure 3–53. *Strongyloides stercoralis.* The center of the field shows rhabditiform larvae developing in characteristic cysts within the epithelium of the duodenal crypts. An ovum is present at *upper left.* Two cross-sections of an adult female worm are present between the epithelial cells of a crypt at *upper left.*

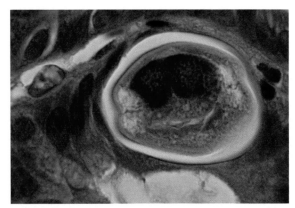

Figure 3–55. *Strongyloides stercoralis.* Cross-section of an adult female shows the external cuticle (which may show striations), and the internal structure includes the paired ovaries.

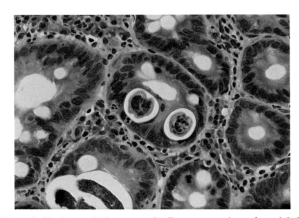

Figure 3–54. *Strongyloides stercoralis.* Two cross-sections of an adult female worm are seen (*center*).

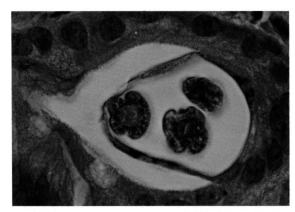

Figure 3–56. *Strongyloides stercoralis.* Rhabditiform larva. The larva is contained within a cyst derived from crypt epithelium, and the cyst itself is bulging into the lumen crypt. Note the characteristic shape and the absence of a cuticle.

WHIPPLE'S DISEASE

Biology of Disease

■ Whipple's disease is a rare systemic infectious disease that may affect virtually any organ in the body but involves the small bowel in the great majority of patients.

■ The causative organism is *Tropheryma whippleii,* a gram-positive actinomycete.

■ Affected organs are infiltrated by histiocytes, which contain phagocytosed bacteria, and the disease probably represents a specific defect of bacterial disposal by macrophages.

Clinical Findings

■ Most patients are middle-aged white men.

■ Presenting features include fever, weight loss, malabsorption, migratory polyarthritis, lymphadenopathy, and increased skin pigmentation.

■ Diarrhea and steatorrhea are common but not always present. Abdominal cramps, anorexia, cachexia, fatigue, lassitude, and weakness may be present.

■ Other extraintestinal manifestations are pleuritis, congestive heart failure, pericarditis, and neurologic manifestations, including personality change and ophthalmoplegia.

Gross Pathology

- Endoscopically, the mucosal folds in the duodenum may display yellowish white plaques or bulbous enlargement of the villi of either diffuse or spotty distribution. In some cases there is no gross abnormality.
- The bowel wall may be thickened and edematous.

Microscopic Pathology

- Macrophages with abundant granular pink cytoplasm expand the lamina propria and widen the villi and may give an impression of a flat mucosa. Lipid droplets are scattered through the lamina propria. Small numbers of neutrophils are often present among the macrophages.
- The macrophages display strong granular PAS positivity after diastase digestion and are negative on Ziehl-Neelsen stain.
- Following treatment, mucosal morphology reverts toward normal but scanty foamy macrophages may remain scattered among the bases of the crypts for a considerable time.
- Crypts are normal or hyperplastic. The brush border is preserved.

Special Diagnostic Techniques

- Small bowel biopsy is the diagnostic procedure of choice.
- Electron microscopy confirms the presence of both intracellular and extracellular bacilli. The macrophages contain membrane-bound phagocytic vacuoles that contain bacilli, either intact or degenerating, or amorphous debris.
- The causative organism can be specifically identified by polymerase chain reaction (PCR).

Differential Diagnosis

Mycobacterium avium-intracellulare or *Histoplasma capsulatum* infection, lipid-storage diseases, macroglobulinemic enteropathy.

Mycobacterium avium-intracellulare (MAI) infection in patients with AIDS resembles Whipple's disease. The lipid vacuoles in lamina propria are absent, however, and MAI is strongly postive on Ziehl-Neelsen stain but only weakly on PAS stain.

Histoplasma capsulatum is recognized by the characteristic morphology of the organisms, which are 3 μm in diameter, PAS positive, and methenamine silver positive.

Tangier disease is a lipid-storage disease resulting from an abnormality of apoprotein A1 that causes it to be rapidly degraded. The lamina propria may be expanded by lipid-rich foamy macrophages. The lipid globules are unstained by the PAS or Ziehl-Neelsen stain. Tangier disease is also distinguished by orange-yellow tonsils, hepatosplenomegaly, peripheral neuropathy, and very low levels of plasma cholesterol and high density lipoproteins. Wolman's disease, an autosomal recessive deficiency of a lysosomal esterase, also causes a diffuse infiltrate of the lamina propria by foamy macrophages. In Gaucher's disease, the characteristic striated macrophages may distend the lamina propria.

Macroglobulinemia may be associated with a distinctive enteropathy comprising lymphangiectasia with strongly eosinophilic proteinaceous material both in the lumens of the dilated lymphatics and in the lamina propria. The proteinaceous material is immunoglobulin-rich fluid. Small numbers of foamy macrophages may also be present.

References

Dobbins WO. Whipple's disease. Mayo Clin Proc 1988;63:623–624.

Fleming JL, Wiesner RH, Shorter RG. Whipple's disease: clinical, biochemical, and histopathologic features and assessment of treatment in 29 patients. Mayo Clin Proc 1988;63:539–555.

Keinath RD, Merrell DE, Vlietstra R, Dobbins WO. Antibiotic treatment and relapse in Whipple's disease: long-term follow-up of 88 patients. Gastroenterology 1985;88:1867–1873.

Relman DA, Schmidt TM, MacDermott RP, Falkow S. Identification of the uncultured bacillus of Whipple's disease. N Engl J Med 1992; 327:293–301.

Wilson KH, Blitchington R, Frothingham R, Wilson JAP. Phylogeny of the Whipple's-disease-associated bacterium. Lancet 1991;338:474–475.

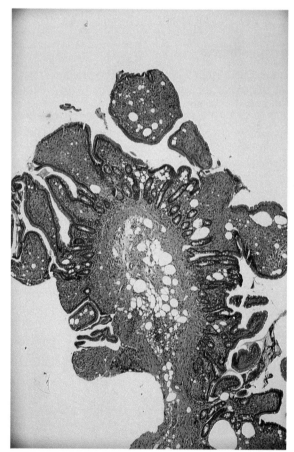

Figure 3–57. Whipple's disease. The villi are greatly expanded by cells and by fatty vacuoles.

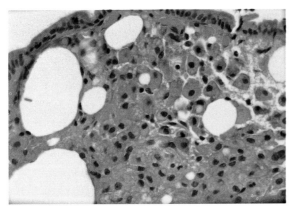

Figure 3–58. The lamina propria contains numerous large macrophages with pink cytoplasm. Fatty vacuoles are also present.

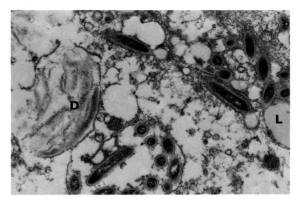

Figure 3–59. Rod-shaped bacilli (*Tropheryma whippleii*) in the cytoplasm of a macrophage and within membrane-bound granules. Note degenerating bacilli (*D*) within a granule and lipid (*L*) (×12,000).

VIRAL GASTROENTERITIS

General Features

- It is estimated that 5 million preschool children throughout the world die annually from the complications of acute, predominantly viral diarrhea.
- Viral gastroenteritis is transmitted by the fecal-oral route and mainly affects children under 5 years. Norwalk virus affects older children and adults.
- Viruses cause nosocomial, institutional, or daycare center outbreaks of gastroenteritis.
- When severe (e.g., rotavirus), diarrhea results in dehydration; it may be life-threatening to infants.
- Rotavirus, enteric adenovirus, and Norwalk virus are well-established pathogens. The importance of astrovirus and of caliciviruses other than Norwalk virus is still being assessed.
- A number of other viruses may produce gastroenteritis but are not yet of proven importance: coronaviruses, pestiviruses, picornaviruses, and togaviruses.
- Enteroviruses have been shown by controlled epidemiologic studies not to be important causes of acute gastroenteritis.
- Most viruses are identified by electron microscopy, immune electron microscopy, immunoassay or nucleic acid hybridization.
- The gastroenteritis viruses may be classified as:
  Rotaviruses
  Enteric adenoviruses
  Small round-structured viruses: astroviruses, caliciviruses, and Norwalk virus

Rotavirus

Biology of Disease

- Rotaviruses are cosmopolitan RNA-viruses 70 nm in diameter. They display a double-walled outer capsid but no envelope. Ultrastructurally, they resemble the spokes of a wheel, whence derives the name. They are members of the Reoviridae family.
- Group A rotavirus is the leading cause of dehydrating diarrhea in infants aged 6 months to 24 months, accounting for about 50% of infants requiring hospitalization for acute diarrhea in developed countries. Adults are occasionally ill, but more often the adult contacts of infected cases are asymptomatic but may excrete virus.
- Worldwide, rotavirus causes an estimated 140 million cases of acute diarrhea annually and 1 million deaths in infants under 2 years of age. Each year in the United States, about 22,000 infants are hospitalized for treatment of dehydration caused by rotavirus diarrhea.
- In temperate climates, rotavirus causes a winter diarrhea, but in the tropics, a year-round infection.
- Rotavirus diarrhea is largely an osmotic diarrhea resulting from nutrient (primarily carbohydrate) malabsorption.
- Breastfeeding protects against infection through transmission of maternal antibodies.
- The incubation period is 1 to 3 days.

Clinical Findings

- Rotavirus produces a wide spectrum of illness ranging from minimally to severely dehydrating diarrhea that may be fatal (especially in underdeveloped countries).
- Initial vomiting is followed by watery diarrhea that lasts from 3 to 5 days on average but may last up to 7 days. Rarely, chronic diarrhea results.
- Low-grade fever is common.

Microscopic Pathology

- In animal studies, rotavirus infects the mature enterocytes on the small bowel villi, causing cell lysis and consequent villous atrophy and crypt hyperplasia.

Special Diagnostic Techniques

- Rapid diagnosis by solid-phase immunoassay for viral antigen in fecal filtrates is the mainstay of diagnosis.

Adenoviruses

Biology of Disease

■ Adenovirus serotypes 40 and 41 are significant causes of infantile diarrhea worldwide, accounting for 4% to 10% of affected cases.

■ Enteric adenoviruses serotypes 40 and 41 rank second in frequency of occurrence to rotavirus in developed countries and account for one sixth of viral diarrhea cases.

■ Adenovirus is a 70-nm DNA virus.

Clinical Findings

■ The incubation period is 8 to 10 days.

■ Spread to adults is uncommon.

■ Illness lasts 5 to 12 days and occasionally up to 2 weeks.

■ Severe dehydration may occur.

■ In immunocompromised patients, particularly those with AIDS or bone marrow transplants, adenovirus gastroenteritis may occur as an opportunistic infection.

Pathology

■ Adenovirus-infected cells may be seen in the surface epithelium in rectal biopsy specimens from patients with AIDS. They show cytoplasmic vacuolization and enlarged, rounded or crescent-shaped, hyperchromatic, amphophilic nuclei. Stromal and endothelial cells are not infected, and the cells are not cytomegalic. The affected cells appear to drop down to the basement membrane level, below the level of the other epithelial nuclei.

■ Ultrastructurally, infected cells show crystalline arrays of viral particles 60 to 80 nm in diameter, with regular hexagonal outlines, within the nuclei. These particles are too large for polyomavirus (40 to 50 nm) or parvovirus (30 to 45 nm) and too small for cytomegalovirus.

Special Diagnostic Techniques

■ A presumptive diagnosis is made if large numbers of adenoviral particles are seen on electron-microscopic examination of stools.

■ Electron microscopy (EM), enzyme-linked immunosorbent assay (ELISA), nucleic acid hybridization, and cell culture techniques are also used for diagnosis.

Astrovirus

■ Astrovirus is a single-stranded, 7.8-kb RNA virus of positive sense.

■ Astrovirus can be grown in cell culture or identified by EM, immunofluorescence, immune electron microscopy (IEM), or ELISA.

■ Unlike caliciviruses, astrovirus has three structural proteins and is immunologically distinct.

■ Large quantities of virus are excreted in stool.

■ Transmission is fecal-oral.

■ Children under 7 years are mainly affected, and the clinical syndrome is not very severe. Nosocomial or institutional outbreaks are most often reported. The elderly may also be affected.

■ Among pediatric outpatients with diarrhea in Thailand, 8.6% of cases and 2% of controls shed astrovirus.

Calicivirus

■ Caliciviruses are single-stranded RNA viruses, 35 to 40 nm in diameter, that have a single major capsid protein and a characteristic morphology that includes cup-shaped surface depressions. They cause gastroenteritis in infants worldwide.

■ Norwalk virus and other small round-structured viruses are similar structurally, immunologically, and in genomic organization and amino-acid sequences to members of the family Caliciviridae and are therefore probably members of that family.

■ The clinical features of some outbreaks closely resemble those of rotavirus, but other outbreaks resemble Norwalk viral disease in which adults are mainly affected.

■ Human calicivirus is not culturable and is detected by EM, IEM, ELISA, or radioimmunoassay.

Norwalk Virus and Norwalk-Like Viruses

Biology of Disease

■ Norwalk virus (named after an outbreak in 1968 in Norwalk, Ohio) is an important cause of outbreaks of diarrhea or "winter vomiting disease." It is transmitted by the fecal-oral route, by person-to-person contact, and by food-borne transmission, especially by undercooked or raw shellfish.

■ Norwalk virus is a round, nonenveloped, 27-μm DNA virus that is identified by electron microscopy of feces. It has an amorphous surface and irregular edges.

■ Norwalk virus infects the proximal small bowel but not the stomach.

■ Norwalk virus infects people of all ages except infants, being most common in older children and young adults.

Clinical Findings

■ Incubation period is 16 to 48 hours.

■ Diarrhea, nausea, crampy abdominal pain, vomiting, and muscle aches are the main symptoms. The diarrhea is watery.

■ The duration of illness is rarely more than 48 hours, often as short as 24 hours.

Microscopic Pathology

■ Volunteer studies have demonstrated villous shortening and crypt hyperplasia, neutrophil infiltration, and increased numbers of mononuclear cells in the lamina propria, vacuolization of the epithelial cell cytoplasm, and higher numbers of epithelial lymphocytes.

Special Diagnostic Techniques

■ Immune electron microscopy using convalescent patient serum to precipitate virus in stool filtrates is the main diagnostic modality.

■ Radioimmunoassay for virus in feces is also possible.

References

Blacklow NR, Greenberg HB. Viral gastroenteritis. N Engl J Med 1991;325:252–264.

Caul EO, Appleton H. The electron microscopical and physical characteristics of small round human fecal viruses: an interim scheme for classification. J Med Virol 1982;9:257–265.

Doane FW, Anderson N. Electron Microscopy in Diagnostic Virology: A Practical Guide and Atlas. Cambridge: Cambridge University Press, 1986.

DuPont HL. Rotavirus gastroenteritis—some recent developments. J Infect Dis 1984;149:663–666.

Elliott EJ. Viral diarrhoeas in childhood. Electron microscopy has improved our understanding. Br Med J 1992;305:1111–1112.

Grey LD. Novel viruses associated with gastroenteritis. Clin Microbiol Newsletter 1991:13:137–144.

Lambden PR, Caul EO, Ashley CR, Clarke IN. Sequence and genome organization of a human small round-structured (Norwalk-like) virus. Science 1993;259:516–519.

Maddox A, Francis N, Moss J, et al. Adenovirus infection of the large bowel in HIV positive patients. J Clin Pathol 1992;45:684–688.

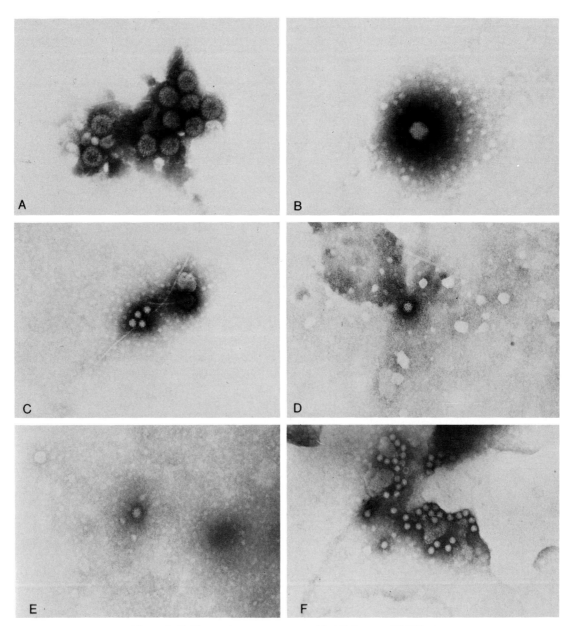

Figure 3–60. Viruses that cause gastroenteritis (all shown ×100,000). *A,* Rotaviruses: 70-nm, round particles resembling wheels with spokes. *B,* Adenovirus; large hexagonal virus 70 nm in diameter. *C,* Astrovirus: 25-nm particles resembling stars. *D,* Calicivirus: 32-nm virus. *E,* Norwalk virus: 32-nm virus, a member of the Calicivirus family. *F,* Parvovirus-like small round virus, 20 nm. (Courtesy of Dr. Paul Hazelton.)

TYPHOID FEVER

Biology of Disease

- *Salmonella typhi* is an invasive organism whose only host is the human.
- Infection is spread by fecal or urinary contamination of water or food. The source is usually a chronic carrier.
- *S. typhi* invades the Peyer's patches and spreads to other viscera via the blood stream.

Clinical Findings

- Disease onset is gradual, with malaise, headache, and a progressive rise in fever.
- Leukopenia is common during the febrile phase.
- Rose-spot rash on the thorax and abdomen, splenomegaly, abdominal distention, and relative bradycardia are typical findings.
- Most patients are constipated, but a minority may have small volume liquid motions ("pea-soup stool").
- Ulcerated Peyer's patches may result in bleeding or perforation.
- Localized *Salmonella* infections such as cholecystitis, osteomyelitis, endocarditis, and meningitis may complicate the disease. Chronic carriers often have persistent low-grade infection of the gallbladder.

Gross Pathology

- For simplicity, the pathologic changes in the Peyer's patches and lymphoid follicles are traditionally described in a weekly sequence. Enlargement of Peyer's patches occurs in the first week, necrosis in the second week, ulceration during the third week, and healing in the fourth week.
- The ulcers are shallow, longitudinal, and located on the antimesenteric border, where Peyer's patches are normally found.

Microscopic Pathology

- During the first week, the Peyer's patches become infiltrated by mononuclear cells, which obliterate the germinal centers. Mesenteric lymph nodes show hyperplastic changes similar to those in the Peyer's patches.
- During the second week, patchy foci of necrosis appear. They enlarge, coalesce, and may cause sloughing of overlying mucosa, resulting in the ulceration that characterizes the third week.
- Neutrophil infiltration is minimal even on ulcerated surfaces. Submucosa shows edema, fibrinous exudation, and infiltrating immunoblasts. Ultimately, the entire patch may undergo necrosis, and perforation can occur.
- Mucosal regeneration begins in the fourth week.

Special Diagnostic Techniques

- Culture of *S. typhi* or of *Salmonella enteritidis* serotype paratyphi A or B from blood or stool is the definitive test. Blood culture results are positive in most patients during the first week. Stool culture results are positive late in the course of illness.
- Widal agglutination test or ELISA assay may show rising antibody titers.

Differential Diagnosis

Other infectious enteritides (e.g., *Yersinia*).

In pathologic specimens other infectious enteritides such as *Yersinia* infection may enter the differential diagnosis. *Yersinia* infection may show bacterial colonies in the ulcers, abundant neutrophils, abscesses in germinal centers, follicular hyperplasia, and granulomatous reaction.

References

Chuttani HK, Jain K, Misra RC. Small bowel in typhoid fever. Gut 1971;12:709–712.

Gonzales A, Vargas V, Guarner L, et al. Toxic megacolon in typhoid fever. Arch Intern Med 1985;145:2120.

Huckstep RL. Pathology. In: Typhoid Fever and Other Salmonella Infections. Edinburgh: Livingstone, 1962;35–43.

Mallory FB. A histological study of typhoid fever. J Exp Med 1898;3:611–638.

Stuart BM, Pullen RL. Typhoid: clinical analysis of three hundred and sixty cases. Arch Intern Med 1946;78:629–661.

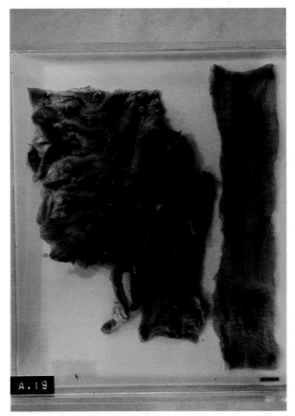

Figure 3–61. Typhoid fever. The *left* specimen shows two ulcerated Peyer's patches. The *right* specimen (terminal ileum, cecum and ascending colon) displays enlarged and ulcerated Peyer's patches and solitary lymphoid follicles. (From the Pathology Museum, University of Manchester, UK. Courtesy of Prof. John McClure.)

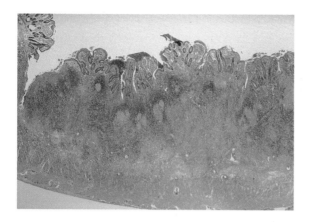

Figure 3–62. Typhoid fever. An ileal Peyer's patch shows ulceration and infiltration by pale-staining histiocytes. Germinal centers are inconspicuous. The lower border of the Peyer's patch, which is usually sharply defined, shows cellular infiltration and fibrinous exudation.

YERSINIA INFECTION

Biology of Disease

■ Enteric infection by either *Yersinia enterocolitica* or *Yersinia pseudotuberculosis* is transmitted by contaminated food or water or through person-to-person contact.

■ *Yersinia* preferentially invades through Peyer's patches and evokes a neutrophil response but resists phagocytosis.

■ *Yersinia* septicemia is a particular risk in patients with iron overload, especially if they are being treated with the siderophore desferrioxamine B, which makes iron available to the bacteria.

Clinical Findings

■ Most symptomatic infections occur in children under 5 years of age.

■ Most patients present with diarrhea and fever. Abdominal pain may be the predominant complaint, and at laparotomy for presumptive appendicitis, either terminal ileitis or mesenteric lymphadenitis is found.

■ Bloody stools are present in less than 10% of affected children.

■ Appendicitis due to *Yersinia* appears to be uncommon. *Yersinia* colitis must be considered in the differential diagnosis of aphthoid ulcers seen colonoscopically.

Gross Pathology

■ The bowel shows congestion, edema, and ulceration of Peyer's patches and solitary lymphoid follicles. Typically, there are no signs of chronicity.

■ The ulcers may extend into the muscle coat, but perforation is an uncommon complication.

■ Mesenteric lymph nodes may be enlarged and matted together and may show microabscesses on cut surface.

■ Rarely, terminal ileum requires excision in the healing phase owing to stricture or continued ulceration.

Microscopic Pathology

■ Gut lymphoid tissue is hyperplastic, with enlarged germinal centers and ulceration. Colonies of gram-negative coccobacilli are seen in the ulcers and are surrounded by neutrophils.

■ Activated lymphoid cells infiltrate the surrounding mucosa and the underlying submucosa and bowel wall (transmural inflammation).

■ Mononuclear cells may form a granulomatous cuff surrounding microabscesses in the germinal centers of Peyer's patches or in the regional lymph nodes.

Special Diagnostic Techniques

■ Culture of the organism from feces or blood is the gold standard for diagnosis.

■ Demonstration of a fourfold rise in antibody titer is also diagnostic in the absence of positive culture.

Differential Diagnosis

Typhoid, tuberculosis, Crohn's disease, idiopathic ulceration.

Culture of the organism and the characteristic tissue reaction distinguish typhoid from yersiniosis.

Suppurating granulomas in yersiniosis are quite different from tuberculous granulomas, which show structureless (caseous) necrosis.

Crohn's disease shows signs of chronicity, including mucosal regeneration, metaplasia, and submucosal fibrosis.

References

Bradford WD, Noce PS, Gutman LT. Pathological features of enteric infection with *Yersinia enterocolitica*. Arch Pathol 1974;93:17–22.

El-Maraghi NRH, Mair NS. The histopathology of enteric infection with *Yersinia pseudotuberculosis*. Am J Clin Pathol 1979;71:631–639.

Gleason TH, Patterson SD. The pathology of *Yersinia enterocolitica* ileocolitis. Am J Surg Pathol 1982;6:347–355.

Robins-Browne RM. *Yersinia enterocolitica*. In: Farthing MJG, Keusch GT (eds). Enteric Infection: Mechanisms, Manifestations and Management. London: Chapman and Hall, 1989;337–349.

Vantrappen G, Agg HO, Ponette E, et al. Yersinia colitis and enterocolitis: gastroenterological aspects. Gastroenterology 1977;72:220–227.

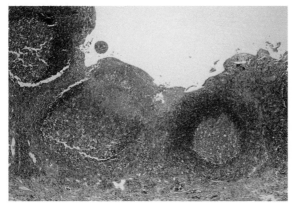

Figure 3–63. *Yersinia enterocolitica* infection. There is ulceration of the mucosa overlying a Peyer's patch.

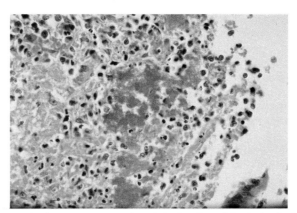

Figure 3–64. *Yersinia enterocolitica* infection. Bacterial colonies in the floor of the ulcer.

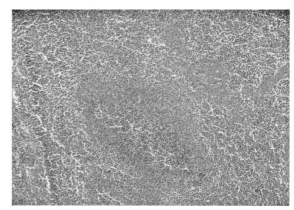

Figure 3–65. *Yersinia enterocolitica* infection. There is an abscess in the germinal center.

TUBERCULOSIS OF BOWEL

Biology of Disease

■ Tuberculosis is primarily a pulmonary disease transmitted by airborne droplets.

■ *Mycobacterium tuberculosis* can infect any part of the gastrointestinal tract secondary to pulmonary involvement. Mycobacteria are coughed up and swallowed and may then directly invade the alimentary tract. Such secondary tuberculosis is usually contained by local immune responses that cause local granulomata and ulceration but relatively little mesenteric lymphadenopathy.

■ Bovine tuberculosis may be transmitted by infected (unpasteurized) milk, producing primary intestinal tuberculosis. In nonimmune hosts, the intestinal lesion is usually inconspicuous, and the mycobacteria spread rapidly to the lymph nodes. Thus, lymphadenopathy may be the dominant component of the infection. Lymphadenopathic abdominal tuberculosis is still prevalent in parts of Africa and the Indian subcontinent.

■ The terminal ileum is the most common GI location, presumably because mycobacteria enter the bowel through membranous enterocytes over Peyer's patches and lymphoid follicles.

■ Complications include stenosis, perforation, and fistula.

■ Tuberculosis is now resurgent in AIDS. Its major manifestations are pulmonary infection, lymphadenopathy, and miliary spread resulting in infection of the liver.

Clinical Findings

■ Only a minority of patients with gastrointestinal tuberculosis have GI symptoms, which include abdominal pain or mass, obstruction, hemorrhage, perforation, fistula, and malabsorption syndrome. The triad of abdominal pain, anorexia, and diarrhea in a patient with active pulmonary tuberculosis is highly suggestive of tuberculous enteritis.

Gross Pathology

■ One typical ileal lesion is an annular circumferential ulcer less than 3 cm in length that results in a napkin-ring stricture. Ulcers may have a ragged appearance, with pseudopolyps or mucosal bridges, or they may be deep and gutterlike. Some ulcers are longitudinal rather than circumferential.

■ Ulcers and strictures may be separated by normal mucosa (skip lesions).
■ The ascending colon may be shortened, and the angle between the terminal ileum and cecum may be obliterated.
■ Large "hypertrophied" ulcers may resemble carcinoma.
■ In "hypertrophic" ileocecal tuberculosis, the bowel, mesenteric fat, and lymph nodes form a large mass with extensive adhesions.

Microscopic Pathology

■ Caseating granulomas in any part of the bowel wall or mesenteric lymph nodes are the hallmark of tuberculosis. Caseation is structureless necrosis.
■ Identification of acid-fast bacilli is required for definite diagnosis.

Special Diagnostic Techniques

■ Culture of *M. tuberculosis* is the gold standard for diagnosis.
■ Organisms may be identified in tissue by acid-fast stains (Ziehl-Neelsen) or by the fluorescent rhodamine-auramine method.
■ Caseating granulomas, without positive culture or stainable organisms, are strongly suggestive of tuberculosis if there are no stainable fungi in the lesion.

Differential Diagnosis

Crohn's disease, yersiniosis.

In Crohn's disease, the granulomas are noncaseating and do not contain acid-fast bacilli. In up to 50% of cases of Crohn's disease, there are no granulomas.

Yersiniosis is an acute infection, not a chronic stricturing one. The granulomas in yersiniosis are typically suppurating, not caseating.

References

Anscombe AR, Keddie NC, Schofield PF. Caecal tuberculosis. Gut 1967;8:337–343.
Case records of the Massachusetts Hospital. Case 35–1988. N Engl J Med 1988;319:564–574.
Gaffney EF, Condell D, Majmudar B, et al. Modification of caecal lymphoid tissue and relationship to granuloma formation in sporadic ileo-caecal tuberculosis. Histopathology 1987;11:691–704.
Howell JS, Knapton PJ. Ileo-caecal tuberculosis. Gut 1964;5:524–529.
Kapoor VK, Sharma LK. Abdominal tuberculosis. Br J Surg 1988;75:2–3.
Palmer KR, Patil DH, Basran GS, et al. Abdominal tuberculosis in urban Britain: a common disease. Gut 1985;26:1296–1305.
Tandon HD, Prakash A. Pathology of intestinal tuberculosis and its distinction from Crohn's disease. Gut 1972;13:260–269.

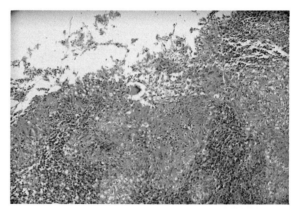

Figure 3–67. Tuberculous ileitis. Granulomatous inflammation in the floor of an ulcer.

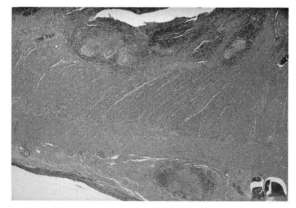

Figure 3–66. Tuberculous ileitis. Granulomas are present in both the submucosa and the serosa.

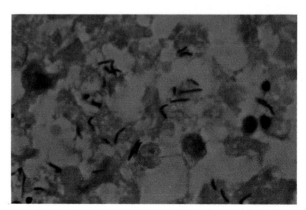

Figure 3–68. Ziehl-Neelsen stain displays several acid-fast bacilli.

MYCOBACTERIUM AVIUM-INTRACELLULARE INFECTION

Biology of Disease

- *Mycobacterium avium-intracellulare* (MAI) infection of the bowel in patients with AIDS may mimic Whipple's disease both endoscopically and histologically.
- In most patients with gastrointestinal MAI infection, the blood CD4 lymphocyte count is below 100×10^6/L.
- The small bowel mucosa is most often involved but the colonic mucosa may be affected either alone or in conjunction with the small bowel.

Clinical Findings

- Patients usually present with diarrhea or steatorrhea.

Gross Pathology

- Endoscopically, multiple yellowish granules or plaques may be seen, but in the early stages, there may be no abnormality.
- The mucosa at autopsy may have an exaggerated villous pattern resembling the pile on a carpet.

Microscopic Pathology

- Large granular macrophages in the lamina propria expand the villi and resemble those of Whipple's disease except for the lack of lipid vacuoles in the lamina propria. The villi may appear blunted.
- The macrophages contain abundant acid-fast bacilli that are typically approximately 12 μm in length but may be much shorter.
- In contrast with Whipple's disease, the macrophages are only weakly PAS-positive. Under oil immersion, the PAS staining is localized in individual bacilli.

- *Mycobacterium avium* can usually be cultured from the stools or peripheral blood in AIDS patients, in whom infection is disseminated throughout the body. Because culture involves a long incubation time, demonstration of acid-fast bacilli in liver or small bowel biopsy specimens is a faster route to presumptive diagnosis.

Special Diagnostic Techniques

- Culture of the mycobacterium is the definitive way to identify the organism.

Differential Diagnosis

Whipple's disease, tuberculosis.

Whipple's disease macrophages are strongly positive to PAS staining and negative to Ziehl-Neelsen staining. In Whipple's disease, there are usually lipid droplets in the lamina propria.

Tuberculosis does not produce such vast numbers of intracellular bacteria or a pattern resembling that seen in Whipple's disease.

References

Gillen JS, Urmacher C, West R, Shike M. Disseminated *Mycobacterium avium-intracellulare* infection in acquired immunodeficiency syndrome mimicking Whipple's disease. Gastroenterology 1983;85:1187–1191.

Guthertz LS, Damster B, Bottone EJ, et al. *Mycobacterium avium* and *Mycobacterium intracellulare* infection in patients with and without AIDS. J Infect Dis 1989;160:1037–1041.

Klatt EC, Jensen DF, Meyer PR. Pathology of *Mycobacterium avium-intracellulare* infection in acquired immunodeficiency syndrome. Hum Pathol 1987;18:709–714.

Strom RL, Gruninger RP, Roth RI, et al. AIDS with *Mycobacterium avium-intracellulare* lesions resembling those of Whipple's disease. N Engl J Med 1983;309:1323–1325.

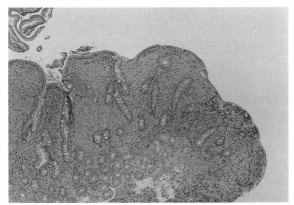

Figure 3–69. *Mycobacterium avium-intracellulare* infection in a patient with AIDS. The lamina propria is expanded by pale-staining histiocytes. The villi appear flattened. The fatty globules seen in Whipple's disease are not present here.

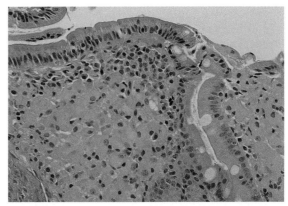

Figure 3–70. *Mycobacterium avium-intracellulare* infection. A large cluster of eosinophilic histiocytes occupies most of the lamina propria.

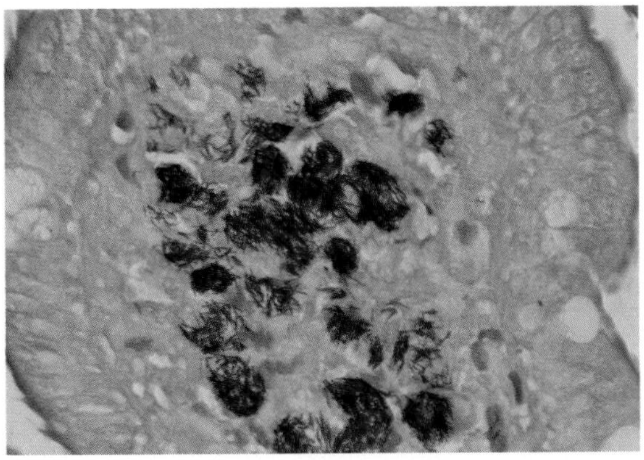

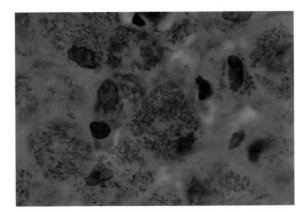

Figure 3–71. *Mycobacterium avium-intracellulare* infection. Ziehl-Neelsen stain reveals innumerable acid-fast bacilli.

Figure 3–72. *Mycobacterium avium-intracellulare* infection. Periodic acid–Schiff method stains the individual mycobacteria weakly.

CLOSTRIDIAL ENTERITIS

Biology of Disease

- *Enteritis necroticans* is a necrotizing condition of the small bowel produced by the beta toxin of *Clostridium perfringens* type C. Occasional cases are due to *C. perfringens* type A. Enteritis due to other strains of clostridia is uncommon.
- Enteritis necroticans was first recognized in Northern Europe after World War II. It regularly followed pig-eating feasts in the Highlands of Papua New Guinea, but active immunization against the beta toxin of *C. perfringens* has resulted in a great decline in incidence. A recent outbreak was reported among Khmer refugee children in Thailand.
- Sporadic cases are reported in western countries, sometimes in the context of bulimia.
- The clostridial toxin is protease sensitive, and in patients with normal pancreatic enzyme secretion, it is rapidly destroyed. In most outbreaks, the diet of those affected has been protein deficient, so that pancreatic protease production may have been diminished.
- Neutropenic enterocolitis primarily involves the cecum (typhlitis) and is due to *Clostridium septicum* or *C. perfringens*. *C. septicum* is a normal commensal. It has been suggested that when neutrophil protease levels are too low to neutralize its toxin, *C. septicum* becomes pathogenic. Occasionally, typhlitis is complicated by metastatic myonecrosis.

Clinical Findings

- Most patients are children. They present with acute abdominal pain, distention, vomiting, shock, and passing of blood per rectum. Milder disease may masquerade as gastroenteritis.

Gross Pathology

- Enteritis necroticans is typically a segmental necrotizing disease of the jejunum with normal areas between the affected areas, but some cases may affect the jejunum and ileum diffusely.
- The jejunum is distended to twice or three times normal diameter.
- Blotchy red areas of hemorrhage are seen on the serosal surface of diseased gut.
- The mucosa initially shows small punched-out grayish ulcers, but later, large flaps of necrotic mucosa are sloughed off.
- Perforation or internal fistula is common.

Microscopic Pathology

- The early lesion is submucosal edema; mucosal necrosis and, ultimately, full-thickness necrosis of a portion of bowel wall follow. Necrosis may extend into or through the muscle coat, and fibrinous peritonitis or frank perforation may be present. Hemorrhage is prominent in the submucosa and subserosa. Gas cysts are a feature of some cases.
- Abundant gram-positive rods may be seen on the surface and within the tissue.
- Obliterative endothelial proliferation of submucosal veins is seen at the junction between necrotic and normal bowel.

Special Diagnostic Techniques

- Culture of *Clostridium* from resected bowel or immunostaining of *Clostridium* may aid diagnosis.

Differential Diagnosis

Ischemic necrosis.

Ischemic necrosis is rarely multisegmental, rarely affects the jejunum, and rarely occurs in children. Secondary bacterial overgrowth after ischemia can confuse the morphology. The mesenteric blood vessels are normal in clostridial enteritis.

References

Cooke RA. The pathology of pig bel. Papua New Guinea Med J 1979;22:35–39.

Devitt PG, Stamp GWH. Acute clostridial enteritis—or pig-bel? Gut 1983;24:678–679.

Johnson S, Echeverria P, Taylor DN, et al. Enteritis necroticans among Khmer children at an evacuation site in Thailand. Lancet 1987;2:496–500.

Lawrence G, Cooke R. Experimental pigbel: the production and pathology of necrotizing enteritis due to *Clostridium welchii* type C in the guinea-pig. Br J Exp Pathol 1980;61:261–271.

Murrell TGC, Roth L. Necrotizing jejunitis: a newly discovered disease in the highlands of New Guinea. Med J Aust 1963;1:61–69.

Murrell TGC, Roth L, Egerton J, et al. Pig-bel: enteritis necroticans. Lancet 1966;1:217–222.

Severin WPJ, de la Fuente AA, Stringer MF. *Clostridium perfringens* type C causing necrotising enteritis. J Clin Pathol 1984;37:942–944.

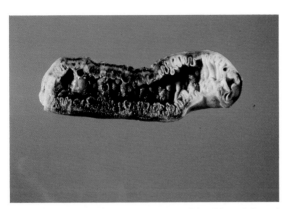

Figure 3–73. Clostridial enteritis. A segment of small bowel shows intramural hemorrhage and mucosal edema and necrosis. This is an example of pigbel. (Courtesy of Dr. Robin Cooke.)

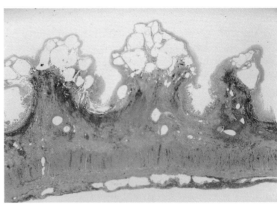

Figure 3–74. Clostridial enteritis. The mucosa shows necrosis and pneumatosis. Pneumatosis is present on the serosa also. (Courtesy of Dr. Rahul Bannerjee.)

CROHN'S DISEASE

Biology of Disease

■ *Crohn's disease* is an idiopathic, chronic, ulceroinflammatory disease of the gastrointestinal tract that most often affects the terminal ileum and colon. Recurrences after resection are the rule.

■ An important criterion for Crohn's disease is persistence. Incidence of focal mucosal inflammation documented months apart are strongly suggestive of Crohn's disease.

■ Hereditary factors play a role in Crohn's disease; there is a higher incidence in Jews than non-Jews and in whites than nonwhites. Crohn's disease is associated with the combination of HLA DR1 and DQw5 in North Americans and with DR4 in Japanese.

■ Cigarette smoking is etiologically associated with Crohn's disease and exacerbates the disease, although some patients never smoked. Paradoxically, smoking is beneficial in ulcerative colitis.

■ Discriminant analysis suggests that Crohn's disease is not a homogeneous entity. This is borne out by the occurrence of Crohn's-like disease in patients with Behçet's disease, neutrophil function defects (chronic granulomatous disease, glycogen storage disease type Ib, and con-genital neutropenia), common variable immunodeficiency, the Hermansky-Pudlak syndrome, and reactive arthritis.

■ Complications of Crohn's disease include bowel obstruction, fistulae, perforation, anal sinuses, and an increased risk of malignancy.

Clinical Findings

■ Diarrhea, abdominal pain, anal fissures or fistulae, intestinal obstruction, internal fistulae, weight loss, and fever are the main manifestations.

■ The onset is insidious, with weight loss, abdominal pain, and low-grade fever.

■ Colonic disease may manifest as perianal disease, moderate diarrhea, and hematochezia.

Gross Pathology

■ The earliest gross lesions are multiple, tiny, randomly scattered "aphthoid" ulcers on otherwise normal mucosa (with a normal pattern of mucosal folds). Ulcers may arise over lymphoid follicles. Ulcers enlarge and coalesce into linear or serpiginous forms, dissecting the mucosa into a cobblestone pattern. Discrete longitudinal or circumferential ulcers may form ragged geographic patterns. Inflamed preulcerated mucosa has been identified in the rectum with the magnifying endoscope.

■ Thickening of the bowel wall occurs owing to submucosal edema and fibrosis of the muscularis mucosae secondary to ulceration. Stenosis or stricture results from submucosal cicatrization after ulceration. The ileocecal valve is often strictured.

■ Regenerated mucosa is grossly flat and granular.

■ Sinuses (blind-ended inflammatory tracts) arise in ulcers, usually at the proximal ends of strictures. Sinuses penetrate into the mesentery and result in inflammatory adhesions to other loops of bowel or viscera. Ultimately a sinus may reach a second epithelial surface to form a fistula. When the ileocecal valve is stenosed, a fistula often penetrates through it from ileum to cecum, an appearance that resembles anal disease.

■ The serosal surface shows fat wrapping, reflecting chronic serositis. Mesenteric lymph nodes are enlarged unless corticosteroid treatment has been given.

■ Jejunal Crohn's disease may show multiple strictures and saccular dilations and must be distinguished from "diaphragm disease" induced by nonsteroidal anti-inflammatory drugs (NSAIDs).

Microscopic Pathology

■ Patchy nonspecific inflammation with adjacent normal mucosa is the most characteristic feature. The inflammation includes increased numbers of lymphocytes, plasma cells, eosinophils, and neutrophils and is seen predominantly in the lower half of the mucosa. Neutrophil or eosinophil cryptitis or crypt abscesses may be present.

■ Noncaseating granulomas strongly suggest the diagnosis. Crypt destruction may be associated with granuloma formation. Granulomas are often seen beneath ulcers. Submucosal granulomas are often beside lymphatic vessels or bulging into dilated lymphatics.

■ Aphthoid ulcers are multiple nonspecific ulcers that arise in inflamed mucosa. They appear to begin as crypt ulcers. They may overlie solitary lymphoid follicles or Peyer's patches. An epithelioid granuloma is sometimes present beneath an aphthoid ulcer in the granulation tissue, in an underlying lymphoid follicle, or in the submucosa.

■ Chronic ulcers display granulation tissue, fibromuscular thickening of muscularis mucosae, submucosal inflammation and lymphangiectasia, and transmural inflammation that includes aggregates of lymphoid cells. Healed ulcers show crypt irregularity, branching, or dropout (i. e., loss of crypts) and associated gastric pyloric metaplasia.

■ Transmural inflammation with lymphoid aggregates in the deep submucosa and serosa are characteristic of Crohn's disease.

■ Strictures are due to hypertrophy and fibrosis of the muscularis mucosae and submucosa in reaction to ulceration.

■ Sinuses and fistulae are initially lined by granulation tissue but may become epithelialized by mucosal regeneration. Sinuses that are cut transversely look like abscesses.

■ Fissures, or narrow microscopic clefts penetrating from the ulcer surface into the muscle coat, may be seen in di-

lated bowel proximal to strictures and also within strictured bowel.

■ Mucosal, submucosal, and serosal lymphangiectasia are often present in the diseased areas. Lymphatics may be surrounded by lymphocytes.

■ Neuroid hypertrophy/hyperplasia in the submucosa is a feature that follows ulceration, presumably owing to destruction of mucosal nerve endings.

■ Hemosiderin deposition is rare.

Special Diagnostic Techniques

■ Upper GI series with barium follow-through may demonstrate ileal disease. Barium enema with air contrast is optimal for delineating colonic disease.

■ Proctosigmoidoscopy or colonoscopy, as indicated by symptoms, allows direct inspection and biopsy of diseased areas. Intact normal-appearing mucosa may show granulomas in 20% of patients if serially sectioned.

Differential Diagnosis

Disorders of neutrophil function, common variable immunodeficiency, Hermansky-Pudlak syndrome, reactive arthritis, ischemia, tuberculosis, yersiniosis, histoplasmosis, NSAID enteropathy, Behçet's disease. See Chapter 4 for distinction from ulcerative colitis.

Chronic granulomatous disease (a disorder of NADPH oxidase) may mimic Crohn's disease, demonstrating patchy ulcers, focal inflammation, and granulomas. Neutrophil numbers are normal, but the nitroblue tetrazolium test result is abnormal. Nucleic acid probes are available for specific molecular defects. Crohn's-like disease may also be seen in children with glycogen storage disease type Ib, congenital neutropenia, Hermansky-Pudlak syndrome, common variable immunodeficiency, and reactive arthritis.

In adults, ischemic strictures, tuberculosis, histoplasmosis, yersiniosis, and NSAID-induced strictures may all need to be considered.

Ischemic strictures follow episodes of acute ischemia that result in mucosal necrosis but leave the wall viable; insults such as cholesterol embolus, thromboembolus, vasculitis, thrombosis, and trauma, including nonpenetrating blunt abdominal trauma. Morphologically, ischemic strictures may show complete circumferential mucosal ulceration, transmural inflammation, fissuring ulceration, and hemosiderin deposition but do not contain granulomas. A crucial finding is mesenteric vessel occlusion or recanalization.

Tuberculosis is characterized by caseating granulomas and the presence of acid-fast bacilli.

The granulomas of histoplasmosis contain the diagnostic 2-μm to 4-μm yeasts.

Colonic amebiasis is characterized endoscopically by ulcers separated by normal mucosa. It is distinguished by identifying Entamoeba histolytica.

Behçet's disease of the intestine may be indistinguishable from Crohn's disease.

References

Abramowsky CR, Sorensen RU. Regional enteritis–like enteropathy in a patient with agammaglobulinemia: histologic and immunocytologic studies. Hum Pathol 1988;19:483–486.

Crohn BB, Ginzburg L, Oppenheimer GD. Regional ileitis. A pathological and clinical entity. JAMA 1932;99:1323–1329.

Hermos JA, Cooper HL, Kramer P, Trier JS. Histological diagnosis by peroral biopsy of Crohn's disease of the proximal intestine. Gastroenterology 1970;59:868–873.

Hywel-Jones J, Lennard-Jones JE, Morson BC, et al. Numerical taxonomy and discriminant analysis applied to non-specific colitis. Q J Med 1973;62:715–732.

Kelly JK, Sutherland LR. The chronological sequence in the pathology of Crohn's disease. J Clin Gastroenterol 1988;10:28–33.

Rappaport H, Burgoyne F, Smetana HF. The pathology of regional enteritis. Milit Surgeon 1951;109:463–502.

Rickert RR, Carter HW. The gross, light microscopic and scanning electron microscopic appearance of the early lesions of Crohn's disease. Scan Electron Micros 1977;2:179–186.

Roe TF, Coates TD, Thomas DW, et al. Treatment of chronic inflammatory bowel disease in glycogen storage disease type Ib with colon stimulating factors. N Engl J Med 1992;326:1666–1669.

Tanaka M, Kimura K, Sakai H, et al. Long-term follow-up for minute gastroduodenal lesions in Crohn's disease. Gastrointest Endosc 1986;32:206–209.

Toyoda H, Wang S-J, Yang H-Y, et al. Distinct associations of HLA class II genes with inflammatory bowel disease. Gastroenterology 1992;104:741–748.

Valdes-Dapena A, Vilardell F. Granulomatous lesions in ileocolitis. Gastroenterologia 1962;97:191–204.

Warren S, Sommers SC. Cicatrizing enteritis (regional ileitis) as a pathologic entity. Analysis of one hundred and twenty cases. Am J Pathol 1948;24:475–497.

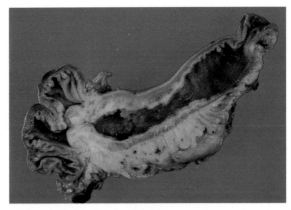

Figure 3–76. Crohn's disease. Ileocecal specimen fixed by distension with formalin. Note the marked thickening of the bowel wall in the terminal ileum and ileocecal valve. On the left side of the specimen, the ileocecal valve bulges into the cecum.

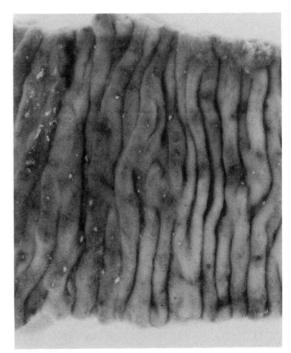

Figure 3–77. Crohn's disease. The ileum shows multiple tiny "aphthoid" ulcers on the mucosal folds. These small ulcers represent the earliest gross manifestation of Crohn's disease.

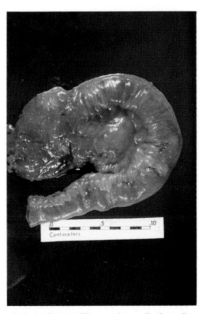

Figure 3–75. Crohn's disease. The specimen displays the terminal ileum and cecum together with mesentery. Note the extension of adipose tissue from the mesentery around the bowel toward the antimesenteric border (creeping fat).

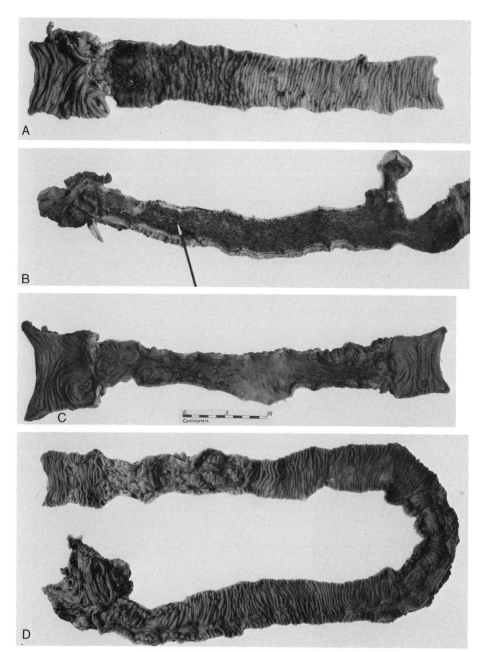

Figure 3–78. Specimens showing Crohn's disease. *A,* Stenosis of the ileo-cecal valve, extensive ulceration of the distal ileum, and proximal aphthoid ulcers. *B,* Extensive serpiginous ulceration and a Meckel's diverticulum. The probe marks a sinus. *C,* Crohn's ileitis with extensive ulceration and flat regenerated mucosa. There is a single round ulcer near the proximal resection margin. *D,* Crohn's ileitis (cecum is at *lower left*). Note ulcerated areas separated by normal mucosa (skip lesions). *E,* Crohn's ileitis with stenosis and marked thickening of the wall. A sinus (or fistula), marked by the orange stick, arises proximal to the point of most severe stenosis. *F,* Ileocolic Crohn's disease. The colon (*left*) shows inflammatory polyps and flat mucosa. There is a fistula through the ileocecal valve (*center*). The terminal ileum shows a stricture, a sinus, and mucosal ulcers (*left*).

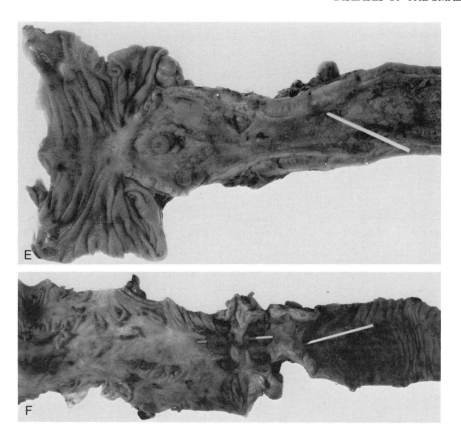

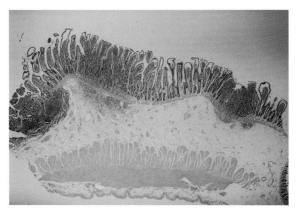

Figure 3–79. Crohn's disease. Three discrete foci of inflammation confined to the mucosa and superficial submucosa represent early microscopic changes of Crohn's disease.

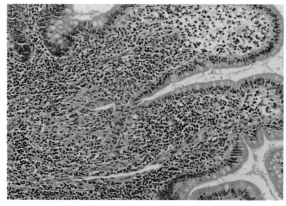

Figure 3–80. Crohn's disease. Focal destruction of a crypt with associated inflammation and granuloma.

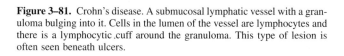

Figure 3–81. Crohn's disease. A submucosal lymphatic vessel with a granuloma bulging into it. Cells in the lumen of the vessel are lymphocytes and there is a lymphocytic cuff around the granuloma. This type of lesion is often seen beneath ulcers.

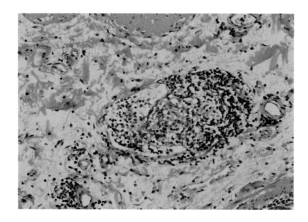

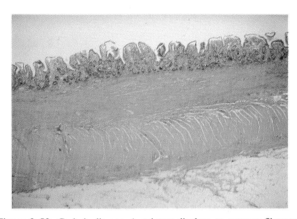

Figure 3–82. Crohn's disease. A stricture displays an extreme fibromuscular thickening in the submucosa that forms a layer as thick as the muscularis propria.

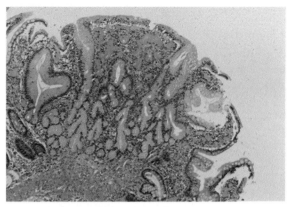

Figure 3–83. Gastric metaplasia in Crohn's disease showing pits and antral-type glands.

NONSTEROIDAL ANTI-INFLAMMATORY DRUG (NSAID) ENTEROPATHY

Biology of Disease

■ Nonsteroidal anti-inflammatory drugs (NSAIDs) may cause intestinal inflammation or ulceration, especially in elderly patients. The ileum and ascending colon are most often affected. Solitary ulcer of the bowel, formerly ascribed to potassium, is most often ascribed to NSAIDs nowadays.

Clinical Findings

■ The clinical findings in NSAID enteropathy consist of blood loss, positive fecal occult blood test results, iron deficiency anemia, intestinal obstruction, and abnormal radiologic findings, including ulcers and ileal diaphragms. NSAIDs are associated with an increased risk of perforation and bleeding from the small bowel and from colonic diverticula. They may exacerbate idiopathic inflammatory bowel disease and may be associated with collagenous colitis.

Gross Pathology

■ NSAID ulcers may be single or multiple and range from tiny linear or punched-out ulcers on the tips of valvulae conniventes to confluent areas of deep ulceration and stricture formation.

■ Ileal mucosal diaphragm disease or ultrashort-segment strictures may be seen. Diaphragms are often multiple and resemble stenosing valvulae conniventes.
■ Diaphragms may also be found in the ascending colon.

Microscopic Pathology

■ NSAID ulcers are entirely nonspecific histologically.
■ Diaphragms have the same components as the plicae circulares, with the addition of a focus of submucosal fibrosis and variable ulceration of the free edges of the diaphragm.

Special Diagnostic Techniques

■ Small bowel radiography and colonoscopy with biopsy may help to establish the diagnosis.

Differential Diagnosis

Crohn's disease of the jejunum.

Jejunal Crohn's disease may cause multiple short strictures and resemble NSAID diaphragm disease. Granulomas, signs of chronic ulceration and regeneration, and typical terminal ileal disease help to make the distinction. Diaphragm disease due to NSAIDs is typically ileal or colonic, not jejunal.

References

Allison MC, Howatson AG, Torrance CJ, et al. Gastrointestinal damage associated with the use of non-steroidal anti-inflammatory drugs. N Engl J Med 1992;327:749–754.

Bjarnason I, Hayllar J, Macpherson AJ, Russell AS. Side effects of non-steroidal antiinflammatory drugs in the small and large intestine in humans. Gastroenterology 1993;104:1832–1847.

Bjarnason I, Price AB, Zanelli G, et al. Clinicopathological features of non-steroidal antiinflammatory drug-induced small intestinal strictures. Gastroenterology 1988;94:1070–1074.

Huber T, Ruchti C, Halter F. Nonsteroidal anti-inflammatory drug–induced colonic strictures: a case report. Gastroenterology 1991;100:1119–1122.

Lang J, Price AB, Levi AJ, et al. Diaphragm disease: pathology of disease of the small intestine induced by non-steroidal anti-inflammatory drugs. J Clin Pathol 1988;41:516–526.

Langman MJS, Morgan L, Worrall A. Use of anti-inflammatory drugs by patients admitted with small or large bowel perforations and haemorrhage. Br Med J 1985;290:347–349.

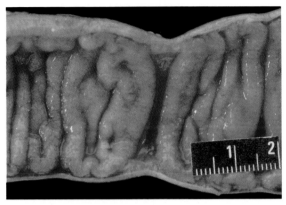

Figure 3–84. NSAID enteropathy. The ileum displays a narrow transverse ulcer. (Courtesy of Dr. Vivian Chang-Poon.)

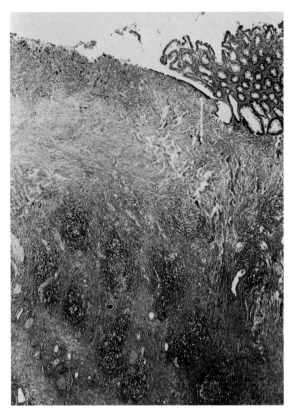

Figure 3–85. NSAID enteropathy. Microscopically, the ulcer shows non-specific features, including surface exudation, submucosal fibrosis, and lymphoid follicles.

POUCHITIS

Biology of Disease

■ Up to a third of patients with ileoanal pouches suffer from intermittent acute pouch diarrhea with watery and/or blood-stained stools and symptoms such as urgency, incontinence, abdominal cramping, and malaise. These symptoms are due to bacterial overgrowth and respond to antibiotic treatment (metronidazole) in most cases.

■ Chronic *ileal pouchitis* is a clinicopathologic syndrome of chronic pouch diarrhea and inflammation unresponsive to antibiotics. Chronic pouchitis occurs in patients who had colectomy for ulcerative colitis but not in those who had familial adenomatous polyposis or other disorders.

■ A minority (2% to 8%) of patients develop chronic pouchitis refractory to antibiotics.

Clinical Findings

■ Patients present with increased pouch effluent, watery or blood stained, and symptoms such as urgency, incontinence, and cramping pain.

Gross Pathology

■ Endoscopically, the pouch may appear friable, erythematous, or focally ulcerated in the chronic pouchitis syndrome. Pseudomembranous pouchitis is rarely seen.

Microscopic Pathology

■ A minority of pouches (13% in one series) may show ileal villi of normal or near normal height with little or no inflammation. Most pouches show increased numbers of mononuclear cells in lamina propria and sometimes a mild neutrophil infiltrate.

■ Acute pouchitis is characterized by a heavy neutrophil infiltrate.

■ Biopsy specimens of chronic pouchitis may resemble those of idiopathic ulcerative colitis. They show active chronic inflammation of the full thickness of the mucosa, neutrophil cryptitis and crypt abscesses, loss of villi, and crypt hyperplasia.

■ If granulomas are present, a diagnosis of Crohn's disease is likely. In excised pouches, ulceration, regeneration, metaplasia, transmural inflammation, and strictures strongly support a diagnosis of Crohn's disease.

■ Increased numbers of goblet cells that may contain sulfomucin of colonic type, constituting a form of colonic metaplasia, are seen in one third of cases.

■ Pyloric metaplasia and features of mucosal prolapse are seen in less than 5% of pouches.

Special Diagnostic Techniques

■ In acute pouchitis, there is decreased fecal concentration of short-chain fatty acids.

■ ^{111}In-labeled granulocyte scanning and fecal excretion represents an objective approach to diagnosis.

Differential Diagnosis

The etiology of chronic pouchitis and its relationship to inflammatory bowel disease are still unclear. In some instances, it appears to represent Crohn's disease, and in others, it resembles recurrence of ulcerative colitis.

References

Clausen MR, Tvede M, Mortensen PB. Short-chain fatty acids in pouch contents from patients with and without pouchitis after ileal pouch–anal anastomosis. Gastroenterology 1992;103:1144–1153.

Di Febo G, Miglioli M, Lauri A, et al. Endoscopic assessment of acute inflammation of the ileal reservoir after restorative ileo-anal anastomosis. Gastrointest Endosc 1990;36:6–9.

Helander KG, Ahren C, Philipson BM, et al. Structure of mucosa in continent ileal reservoirs 15 to 19 years after construction. Hum Pathol 1990;21:1235–1238.

Kmiot WA, Hesselwood SR, Smith N, et al. Evaluation of the inflammatory infiltrate in pouchitis with ^{111}In-labelled granulocytes. Gastroenterology 1993;104:981–988.

Lohmuller JL, Pemberton JH, Dozois RR, et al. Pouchitis and extraintestinal manifestations of inflammatory bowel disease after ileal pouch–anal anastomosis. Ann Surg 1990;211:622–629.

Shepherd NA, Jass JR, Duval I, et al. Restorative proctocolectomy with ileal reservoir: pathological and histochemical study of mucosal biopsy specimens. J Clin Pathol 1987;40:601–607.

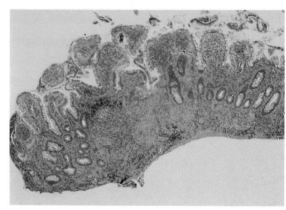

Figure 3–86. Mild chronic pouchitis. The villi are shortened and widened, and the density of cells in the lamina propria is increased.

INTESTINAL LYMPHANGIECTASIA

Biology of Disease

■ *Intestinal lymphangiectasia* describes dilated lymphatic vessels in the small bowel mucosa. Primary lymphangiectasia is a rare sporadic, congenital or acquired disorder in which mucosal lymphatics are widely distended and leak protein and lymphocytes into the intestinal lumen, resulting in hypoalbuminemia and lymphopenia. Primary lymphangiectasia may solely affect the bowel and its mesentery or may be one component of Milroy's disease (familial lymphedema). Blood loss occurs rarely.

■ Secondary lymphangiectasia may result from retroperitoneal lymph node obstruction by neoplasm, retroperitoneal fibrosis, tuberculosis, lymphoma, macroglobulinemia, systemic sclerosis, radiation, or Crohn's disease.

■ Constrictive pericarditis or chronic congestive heart failure may also cause secondary intestinal protein loss.

■ In young women, acquired lymphangiectasia may be a manifestation of early systemic lupus erythematosus. In this context, the protein loss is not accompanied by loss of lymphocytes.

Clinical Findings

■ Patients present with severe peripheral edema, abdominal complaints, diarrhea or steatorrhea, chylous ascites, hypoalbuminemia, yellow nails, or immunodeficiency. Steatorrhea may result from loss of fat in the lymph.

Gross Pathology

■ Endoscopically, multiple tiny white flecks may be seen on the duodenal mucosa as are seen in Waldenström's macroglobulinemia and sometimes in Whipple's disease.

■ At laparotomy, the bowel has a brown color (brown bowel syndrome) owing to lipofuscinosis of the muscle coat.

Microscopic Pathology

■ The lacteals in the intestinal villi are greatly dilated, with consequent distention of the villi and edema of the lamina propria. Serial sections show edema of villous lamina propria at one level and lymphangiectasia at others, so that in any one section there may only be one or two dilated lymphatics. The diagnosis often depends on examination of serial sections.

- Foamy macrophages, negative to PAS staining but positive to oil red–O staining, may be present in the lamina propria.
- Sometimes there is distention of lymphatics of the submucosa, serosa, and mesentery.
- Brown bowel due to lipofuscin pigmentation of the muscle coat may result from vitamin E deficiency.

Special Diagnostic Techniques

- Protein loss in feces may be demonstrated either by measurement of alpha$_1$-antitrypsin or of radiolabeled albumin and ceruloplasmin in feces.
- In the congenital disease, lymphangiography may demonstrate hypoplastic peripheral lymphatics and abnormal central lymphatics.

Differential Diagnosis

Local lymphatic dilation, normal duodenum.

Local lymphatic dilation as part of a lymphangioma may look like lymphangiectasia on biopsy.

Occasionally dilated lymphatics may be seen in otherwise normal duodenal biopsies in patients who do not have protein loss from the bowel.

References

Browse NL, Wilson NM, Russo F, et al. Aetiology and treatment of chylous ascites. Br J Surg 1992;79:1145–1150.
Edworthy SM, Fritzler MJ, Kelly JK, et al. Protein-losing enteropathy in systemic lupus erythematosus associated with intestinal lymphangiectasia. Am J Gastroenterol 1990;85:1398–1402.
Fleisher TA, Strober W, Muchmore AV, et al. Corticosteroid-responsive intestinal lymph-angiectasia secondary to an inflammatory process. N Engl J Med 1979;300:605–606.
Harris M, Burton IE, Scarffe JH. Macroglobulinemia and intestinal lymphangiectasia: a rare association. J Clin Pathol 1983;36:30–36.
Schwartz M, Jarnum S. Protein-losing gastroenteropathy: hypoproteinemia due to gastrointestinal protein loss of varying etiology diagnosed by means of ^{131}I-albumin. Dan Med Bull 1961;8:1–10.
Strober W, Wochner RD, Carbone PP, Waldmann TA. Intestinal lymphangiectasia: a protein-losing enteropathy with hypo-gammaglobulinemia, lymphocytopenia and impaired homograft rejection. J Clin Invest 1967;48:1643–1656.

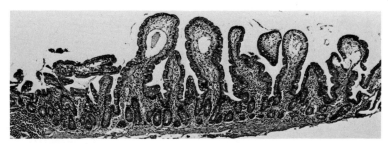

Figure 3–87. Intestinal lymphangiectasia. Three villi display dilated lymphatics in this plane of section. Other villi showed edema in this plane and lymphangiectasia in deeper sections.

CHYLOUS CYST AND CYSTIC LYMPHANGIOMA

Biology of Disease and Clinical Findings

- Chylous (lymphangiectatic) cyst is usually an incidental finding in a resected specimen, at autopsy, or at endoscopy in an adult patient. Chylous cysts may be single or multiple. They do not produce symptoms and do not cause protein loss.
- *Cystic lymphangioma* is an uncommon unilocular or multilocular cystic lesion of the mesentery that may be asymptomatic or may present in childhood with abdominal pain, bowel obstruction, torsion or infection.

Gross Pathology

- Chylous cysts are cream colored, up to 1 cm in diameter, and located in the distal duodenum or jejunum.

- Cystic lymphangiomas of the mesentery are usually multilocular and may be several centimeters in diameter. They contain milky chyle. The internal lining of the cysts is smooth.

Microscopic Pathology

- Chylous cysts comprise unilocular or multilocular, thin-walled lymphatic cysts in the submucosa and mucosa. They contain amorphous, weakly eosinophilic material, foamy macrophages, and scanty lymphocytes. The lymphatics in the overlying mucosa may be dilated, similar to those in intestinal lymphangiectasia.
- Cystic lymphangiomas of mesentery are lined by flattened endothelium, and the cyst walls are usually thin and contain focal lymphocytic aggregates. In some cases, the walls may be thicker and may contain collagen or smooth muscle.

Differential Diagnosis

Lymphangiectasia, cystic mesothelioma.

Endoscopic biopsy histology of a lymphangiectatic cyst may be identical to that of lymphangiectasia, and the distinction is based on the endoscopic appearances and normal serum albumin.

The distinction of cystic lymphangiomas from cystic mesotheliomas is based on the characteristic multilocular cystic morphology of the mesothelioma and the positive staining of mesothelial cells for cytokeratin.

References

Carpenter HA, Lancaster JR, Lee RA. Multilocular cysts of the peritoneum. Mayo Clin Proc 1982;57:634–638.

Shilkin KB, Zerman BJ, Blackwell JB. Lymphangiectatic cysts of the small bowel. J Pathol Bacteriol 1968;96:353–358.

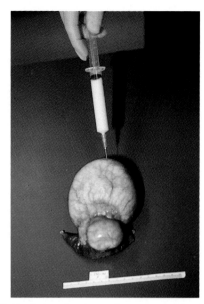

Figure 3–89. Cystic lymphangioma of mesentery encroaching on small bowel of a 3-year-old child. Note the creamy chyle in the syringe. (Courtesy of Dr. Michael O'Connor.)

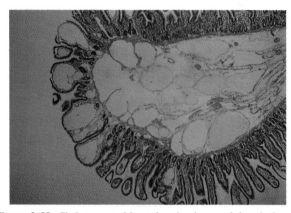

Figure 3–88. Chylous cyst. Mucosal and submucosal lymphatics are dilated.

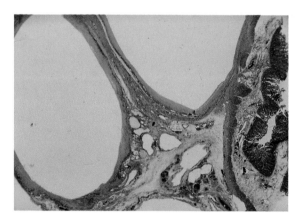

Figure 3–90. Cystic lymphangioma. The cyst walls are thick and collagenous.

ABETALIPOPROTEINEMIA AND RELATED DISORDERS

Biology of Disease and Clinical Findings

■ *Abetalipoproteinemia, hypobetalipoproteinemia,* and *chylomicron retention disease* (Andersen's disease) are members of a group of rare hereditary disorders of chylomicron formation. Normally, chylomicrons are formed in the enterocytes and carry fats into the lymphatics and thence into the blood. In the first two conditions, betalipoprotein is absent or diminished, preventing chylomicron forma-

tion. In the last condition, the defect may be either in the assembly or release of chylomicrons.

■ In abetalipoproteinemia, microsomal triglyceride transfer protein, which is normally located in the lumen of microsomes, is absent, and this is probably the basic abnormality.

■ In all three disorders, the enterocytes are replete with fat and there is fat malabsorption and steatorrhea, resulting in failure to thrive in infancy or growth retardation in childhood.

■ In abetalipoproteinemia, secondary sensory neuropathy, ataxia, and retinitis pigmentosa develop in later life. Acanthocytosis (spiny projections from the red blood cells) is seen on blood films in abetalipoproteinemia but not in the other two disorders.

■ About a third of patients affected with any of these disorders have consanguineous parents. Heterozygotes are phenotypically normal.

Gross Pathology

■ Endoscopically, the mucosa of the duodenum may have a grayish appearance.

Microscopic Pathology

■ Villous architecture is normal, but there is lipid vacuolation of the absorptive epithelial cells. Fat can be demonstrated in enterocytes by oil red–O staining of frozen sections or by examination of osmium-fixed tissue.

Special Diagnostic Techniques

■ Serum apolipoprotein B may be measured by radioimmunoassay.

References

Black DD, Hay RV, Rohwer-Nutter PL, et al. Intestinal and hepatic apolipoprotein B gene expression in abetalipoproteinemia. Gastroenterology 1991;101:520–528.
Bouma ME, Bellcler I, Pessah M, et al. Description of two different patients with abetalipoproteinemia: synthesis of a normal-sized apolipoprotein B-48 in intestinal organ culture. J Lipid Res 1990;31:1–15.
Cotrill C, Glueck CJ, Lauba V, et al. Familial homozygous hypobeta-lipoproteinemia. Metabolism 1974;23:779–791.
Isselbacher KJ, Scheig R, Plotkin GR, Caulfield JB. Congenital beta-lipoprotein deficiency: an hereditary disorder involving a defect in the absorption and transport of lipids. Medicine 1964;43:347–361.
Roy CC, Levy E, Green PHR, et al. Malabsorption, hypocholesterolemia, and fat-filled enterocytes with increased intestinal apoprotein B: chylomicron retention disease. Gastroenterology 1987;92:390–399.
Wetteran JR, Aggerbeck LP, Bouma M-E, et al. Absence of microsomal triglyceride transfer protein in individuals with abetalipoproteinemia. Science 1992;258:999–1001.

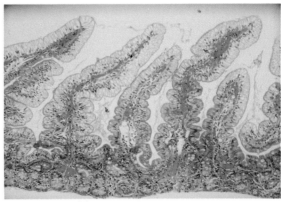

Figure 3–91. Abetalipoproteinemia. Villi are of normal height, and crypts are of normal depth. The enterocytes show cytoplasmic vacuolization, giving an extremely pale color to the picture. (Original microscope slide courtesy of Dr. Laurence Jewell.)

MACROGLOBULINEMIC ENTEROPATHY

Biology of Disease

■ *Macroglobulinemia* is a great excess of IgM in the blood produced by a lymphoplasmacytic lymphoma of the bone marrow or lymph nodes.
■ Rarely, macroglobulinemia manifests as steatorrhea. Affected patients have secondary lymphangiectasia and deposition of macroglobulin in the small bowel mucosa. Protein-losing enteropathy is a feature of some cases, too. These features are thought to be due to lymphatic stasis secondary to increased viscosity caused by complexes of IgM and phospholipid.
■ After chemotherapy or plasmapheresis, the malabsorption may disappear and the intestinal lymphangiectasia may regress.

Clinical Findings

■ In addition to the usual findings in macroglobulinemia—anemia, splenomegaly, hemorrhagic tendency, and weight loss—patients may manifest abdominal distention, diarrhea, or steatorrhea.

■ Affected patients are usually in the seventh to the ninth decades of life.

Gross Pathology

■ Endoscopically or at autopsy, the small bowel mucosa may show innumerable tiny white or yellowish flecks or granules, each representing a dilated mucosal lymphatic. These flecks begin abruptly beyond the pylorus, cover the entire mucosal surface, and gradually disappear in the ileum.
■ Serosal lymphatics may also be dilated, nodular, and filled with firm white material. Mesenteric lymph nodes are enlarged and contain cheesy material.

Microscopic Pathology

■ Small bowel mucosa shows expanded, clubbed villi with dilated lymphatics filled with amorphous eosinophilic proteinaceous material. Similar proteinaceous material is present also in the lamina propria. This material is PAS-positive and diastase-resistant. Foamy macrophages may also be present. There is no evidence of lymphoma in the bowel itself.

■ Mesenteric lymph node sinusoids are distended by eosinophilic material and foamy histiocytes. There may be no evidence of lymphoma in the mesenteric nodes, or else there may be combined lymphoma and lymphangiectasia.

Special Diagnostic Techniques

■ The proteinaceous material reacts positively to immunostaining for IgM and either lambda or kappa light chains.

Differential Diagnosis

Intestinal lymphangiectasia, Whipple's disease, *Mycobacterium avium-intracellulare* infection.

Intestinal lymphangiectasia is distinguished by the absence of the proteinaceous coagulum in the dilated capillaries and in lamina propria.

Whipple's disease and *Mycobacterium avium* infection are characterized by accumulation of granular macrophages in the lamina propria.

References

Bedine MS, Yardley JH, Elliott HL, et al. Intestinal involvement in Waldenström's macroglobulinemia. Gastroenterology 1973;65:308–315.

Cabrera A, de la Pava S, Pickren JW. Intestinal localization of Waldenström's disease. Arch Intern Med 1964;114:399–407.

Harris M, Burton IE, Scarffe JH. Macroglobulinaemia and intestinal lymphangiectasia: a rare association. J Clin Pathol 1983;36:30–36.

Pruzanski W, Warren RE, Goldie JH, Katz A. Malabsorption syndrome with infiltration of the intestinal wall by extracellular monoclonal macroglobulin. Am J Med 1973;54:811–818.

Tubbs RR, McLaughlin JP, Winkelman EI, et al. Macroglobulinemia and malabsorption. Clev Clin Q 1977;44:189–197.

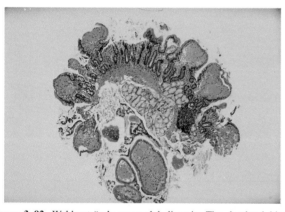

Figure 3–92. Waldenström's macroglobulinemia. The duodenal biopsy specimen displays several villi that are widely distended by pink proteinaceous material. (Courtesy of Dr. Scott Saul.)

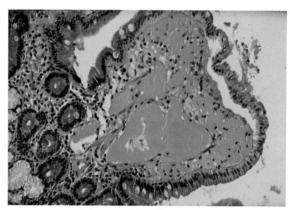

Figure 3–93. Macroglobulinemia. The villus displays lymphangiectasia. The lymphatic lumen and the lamina propria of the villus contain large quantities of pink proteinaceous material.

PRIMARY HYPOGAMMAGLOBULINEMIA

Biology of Disease

■ Primary hypogammaglobulinemia encompasses two main diseases, X-linked agammaglobulinemia and common variable immunodeficiency (CVID). Two other entities, thymoma with hypogammaglobulinemia occurring in patients over the age of 40 years and X-linked immunodeficiency with hyper-IgM (HIGM1), are also included.

■ Several different molecular or cellular abnormalities may give rise to CVID, including defects of T-cell immunoregulation, an intrinsic B-cell defect, and autoantibodies to T and B cells. X-linked immunodeficiency is a block in development of B-cell precursors due to mutations in the gene encoding a protein-tyrosine kinase.

HIGM1 is caused by defective expression of a CD40 ligand on T cells.

■ The criteria for diagnosis of X-linked hypogammaglobulinemia are: serum IgG below 2.0 g/L, absence of circulating B cells, and an affected male relative on the maternal side. Patients with CVID are of either sex, have circulating B cells, and have persistently low levels of one or more class of immunoglobulins (IgG < 7.2 g/L, IgM < 2.0 g/L, IgA < 0.8 g/L).

■ The risk of pernicious anemia, gastrointestinal carcinoma, and lymphoma is increased.

Clinical Findings

■ X-linked agammaglobulinemia presents as recurrent infections in boys. The peak incidence of onset is at 6 months, but cases manifest up to 5 years of age. Common variable immunodeficiency has two peaks for onset of symptoms, the first at 1 to 5 years and the second at 16 to 20 years. There may be a long delay before diagnosis, however.

■ Symptoms include sinusitis, bronchiectasis, recurrent respiratory infections, chronic diarrhea, and malabsorption.
■ *Giardia lamblia, Cryptosporidium,* or persistent infection with a common pathogen such as *Campylobacter jejuni* or *Salmonella* may contribute to diarrhea and malabsorption.
■ Current treatment is intravenous immunoglobulin.

Gross Pathology

■ Lymphoid hyperplasia may be visible endoscopically in the duodenum as multiple tiny mucosal nodules.

Microscopic Pathology

■ Plasma cells are scanty or absent from the lamina propria, and nodular hyperplasia of the solitary lymphoid follicles is present in at least 20% of cases.
■ Villous morphology may be normal. A small number of patients have classic celiac disease, with villous atrophy and crypt hyperplasia responsive to gluten withdrawal.
■ Giardiasis with associated mucosal inflammation, villous atrophy, and crypt hyperplasia is common.
■ Atrophic gastritis and achlorhydria may occur in common variable immunodeficiency.
■ Chronic inflammatory bowel disease that may resemble Crohn's disease and that responds rapidly to an elemental diet has been described in CVID.

Special Diagnostic Techniques

■ Immunostaining for immunoglobulin heavy chains confirms the absence or extreme paucity of plasma cells.

Differential Diagnosis

Secondary hypogammaglobulinemia.

Hypogammaglobulinemia may also occur secondary to intestinal lymphangiectasia, other protein-losing enteropathies, and renal protein loss.

References

Abramowsky CR, Sorensen RU. Regional enteritis–like enteropathy in a patient with agammaglobulinemia: histologic and immunocytologic studies. Hum Pathol 1988;19:483–486.

Gryboski JD, Self TW, Clemett A, Herskovic T. Selective immunoglobulin A deficiency and intestinal nodular lymphoid hyperplasia: correction of diarrhea with antibiotics and plasma. Pediatrics 1968;42:833–837.

Herman PE, Huizenga KA, Hoffman HN, et al. Dysgammaglobulinemia associated with nodular lymphoid hyperplasia of the small intestine. Am J Med 1966;40:78–79.

Hermaszewski RA, Webster ADB. Primary hypogammaglobulinemia: a survey of clinical manifestations and complications. Q J Med 1993;86:31–42.

Kopp WL, Trier JS, Stiehm ER, Foroozan P. "Acquired" agammaglobulinemia with defective delayed hypersensitivity. Ann Intern Med 1968;69:309–317.

Korthauer U et al. Defective expression of T-cell CD 40 ligand causes X-linked immunodeficiency with hyper-IgM. Nature 1993;361:539–541.

Perlmutter DH, Leichtner AM, Goldman H, Winter HS. Chronic diarrhea associated with hypogammaglobulinemia and enteropathy in infants with children. Dig Dis Sci 1985;30:1149–1155.

Sloper KS, Dourmashkin RR, Bird RB, et al. Chronic malabsorption due to cryptosporidiosis in a child with immunoglobulin deficiency. Gut 1982;23:80–82.

Vetrie D, Vorechovsky J, Sideras P, et al. The gene involved in X-linked agammaglobulinemia is a member of the *Src* family of protein-tyrosine kinases. Nature 1993;361:226–233.

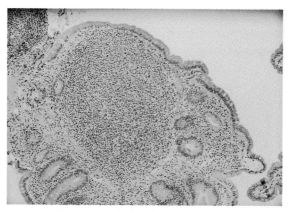

Figure 3–94. Hypogammaglobulinemia. Duodenal biopsy displays a hyperplastic lymphoid follicle that lacks a germinal center. There are no plasma cells.

TANGIER DISEASE

Biology of Disease

■ *Tangier disease* is an autosomal recessive disorder of apoprotein A1 (ApoA1), the main protein of high-density lipoproteins (HDLs).
■ An abnormality in post-translational processing of ApoA1 is believed to result in rapid degradation. The precise molecular defect has not yet been identified. Patients have very low plasma levels of HDLs and cholesterol, hypoalphalipoproteinemia, hypertriglyceridemia, and accumulation of cholesteryl esters in macrophages.

Clinical Findings

■ Diarrhea and steatorrhea are usual presenting features. The patients are adults. Despite the extremely low HDL, they do not develop atherosclerosis.
■ Tonsils are enlarged and show yellow-orange streaking.
■ Liver and spleen are enlarged.
■ Peripheral neuropathy and corneal opacities are commonly present.

Gross Pathology

■ On colonoscopy or duodenoscopy, orange-brown mucosal spots are seen.

■ At laparotomy or autopsy, the liver has an orange-yellow appearance.

Microscopic Pathology

■ Macrophages are distended by lipid, giving a pale eosinophilic or foamy appearance. The macrophages are located in bowel mucosa and submucosa, lymph nodes, tonsils, thymus, liver, and spleen.

Special Diagnostic Techniques

■ High-density lipoprotein levels are greatly reduced in serum: HDL cholesterol levels are low, and the LDL-cholesterol-to-HDL-cholesterol ratio is greatly increased.

Differential Diagnosis

Whipple's disease, *Mycobacterium avium-intracellulare* infection.

On duodenal mucosal biopsy, Tangier disease must be distinguished from Whipple's disease and *Mycobacterium avium-intracellulare* infection. In Tangier disease, the macrophages are PAS negative, oil red–O positive on frozen section and Ziehl-Neelsen negative.

References

Frohlich J, Westerlund J, Sparks D, Pritchard PH. Familial hypoalphalipoproteinemias. Clin Invest Med 1990;13:202–210.

Law SW, Brewer HB Jr. Tangier disease. The complete mRNA sequence encoding for preproapo-A1. J Biol Chem 1985;260:12810–12814.

Malloy MJ, Kane JP. Hypolipidemia. Med Clin North Am 1982;66:469–484.

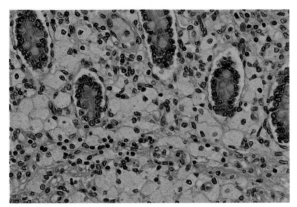

Figure 3–95. Tangier disease. Numerous foamy macrophages occupy the lamina propria.

PSEUDOMELANOSIS AND HEMOSIDEROSIS DUODENI

Biology of Disease

■ *Pseudomelanosis of the duodenum* is the term applied to pigment spots that are variably slate gray, black, or brown and scattered throughout the first and second parts of the duodenum. Anthracene purgatives are not associated with pseudomelanosis duodeni, but hydralazine and propranolol were used by several reported patients.

■ *Hemosiderosis of the duodenal mucosa* is an accumulation of hemosiderin in macrophages in lamina propria. It is associated with oral iron therapy.

Clinical Findings and Gross Pathology

■ Speckled black, brown, or gray pigmentation of the duodenal mucosa is typically seen in pseudomelanosis. Hemosiderosis may not be visible grossly or endoscopically.

■ Most patients are women more than 50 years old.

Microscopic Pathology

■ Brown or black pigment granules are seen in macrophages in the lamina propria of patients with pseudomelanosis. Pigment may also be free in the lamina propria or rarely in epithelial cells. The pigment may stain positively for melanin by the Masson-Fontana method and positively for iron by Perl's stain.

■ Hemosiderin has a golden brown appearance and is Perl's positive and Masson-Fontana negative.

Special Diagnostic Techniques

■ Ultrastructurally angular, membrane-bound, electron-dense bodies, some within lysosomes, are characteristic.

■ Electron probe analysis reveals high iron and sulphur content.

References

Castellano G, Canga F, Lopez I, et al. Pseudomelanosis of the duodenum: endoscopic, histologic, and ultrastructural study of a case. J Clin Gastroenterol 1988;10:150–154.

Kang JY, Wu AYT, Chia JLS, et al. Clinical and ultrastructural studies in duodenal pseudomelanosis. Gut 1987;28:1673–1681.

Kuo Y-C, Wu C-S. Duodenal melanosis. J Clin Gastroenterol 1988;10:160–164.

Lin H-J, Tsay S-H, Chiang H, et al. Pseudomelanosis duodeni: case report and review of literature. J Clin Gastroenterol 1988;10:155–159.

Rex DK, Jersild RA Jr. Further characterization of the pigment in pseudomelanosis duodeni in three patients. Gastroenterology 1988;95:177–182.

Sharp JR, Insalaco SJ, Johnson LF. "Melanosis" of the duodenum associated with a gastric ulcer and folic acid deficiency. Gastroenterology 1980;78:366–369.

West B. Pseudomelanosis duodeni. J Clin Gastroenterol 1988;10:127–129.

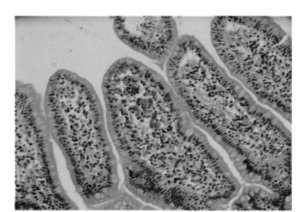

Figure 3–96. Hemosiderosis. The small-bowel villi show golden brown pigment within macrophages in the lamina propria.

PEUTZ-JEGHERS SYNDROME

Biology of Disease

■ *Peutz-Jeghers syndrome* is an autosomal dominant syndrome of gastrointestinal polyposis and brown macules (lentigines) on the lips, oral mucosa, digits, palms and soles. The polyps are hamartomas composed of differentiated tissues native to the location but present in abnormal proportions to one another. Polyps may arise in the stomach, small bowel, or large bowel.

Clinical Findings

■ Affected patients most often present in their teens but may present as young as 2 years or older than 40 years. The usual symptoms are abdominal pain and blood in the stools due to intussusception.

■ Ovarian tumors of ordinary types may complicate the syndrome. Two distinctive tumors associated with the syndrome are sex cord tumor with annular tubules of the ovary and adenoma malignum of the cervix uteri. Adenocarcinomas of the GI tract, pancreas, breast, or lung have also been reported in association with the syndrome.

Gross Pathology

■ Polyps with cerebriform convolutions or lobations are found mainly in the small bowel but also in stomach and colon. Polyps measure up to several centimeters in diameter. The total number of polyps rarely exceeds 20.

■ Intussusception with a leading polyp is a common finding.

Microscopic Pathology

■ Polyps have an arborizing core of muscularis mucosae covered by cytologically normal mucosa. The latter includes villi and crypts with normal endocrine, Paneth's, goblet, and absorptive epithelial cells in normal relationship to one another.

■ Reactive epithelial changes may be mistaken for adenoma. Rarely, dysplastic epithelium or carcinoma is found in these polyps.

■ Within polyps, mucosal glands are commonly displaced into the stalk, giving a pseudoinvasive appearance.

Differential Diagnosis

Adenomatous polyps.

Peutz-Jeghers polyps are distinguished from adenomatous polyps by the characteristic branching core of muscularis mucosae covered by normally maturing mucosa. Uncommonly, however, dysplasia does arise focally in Peutz-Jeghers polyps.

References

Bolwell JS, James PD. Peutz-Jeghers syndrome with pseudo-invasion of hamartomatous polyps and multiple epithelial neoplasms. Histopathology 1979;3:39–50.

Foley TR, McGarrity TJ, Abt AB. Peutz-Jeghers syndrome: a clinicopathologic survey of the "Harrisburg Family" with a 49 year follow-up. Gastroenterology 1988;95:1535–1540.

Giardiello FM, Welsh SB, Hamilton SR, et al. Increased risk of cancer in the Peutz-Jeghers syndrome. N Engl J Med 1987;316:1511–1514.

Narita T, Tadashi E, Ito T. Peutz-Jeghers syndrome with adenomas and adenocarcinomas in colonic polyps. Am J Surg Pathol 1987;11:76–81.

Patterson MJ, Kernen JA. Epithelioid leiomyosarcoma originating in a hamartomatous polyp from a patient with Peutz-Jeghers syndrome. Gastroenterology 1985;88:1060–1064.

Perzin KH, Bridge MF. Adenomatous and carcinomatous changes in hamartomatous polyps of the small intestine (Peutz-Jeghers syndrome): report of a case and review of the literature. Cancer 1982;49:971–983.

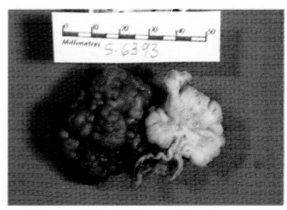

Figure 3–97. Peutz-Jeghers polyp. The surface is lobated.

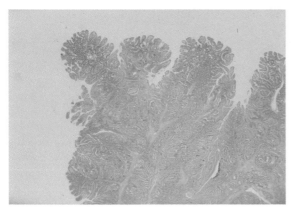

Figure 3–98. Peutz-Jeghers polyp. There is a branching core of muscularis mucosae covered by normal villi.

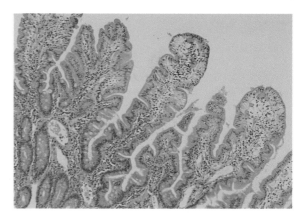

Figure 3–99. Peutz-Jeghers polyp. The villi are normal in appearance.

CARCINOID TUMORS AND NEUROENDOCRINE CARCINOMAS

Biology of Disease

- *Carcinoid tumors* are neoplasms of the endocrine cells of the gut. Carcinoid is the most common tumor of the ileum. Most carcinoids are slow growing and indolent. Less well-differentiated variants are more aggressive.
- Carcinoids are all potentially malignant, but many do not metastasize and are incidental findings at autopsy. The risk of metastasis increases with increasing size of the primary tumor. Tumors more than 2 cm in diameter have a greater risk of metastasis.
- Duodenal carcinoids have several peculiarities. Many occur in the periampullary region, including those complicating neurofibromatosis. Some are somatostatinomas and may show psammoma bodies. Gastrinomas of the duodenum may be seen in multiple endocrine adenomatosis type 1. Zollinger-Ellison syndrome may complicate duodenal gastrinoma. About 20% of duodenal carcinoids metastasize. Features associated with metastatic risk include involvement of muscularis propria, size greater than 2 cm, and the presence of mitotic figures. Rarely, small cell neuroendocrine carcinomas arise in the periampullary region.
- Carcinoids vary in morphology and behavior with location in the GI tract. Embryologic origin or tissue differentiation has been invoked to account for the differences. Foregut carcinoids are mainly argyrophilic (require an external reducing agent in silver stains), midgut carcinoids are argentaffinic, and hindgut carcinoids are often nonreactive with silver. Classic ileal carcinoids produce serotonin or 5-hydroxytryptophane.

Clinical Findings

- Sex incidences are nearly equal, and most cases occur in adults. Jejunoileal carcinoids are most often seen in patients in the sixth and seventh decades of life.
- Carcinoids may manifest as small bowel obstruction, metastases, bowel ischemia, or carcinoid syndrome from liver metastases, or they may be found incidentally at autopsy or at surgery.
- Liver or lung metastases may be associated with the carcinoid syndrome owing to release of serotonin (5-hydroxytryptamine), 5-hydroxytryptophan, histamine, prostaglandins, and kinins or other peptides by the tumor. The main features of the syndrome comprise episodes of flushing of the face and upper limbs, diarrhea, abdominal pain, bronchospasm, and palpitations. Only 7% of patients had the syndrome in one reported series.

Gross Pathology

- Seventy percent of ileal carcinoids are less than 1.5 cm in diameter, but some measure 5 cm or more in diameter.
- Mesenteric lymph node metastases often are much larger than the primary tumor.
- Approximately 30% of ileal carcinoids are multiple, and this subgroup is associated with intramucosal endocrine cell hyperplasia.
- Ileal carcinoids are usually sessile, umbilicated nodules or polyps or ulcerating tumors that may thicken and kink the bowel wall. Kinking of the bowel may cause obstruction.
- The cut surface is yellowish in color, and the tumor is located in the submucosa and muscle coat, which is thickened and rigid.

Microscopic Pathology

- Carcinoids are distinctive tumors of small regular cells that grow in nests, trabeculae, cords, tubules, or sheets and may form rosettes.
- Carcinoids of the ileum and appendix are "classic" carcinoids composed of nests of cells that show retraction artifact spaces around the margin after formalin fixation.
- Classic carcinoids stain positively with argyrophil stains and immunostains for chromogranin and serotonin.

- Carcinoids of the duodenum, jejunum, or rectum are more often nonclassic glandular carcinoids that grow in tubules, cords, glands, or rosettes.
- Individual cells may be columnar or polygonal, and their nuclei are rounded to oval, and uniform in shape and size.
- Atypical carcinoids, or neuroendocrine carcinomas, are composed of intermediate-sized cells with large nuclei and prominent nucleoli. They may show areas of necrosis and a sheetlike growth pattern in addition to cell nests or carcinoid-like features. In the extreme, these tumors may assume a small cell, undifferentiated appearance and extremely aggressive behavior.
- Psammoma bodies are seen in duodenal somatostatinomas and appear to result from calcification in the luminal secretions of tumor acini.

Special Diagnostic Techniques

- Silver stains (argyrophil and argentaffin) and immunoperoxidase stains for serotonin or chromogranin.
- A variety of peptide hormones may be identified by immunocytochemistry.
- Ultrastructural demonstration of neurosecretory granules may be essential to diagnosis of some tumors as carcinoids.

- Urinary excretion of 5-hydroxyindole acetic acid, a breakdown product of 5-hydroxytryptamine, is a test for carcinoid tumor.

References

Burke AP, Sobin LH, Federspiel BH, et al. Carcinoid tumors of the duodenum. A clinicopathologic study of 99 cases. Arch Pathol Lab Med 1990;114:700–704.
Dayal Y, Tallberg KA, Nunnemacher G, et al. Duodenal carcinoids in patients with and without neuro-fibromatosis: a comparative study. Am J Surg Pathol 1986;10:348–357.
Griffiths DFR, Jasani B, Newman GR, et al. Glandular duodenal carcinoid—a somatostatin rich tumour with neuroendocrine associations. J Clin Pathol 1984;37:163–169.
Johnson LA, Lavin P, Moertel CG, et al. Carcinoids: the association of histologic growth pattern and survival. Cancer 1983;51:882–889.
McNeal JE. Mechanism of obstruction in carcinoid tumors of the small intestine. Am J Clin Pathol 1971;56:452–458.
Moertel CG, Sauer WG, Dockerty MB, Baggenstoss AH. Life history of the carcinoid tumor of the small intestine. Cancer 1961;14:901–912.
Moyana TN, Sutkunam N. A comparative immunohistochemical study of jejunileal and appendiceal carcinoids. Implications for histogenesis and pathogenesis. Cancer 1992;70:1081–1088.
Zakariai YM, Quan SHQ, Hajdu SI. Carcinoid tumors of the gastrointestinal tract. Cancer 1975;35:588–591.
Zamboni G, Granzin G, Bonetti F, et al. Small-cell neuroendocrine carcinoma of the ampullary region. Am J Surg Pathol 1990;14:703–713.

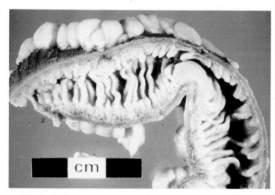

Figure 3–100. An ileal carcinoid tumor has kinked the bowel. This pattern of kinking, the most common cause of ileal obstruction due to carcinoid tumor, is a common mode of presentation. Note the homogeneous yellow appearance of the cut surface of the tumor. (From the Pathology Museum, University of Manchester, UK. Courtesy of Prof. John McClure.)

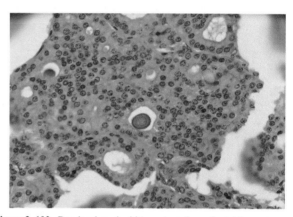

Figure 3–102. Duodenal carcinoid (somatostatinoma) contains psammoma bodies.

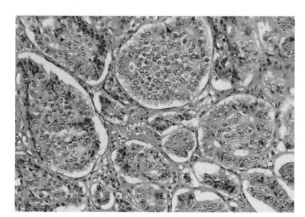

Figure 3–101. Ileal carcinoid tumor. This classic carcinoid displays nests of regular endocrine cells with rounded nuclei. The nests also show the characteristic retraction artifact seen in formalin-fixed carcinoids.

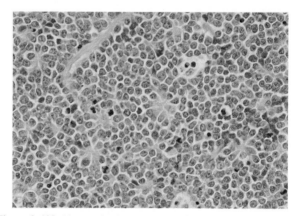

Figure 3–103. Neuroendocrine carcinoma of small bowel shows poorly differentiated small cells and rosettes.

GANGLIOCYTIC PARAGANGLIOMA

Biology of Disease

■ *Gangliocytic paraganglioma* is a rare tumor, virtually unique to the duodenum, that contains ganglion-like cells, carcinoid-like epithelial cells, and spindle cells of nerve sheath (Schwann) type.

Clinical Findings

■ Patient age at presentation ranges from 23 to 83 years, with the average 54 years.
■ Presenting complaints include abdominal pain and bleeding. The findings may consist of gastric outlet obstruction and biliary obstruction.
■ Some gangliocytic paragangliomas are incidental findings at autopsy.

Gross Pathology

■ The behavior is benign despite an infiltrative growth pattern.
■ Most gangliocytic paragangliomas are polyps or nodules in the second portion of the duodenum or near the ampulla. They usually involve the submucosa and muscularis propria.
■ These tumors range from 1.2 to 10 cm in diameter, most measuring between 2 and 4 cm.

Microscopic Pathology

■ Gangliocytic paraganglioma is composed of a mixture of epithelioid cells, ganglion cells, and Schwann cells.
■ The epithelioid cells have finely granular cytoplasm and form rounded or oval cell balls, ribbons, or festoons resembling carcinoids.
■ The ganglion cells are large, polygonal cells with acidophilic cytoplasm and large round nuclei.

■ The spindle cells resemble nerve sheath cells, with central elongated, wavy, tapering nuclei and amphophilic, nonfilamentous cytoplasm, and they form the matrix in which the ganglion cells and epithelioid cells are found.
■ Despite being benign in behavior, these tumors infiltrate the muscle coat.

Special Diagnostic Techniques

■ Immunostaining shows S100 positivity in the spindle cells, synaptophysin, and neuron-specific enolase in all cell types. A variety of peptides may be demonstrable in the epithelioid (carcinoidal) areas, pancreatic polypeptide being the most common.

Differential Diagnosis

Carcinoid, adenocarcinoma.

Carcinoid tumors do not show ganglion-like cells. Schwann-like cells are not seen in jejunoileal carcinoids although they are present in appendiceal carcinoids and paragangliomas (S100-positive sustentacular cells).

Adenocarcinomas secrete mucin, which gangliocytic paragangliomas do not.

References

Burke AP, Helwig EB. Gangliocytic paraganglioma. Am J Clin Pathol 1989;92:1–9.

Hamid QA, Bishop AE, Rode J, et al. Duodenal gangliocytic paragangliomas: a study of 10 cases with immunocytochemical neuroendocrine markers. Hum Pathol 1986;17:1151–1157.

Perrone T, Sibley RK, Rosai J. Duodenal gangliocytic paraganglioma: an immunohistochemical and ultrastructural study and a hypothesis concerning its origin. Am J Surg Pathol 1985;9:31–41.

Reed RJ, Daroca PJ, Harkin JC. Gangliocytic paraganglioma. Am J Surg Pathol 1977;1:207–216.

Scheithauer BW, Nora FE, Lechago J, et al. Duodenal gangliocytic paraganglioma: clinicopathologic and immunocytochemical study of 11 cases. Am J Clin Pathol 1986;86:559–565.

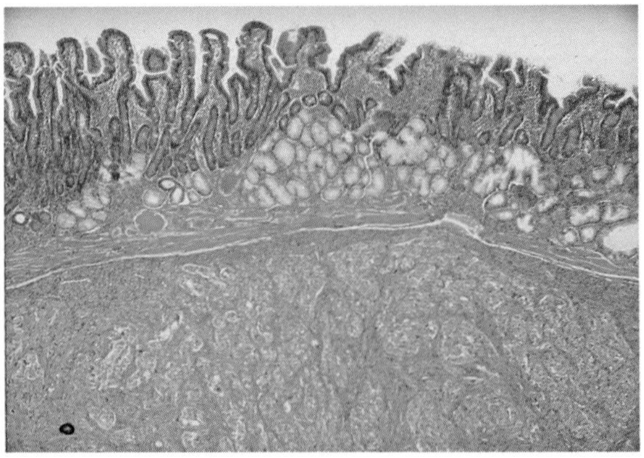

Figure 3–104. Gangliocytic paraganglioma of duodenum. Low-power view shows the tumor in the submucosa.

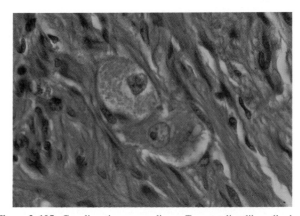

Figure 3–105. Gangliocytic paraganglioma. Two ganglion-like cells show abundant cytoplasm and large open nuclei.

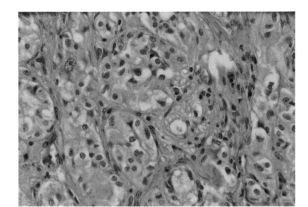

Figure 3–106. Gangliocytic paraganglioma. Carcinoid-like epithelial elements form nests and trabeculae separated by spindle cells.

ADENOMAS OF SMALL BOWEL

Biology of Disease

- *Adenomas* are benign neoplasms of mucosal crypts that may occur throughout the small bowel.
- They may complicate familial polyposis coli, Crohn's disease, and Peutz-Jeghers syndrome.
- Most adenocarcinomas appear to arise in adenomas.

Clinical Findings

- Adenomas may manifest as bleeding, anemia, obstruction, or intussusception. Jejunal and ileal tumors manifest only if they are large and symptomatic; they are then surgically excised.
- Duodenal periampullary adenomas may be troublesome in practice. Large adenomas have an invasive component in upwards of 15% of cases but these elements may not be present on biopsy. Some tumors are resectable by duodenotomy without pancreatectomy. Tumors may be removed piecemeal through the endoscope or pancreatico-duodenectomy may be performed, depending on the individual clinical circumstances.

Gross Pathology

- Adenomas vary in size from barely visible to 10 cm or more. They may be flat, sessile, or pedunculated. They tend to be paler than the surrounding mucosa.

Microscopic Pathology

- Like their counterparts in colon, small bowel adenomas may be tubular, villous, or tubulovillous. They may be of

low-grade or high-grade dysplasia (see discussion of adenomas in Chapter 4), and dysplasia is an essential diagnostic feature.

References

Blackman E, Nash SV. Diagnosis of duodenal and ampullary epithelial neoplasms by endoscopic biopsy: a clinical, pathologic and immunohistochemical study. Hum Pathol 1985;16:901–910.

Van Stolk BJ, Sivak MV, Petrini JL, et al. Endoscopic management of gastrointestinal polyps and periampullary lesions in familial adenomatous polyposis and Gardner's syndrome. Endoscopy 1987;19:19–22.

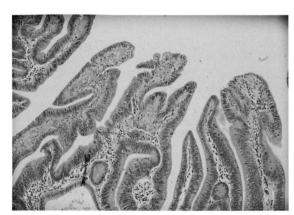

Figure 3–107. Adenoma of duodenum. Higher-magnification shows several adenomatous villi lined by hyperchromatic epithelium.

ADENOCARCINOMA

Biology of Disease

- *Adenocarcinoma* is a malignant tumor of mucosal origin that contains mucin-secreting, absorptive, and sometimes endocrine or Paneth's cells.
- Adenocarcinoma of the small bowel is a rare primary neoplasm. It arises most often in the duodenum.
- Duodenal and periampullary adenocarcinomas are sometimes associated with familial polyposis coli. Duodenal and jejunal adenocarcinomas may complicate celiac disease, and ileal adenocarcinomas may complicate Crohn's disease. An increased risk of adenocarcinoma is reported in Peutz-Jeghers syndrome as well.
- Prognosis relates to depth of invasion and presence or absence of metastatic spread.

Clinical Findings

- Adenocarcinomas present with iron deficiency anemia, biliary obstruction, small bowel obstruction, weight loss, and sometimes a palpable abdominal mass.

Gross Pathology

- Adenocarcinoma is usually an ulcerating tumor that invades the bowel wall. The tumor margins are typically raised and rolled, but polypoid or combined polypoid and ulcerating variants are seen. Exophytic growth usually implies a well-differentiated component of the tumor or residual benign adenoma.

Microscopic Pathology

- Severely dysplastic glands or epithelium is present in a desmoplastic stroma and invades the bowel wall.
- The cells display oval or rounded nuclei, clumped chromatin, clearing of the nucleoplasm, chromatin condensation around the nuclear membrane, and nuclear pleomorphism. Nucleoli may be large or irregular.
- Mucin secretion varies from minimal to abundant. Mucin lakes may result from distention of individual glands or from secretion by the glands into the stroma. Signet-ring primary small bowel adenocarcinomas are rare.
- An endocrine cell component is common in these tumors.
- Residual adenoma or dysplasia establishes that the tumor is primary rather than secondary. Invasion to various depths of the muscle coat is usual. If tumor reaches the peritoneal surface, there is a high risk of intraperitoneal recurrence or transcoelomic spread.
- Lymph node metastases are commonly present, and blood-borne spread to the liver occurs in some cases.

Special Diagnostic Techniques

- Barium swallow may show an apple core lesion, duodenoscopy may allow direct vision and biopsy of a tu-

mor, and ultrasonography or CT scan may show bile duct dilatation.

Differential Diagnosis

Adenoma, carcinoid, metastasis from other primary tumor.
Adenoma shows no desmoplasia or invasion.
Carcinoids are devoid of mucin and show a characteristic morphology.
Metastases show no residual adenoma or carcinoma in situ and usually invade from the outside. Known primary tumors elsewhere are usually present.

References

Barclay THC, Schapira DV. Malignant tumors of the small intestine. Cancer 1983;51:878–881.

Bridge MF, Perzin KH. Primary adenocarcinoma of the jejunum and ileum: a clinicopathologic study. Cancer 1975;36:1876–1887.

Iwafuchi M, Watanabe H, Ishihara N, et al. Neoplastic endocrine cells in carcinomas of the small intestine: histochemical and immunohistochemical studies of 24 tumors. Hum Pathol 1987;18:185–194.

Laws HL, Han SY, Aldrete JS. Malignant tumors of the small bowel. South Med J 1984;77:1087–1090.

Lien G-S, Mori M, Enjoji M. Primary carcinoma of the small intestine. A clinicopathologic and immunohistochemical study. Cancer 1988;61:316–323.

Lundqvist M, Wilander E. Exocrine and endocrine cell differentiation in small intestinal adenocarcinomas. Acta Path Microbiol Immunol Scand (A) 1983;91:469–474.

Williamson RCN, Welch C, Malt RA. Adenocarcinoma and lymphoma of the small intestine: distribution and etiologic associations. Ann Surg 1983;197:172–178.

Wilson JM, Melvin DB, Gray GF, Thorbjarnason B. Primary malignancies of the small bowel: a report of 96 cases and review of the literature. Ann Surg 1974;180:175–179.

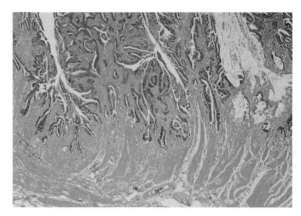

Figure 3–108. Primary adenocarcinoma of the small intestine. Adenocarcinomatous glands infiltrate the muscularis propria.

TUMORS OF AMPULLA OF VATER

Biology of Disease

■ *Periampullary tumors* are tumors arising from the duodenal mucosa around the ampulla, from the ampulla itself, from the common bile duct, or from the main pancreatic duct.

■ Adenomas and adenocarcinomas are the most common tumors. Both may be associated with familial adenomatous polyposis. Carcinomas confined within the muscle of Oddi carry an excellent prognosis, whereas tumors extension beyond the muscle coat lowers the 5-year survival rate to 25%.

■ Benign tumors of the ampulla include granular cell myoblastoma, neurofibroma, leiomyoma, hemangioma, adenomyoma, and hamartoma.

■ Rarely, carcinoid tumors or small cell carcinomas of the ampulla occur. Ampullary carcinoids and neurofibromas may be associated with von Recklinghausen's disease.

Clinical Findings

■ Jaundice (50%), abdominal pain (72%), weight loss, anemia, and, rarely, pancreatitis are the clinical findings.

Gross Pathology

■ Grossly, ampullary tumors may be polypoid, ulcerating, or infiltrating. Polypoid tumors are usually adenomas, whereas ulcerating and infiltrating tumors are usually carcinomas.

Microscopic Pathology

■ Adenomas may be tubular, villous, or tubulovillous. Severe cytologic dysplasia is characterized by large, open nuclei reaching the surface without maturation. Secondary gland formation is an architectural feature of severe dysplasia.

■ Invasive carcinoma is signified by the combination of invasion and severe dysplasia. Lymphatic invasion may be present. Residual benign adenomas are found in 90% of carcinomas.

■ Biopsy performed within 48 hours of sphincterotomy may show reactive cellular atypia and pseudomalignancy.

Special Diagnostic Techniques

■ Diagnostic investigations used to identify tumors of the ampulla of Vater include endoscopic retrograde cholangiopancreatography, computed tomography, endosonography, fine-needle aspiration cytology, and percutaneous transhepatic cholangiography. Biopsy at endoscopy is the mainstay of diagnosis. Piecemeal removal of tumor may also be attempted.

Differential Diagnosis

The distinction of invasive carcinomas from severely dysplastic adenomas may be difficult, especially because carcinomas arise from adenomas. Superficial biopsies may reveal only an adenoma and miss the more deeply located malignancy. The presence of jaundice favors a diagnosis of malignancy.

References

Baczako K, Buchler M, Beger H-G, et al. Morphogenesis and possible precursor lesions of invasive carcinoma of the papilla of Vater: epithelial dysplasia and adenoma. Hum Pathol 1985;16:305–310.

Blackman E, Nash SV. Diagnosis of duodenal and ampullary epithelial neoplasms by endoscopic biopsy: a clinicopathologic and immunohistological study. Hum Pathol 1985;16:901–910.

Komorowski RA, Beggs BK, Geenan JE, Venu RP. Assessment of ampulla of Vater pathology: an endoscopic approach. Am J Surg Pathol 1991;15:1188–1196.

Seifert E, Schulte F, Stolte M. Adenoma and carcinoma of the duodenum and papilla of Vater: a clinicopathologic study. Am J Gastroenterol 1992;87:37–41.

Yamaguchi K, Enjoji M. Carcinoma of the ampulla of Vater: a clinicopathologic study and pathologic staging of 109 cases of carcinoma and 5 cases of adenomas. Cancer 1981;59:506–515.

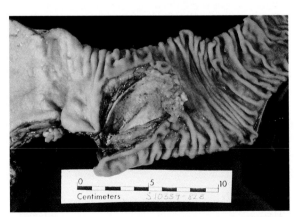

Figure 3–109. Papillary adenoma of the ampulla of Vater with dilated common bile duct.

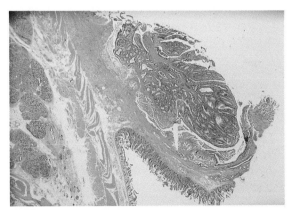

Figure 3–110. Ampulla of Vater. Tubular adenoma.

SECONDARY NEOPLASMS

Biology of Disease

■ Metastatic carcinoma of the small bowel is most often secondary to an intra-abdominal or pelvic primary tumor of the colon, pancreas, ampulla, stomach, ovary, uterus, or kidney.

■ Extra-abdominal primary tumors associated with small bowel metastasis include breast and lung carcinomas, and melanoma.

Clinical Findings

■ Metastases to the small bowel most often manifest as obstruction. Perforation or hemorrhage may also occur. More often, metastases are incidental findings at surgery or autopsy.

Gross Pathology

■ Direct invasion from the colon, stomach, pancreas, or other organ may be obvious at surgery. Alternatively, a primary tumor may have been diagnosed previously, and the metastases may be multiple, with predominantly serosal involvement. Direct growth in continuity from the colon or stomach to the small bowel may produce a malignant fistula.

■ Metastases may produce numerous small serosal nodules or plaques and also stud the omentum, mesentery, and peritoneum. A common appearance is an elevated, mucosal plaque that shows targetoid central ulceration but predominantly submucosal growth.

Microscopic Pathology

■ Secondary carcinomas may not involve the mucosa and always lack a component of adenoma or carcinoma in situ at the margin of the tumor.

■ Secondary lobular carcinoma of the breast often shows a pattern like linitis plastica and may include signet-ring cells. These tumor cells contain intracytoplasmic lumina, which may show a rim of alcian blue positivity and a PAS-positive blob in the lumen.

■ Squamous cell carcinoma is usually secondary to carcinoma of the cervix uteri or of the lung.

■ Clear cell morphology may indicate a renal origin, melanoma or, rarely, hepatocellular carcinoma.

■ Melanomas show positive staining for HMB45, S100, and vimentin.

■ Mucin secretion may indicate primaries in stomach, colon, pancreas, ovary, or breast.

■ Lymphomatous or leukemic deposits in bowel are not uncommon at autopsy.

Special Diagnostic Techniques

■ Positive immunostaining for cytokeratin indicates an epithelial tumor. Vimentin is a mesenchymal marker. HMB45 is a melanoma marker, S100 and neuron-specific enolase are neural markers.

Differential Diagnosis

Primary tumor of colon.

The distinction from primary tumors depends on demonstrating (1) morphology different from that of primary tumors, (2) multiplicity, (3) lack of a preexistent adenoma, (4) distinctive morphology or immunostaining, and (5) existence of a compatible primary neoplasm elsewhere in the body.

Primary anaplastic sarcomatoid carcinoma may be hard to distinguish from metastases.

References

De Castro CA, Dockerty MB, Mayo CW. Metastatic tumors of the small intestines. Surg Gynecol Obstet 1957;105:159–165.

Hansen RM, Lewis JD, Janjan NA, Komorowski RA. Occult carcinoma of the breast masquerading as primary adenocarcinoma of the small intestine. J Clin Gastroenterol 1988;10:213–217.

McNeill PM, Wagman LD, Neifeld JP. Small bowel metastases from primary carcinoma of the lung. Cancer 1987;59:1486–1489.

Robey-Cafferty SS, Silva EG, Cleary KR. Anaplastic and sarcomatoid carcinoma of the small intestine: a clinicopathological study. Hum Pathol 1989;20:858–863.

Sweetenham JW, Whitehouse JM, Williams CJ, Mead GM. Involvement of the gastrointestinal tract by metastases from germ cell tumors of the testis. Cancer 1988;61:2566–2570.

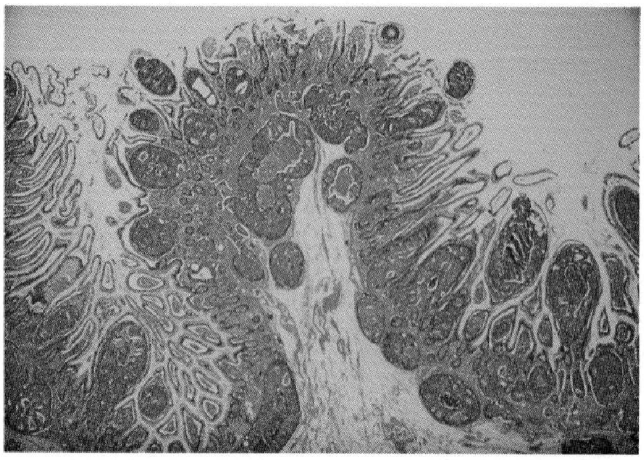

Figure 3–111. Lymphatic spread of cecal adenocarcinoma into the terminal ileum gave a radiologic picture resembling that of Crohn's disease.

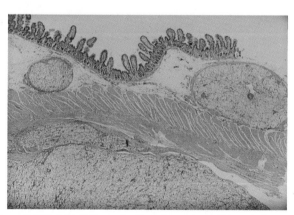

Figure 3–112. Metastatic renal cell carcinoma in small bowel. The tumor has the typical clear cell appearance of renal cell carcinoma.

MALIGNANT MELANOMA

Biology of Disease

■ Malignant melanoma of the bowel is usually metastatic. Primary melanoma of small bowel is exceedingly rare. Melanoma of the anorectum and esophagus is usually primary (see Chapter 6).

Clinical Findings

■ Secondary melanoma may manifest as obstruction, hemorrhage, intussusception, or abdominal mass.

Gross Pathology

■ Metastatic melanomas may be solitary but are usually multiple. They may be visibly pigmented or pale. They are fleshy, well-defined, rounded, nodules that protrude from the serosa or into the lumen. About one third of patients dying from disseminated melanoma have small bowel involvement.

Microscopic Pathology

■ Definitive diagnosis of primary malignant melanoma in any location requires demonstration of in situ melanoma and junctional activity in the mucosa at the margin of the tumor.
■ The predominant cell type may be epithelioid, but spindle cells, clear (balloon) cells, or pleomorphic sarcomatoid cells may be present or prominent.
■ Huge inclusion-like nucleoli are commonly present.

■ Mucin is absent. The Masson-Fontana method stains melanin black. Rare cases are amelanotic.

Special Diagnostic Techniques

■ Immunostains for S100 protein and HMB45 are at least focally positive, and stains for cytokeratins are negative.

Differential Diagnosis

Carcinoma, lymphoma, mesothelioma.
   Carcinomas of poorly differentiated type are generally cytokeratin positive and may include mucin-secreting areas.
   Lymphoma of the rectum should always be confirmed to be of lymphoid origin by leukocyte common antigen and lymphocyte-specific immunostains and also by gene rearrangement studies.
   Primary mesothelioma of peritoneum may involve the small bowel and masquerade as a primary or secondary neoplasm. It may show epithelioid and sarcomatoid areas. It is cytokeratin positive and S100 negative.

References

DeCastro CA, Dockerty MB, Mayo CW. Metastatic tumors of the small intestines. Surg Gynecol Obstet 1957;105:159–165.
Geboes K, de Jaeger E, Rutgeerts P, Vantrappen G. Symptomatic gastrointestinal metastases from malignant melanoma. J Clin Gastroenterol 1988;10:64–70.
Goldman S, Glimelius B, Pahlman L. Anorectal malignant melanoma in Sweden: report of 49 patients. Dis Colon Rectum 1990;33:874–877.
Goodman PL, Karakousis CP. Symptomatic gastrointestinal metastases from malignant melanoma. Cancer 1981;48:1058–1059.
Willbanks OL, Fogelman MJ. Gastrointestinal melanosarcoma. Am J Surg 1970;120:603–606.

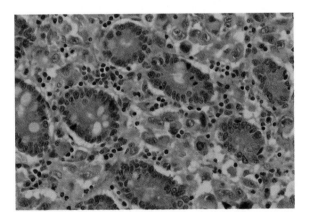

Figure 3–113. Secondary malignant melanoma infiltrating small-bowel mucosa. The melanoma cells are large pleomorphic epithelioid cells.

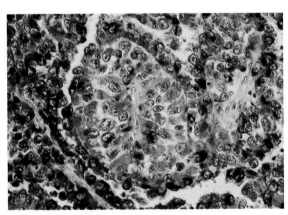

Figure 3–114. Malignant melanoma. Positive immunostaining for HMB45, a melanoma-specific antigen.

VISCERAL NEUROPATHY

Biology of Disease

- Familial visceral neuropathies comprise several rare distinct disease entities that cause chronic primary intestinal pseudo-obstruction.
- One form is recessively inherited and associated with intranuclear neuronal inclusions. Another recessively inherited form is associated with mental retardation and calcification of basal ganglia.
- An autosomal dominant form of visceral neuropathy affecting predominantly the small bowel has been rarely reported.
- Sporadic visceral neuropathies without a clear pattern of inheritance are also described.
- Degenerative or inflammatory acquired visceral neuropathy may also occur. A paraneoplastic form is described with small cell carcinoma of the lung.

Clinical Findings

- Chronic intestinal pseudo-obstruction is a syndrome of abdominal pain and distention with weight loss and sometimes vomiting, steatorrhea, or diarrhea. Colonic pseudo-obstruction is characterized by abdominal pain and distention with constipation.

Gross Pathology

- Bowel dilatation, thinning of the wall, diverticulosis, idiopathic megacolon, and megaduodenum may be manifestations of visceral neuropathy.

Microscopic Pathology

- Neuronal intranuclear inclusion disease displays large, single or double, rounded, eosinophilic intranuclear inclusions in about a third of ganglion cells in the submucosal and myenteric plexuses and also in the brain and spinal cord.
- Decreased numbers of neurons may be seen within the myenteric plexus.
- One form of sporadic visceral neuropathy is characterized by loss of the normal staining within the center of the nerve cells, such that only a rim of cytoplasm remains along the margins.
- In paraneoplastic neuropathy secondary to small cell carcinomas, there may be infiltration of the myenteric plexus with plasma cells and lymphocytes. The submucosal plexus may be spared. Silver stains may show a decrease of both argyrophilic and argyrophobic neurons in all areas of the gastrointestinal tract. Many of the remaining neurons are vacuolated and display cytoplasmic irregularity and a reduced number of processes; a few normal neurons remain. Swelling, fragmentation, and dropout of axons and glial cell proliferation occur secondarily. This condition may be autoimmune and due to cross-reactive lymphocytes elicited by tumor neoantigens.

- Idiopathic visceral neuropathy with inflammatory cell infiltration and axonal degeneration, similar to findings in the paraneoplastic form, are rarely seen. One case was reported with progressive brain-stem dysfunction.

Special Diagnostic Techniques

- Smith's technique involves fixing the opened bowel flat. Blocks are embedded with the serosal surface on the face and sectioned at 50 μm until a section is reached that includes the plane of the plexus. Sections are stained with silver, which impregnates neurons and axons.
- Silver stains show patchy abnormalities—swelling, fragmentation, and dropout of argyrophilic and argyrophobic neurons; fragmentation and loss of axons and proliferation of glial cells.

Differential Diagnosis

Chagas's disease, cytomegalovirus infection of neurons.

Chagas's disease due to *Trypanosoma cruzi* is a common condition in South America. *T. cruzi* can infect any part of the alimentary tract, destroying the ganglia and causing megaesophagus or visceral dilatation. The affected part shows smooth muscle thickening and lymphoplasmacytic infiltration of the myenteric plexus. Silver stains show degeneration and loss of argyrophilic and argyrophobic neurons, degeneration of nerve fibers, and only an occasional remnant of an axon in some nerve tracts. Glial cell proliferation is not prominent. (The predominant neural destruction is curious, because *T. cruzi* colonizes muscle cells, not nerve cells.)

Cytomegalovirus has rarely been reported to infect the myenteric plexus and is diagnosed on finding the characteristic inclusions. Degeneration of neurons and inflammatory cell infiltration also occur.

References

Chinn JS, Schuffler MD. Paraneoplastic visceral neuropathy as a cause of severe gastrointestinal motor dysfunction. Gastroenterology 1988;95:1279–1286.

Howard ER, Garrett JR, Kidd A. Constipation and congenital disorders of the myenteric plexus. J Roy Soc Med 1984; 77(suppl 3):13–19.

Krishnamurthy S, Schuffler MD, Belic L, Schweid AI. An inflammatory axonopathy of the myenteric plexus producing a rapidly progressive intestinal pseudoobstruction. Gastroenterology 1986;90:754–758.

Schuffler MD, Baird HW, Fleming CR, et al. Intestinal pseudoobstruction as the presenting manifestation of small-cell carcinoma of the lung: a paraneoplastic neuropathy of the gastrointestinal tract. Ann Intern Med 1983;98:129–133.

Schuffler MD, Bird TD, Sumi SM, Cook A. A familial neuronal disease presenting as intestinal pseudoobstruction. Gastroenterology 1978;75:889–898.

Schuffler MD, Jonas Z. Chronic idiopathic intestinal pseudo-obstruction caused by a degenerative disorder of the myenteric plexus: the use of Smith's method to define the neuropathology. Gastroenterology 1982;82:476–886.

Schuffler MD, Leon SH, Krishnamurthy S. Intestinal pseudoobstruction caused by a new form of visceral neuropathy: palliation by radical small bowel resection. Gastroenterology 1985;89:1152–1156.

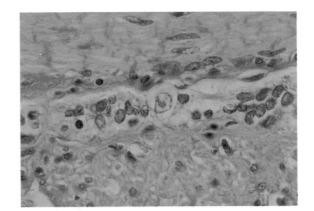

Figure 3–115. Neuronal inclusion body disease. An eosinophilic inclusion body is present in the ganglion cell in the central field.

VISCERAL MYOPATHY

Biology of Disease

■ The *visceral myopathies* are disorders of visceral smooth muscle that cause pseudo-obstruction, bowel dilatation, and muscle coat atrophy. They may be either familial or acquired.

■ Scleroderma or systemic sclerosis is the most common acquired cause of muscle coat atrophy with pseudo-obstruction. The surviving muscle fibers are usually not vacuolated or degenerate as they are in primary visceral myopathy.

■ Visceral myopathy may also occur in myotonic dystrophy, progressive muscular dystrophy, amyloidosis, and diffuse lymphoid infiltration.

Clinical Findings

■ The patient with familial visceral myopathy presents usually with symptoms of intestinal pseudo-obstruction.

Gross Pathology

■ As in visceral neuropathy, the typical case shows dilatation of the bowel, thinning of the muscle coat, wide-mouthed diverticula, and intact mucosa.

Microscopic Pathology

■ Histologically, there is degeneration, atrophy, and fibrous replacement of one or both layers of the muscle coat and sometimes of the muscularis mucosae.

■ Smooth muscle cells may have poorly staining cytoplasm and indistinct cell margins, producing a smudged appearance. Muscle cell degeneration gives a vacuolated appearance.

■ Collagen deposition follows cell dropout, giving a distinctive honeycomb pattern. Occasionally, histologic distinction from systemic sclerosis may not be possible.

Special Diagnostic Techniques

■ Ultrastructural and immunocytochemical studies may aid in defining specific abnormalities in these disorders.

Differential Diagnosis

Visceral neuropathy.
    Visceral neuropathy is signified by abnormalities of the myenteric or submucosal plexus.

References

Alstead EM, Murphy MN, Flanagan AM, et al. Familial autonomic visceral myopathy with degeneration of muscularis mucosae. J Clin Pathol 1988;41:424–429.

Anuras S, Mitros FA, Milano A, et al. A familial visceral myopathy with dilatation of the entire gastrointestinal tract. Gastroenterology 1986;90:385–390.

Jayachandar J, Frank JL, Jonas MM. Isolated intestinal myopathy resembling progressive systemic sclerosis in a child. Gastroenterology 1988;95:1114–1118.

Leon SH, Schuffler MD, Kettler M, Rohrmann CA. Chronic intestinal pseudoobstruction as a complication of Duchenne's muscular dystrophy. Gastroenterology 1986;90:455–459.

Mitros FA, Schuffler MD, Teja K, Anuras S. Pathologic features of familial visceral myopathy. Hum Pathol 1982;13:825–833.

Schuffler MD, Beegle RD. Progressive systemic sclerosis of the gastrointestinal tract and hereditary hollow visceral myopathy: two distinguishable disorders of gastrointestinal smooth muscle. Gastroenterology 1979;77:664–671.

Schuffler MD, Pagon RA, Schwartz R, Bill AH. Visceral myopathy of the gastrointestinal and genitourinary tracts in infants. Gastroenterology 1988;94:892–898.

Smith JA, Hauser SC, Madara JL. Hollow visceral myopathy: a light- and electron-microscopic study. Am J Surg Pathol 1982;6:269–275.

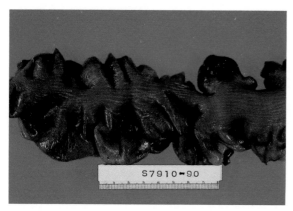

Figure 3–116. Chronic intestinal pseudo-obstruction. The small bowel displays multiple saccular dilatations exempting only the antimesenteric border, which looks somewhat like a taenia coli. The muscularis propria was diffusely atrophied and was preserved only along the antimesenteric border in this specimen.

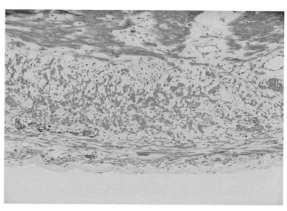

Figure 3–118. Trichrome stain demonstrates smooth muscle vacuolization and intercellular collagen deposition.

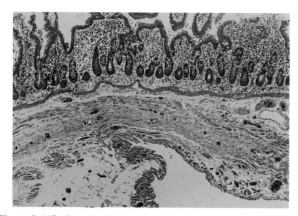

Figure 3–117. Chronic primary intestinal pseudo-obstruction. Trichrome stain demonstrates atrophy of the muscularis propria. The muscularis mucosae is normal.

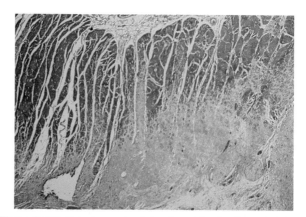

Figure 3–119. Colonic pseudo-obstruction with scleroderma. Trichrome stain demonstrates considerable fibrosis of the muscularis propria.

CHAPTER ■ 4

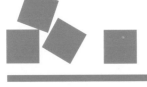

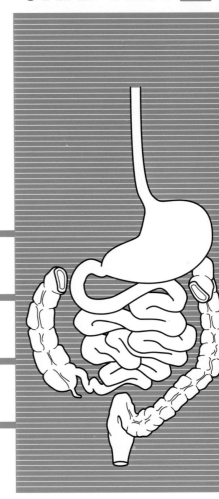

DISEASES OF THE
APPENDIX

ACUTE APPENDICITIS

Biology of Disease

- The peak age incidence is 10 to 25 years, but no age group, even the very young or very old, is exempt.
- The etiology is not clear. A "westernized" diet has been implicated, including a reduction in dietary fiber.
- The pathogenesis appears to involve a two-stage reaction, with initial mucosal damage followed by a bacterial infection that spreads from the mucosa through the appendix wall.
- The cause of the initial mucosal damage is uncertain, but luminal obstruction has been implicated. Obstruction may be due to the presence of a fecalith, fragments of undigested food, or lymphoid hyperplasia of the mucosa.
- Infection usually results from a mixed intestinal flora and is clearly responsible for the suppurative reaction seen microscopically.

Clinical Features

- Symptoms usually commence with pain in the periumbilical region, which later spreads to the left iliac fossa. This change in location is thought to coincide with the development of localized peritonitis.
- On examination, there is guarding and rigidity, which is initially located in the left iliac fossa but this may spread if peritoneal inflammation becomes generalized.
- Complications, generally secondary to appendix rupture, include local abscess formation, diffuse peritonitis, and septicemia.

Gross Pathology

- In the early stages, when inflammation is localized to the mucosa and submucosa, the appendix may appear normal.

- Once the muscularis propria is involved, the appendix becomes swollen and plum colored.
- With serosal involvement, the peritoneum becomes dull gray. Later, a purulent exudate forms on the surface.
- Ultimately, there is perforation secondary to necrosis of the wall (gangrenous appendicitis).

Microscopic Pathology

- The initial lesion is a mucosal erosion with exudation of neutrophils and formation of crypt abscesses.
- Crypt abscesses burst into the lamina propria, and pus enters the appendiceal lumen.
- With disease progression, pus spreads through the muscularis propria, resulting in perforation.
- Resolved acute appendicitis may show extensive fibrosis of the wall and even a fibrous obliteration of the lumen.

Differential Diagnosis

Perioperative serosal inflammation, peritonitis secondary to rupture of another abdominal viscus.

Operative manipulation of the serosa of the appendix can result in vascular dilatation and congestion with exudation of neutrophils. The neutrophils rarely form a layer more than one or two cells thick, and there is no corresponding inflammation in the wall of the appendix.

The appendiceal serosa may occasionally be involved by pus spreading from another site. In this case, the layer of pus is generally thick and is not accompanied by marked vascular dilatation. The wall of the appendix is not inflamed.

References

Butler C. Surgical pathology of acute appendicitis. Hum Pathol 1981;12:870–878.

Cheng AR. An analysis of the pathology of 3,003 appendices. Aust NZ J Surg 1981;61:169–178.

Seal A. Appendicitis: a historical review. Can J Surg 1981;24:427–433.

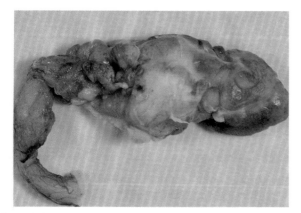

Figure 4–1. Acute appendicitis showing serosal congestion and purulent exudate.

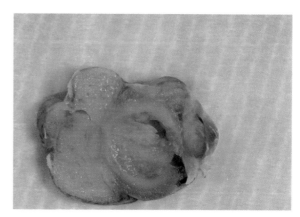

Figure 4–2. Perforation of appendix.

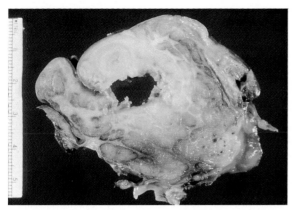

Figure 4–3. Appendix abscess. Pus has drained from the abscess cavity.

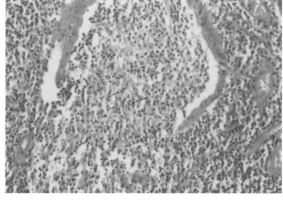

Figure 4–5. Crypt abscess with rupture into the lamina propria.

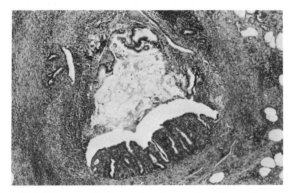

Figure 4–4. Transmural inflammation of appendix and extensive mucosal ulceration.

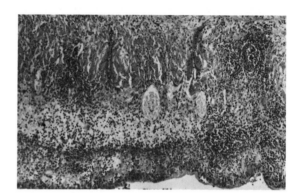

Figure 4–6. Acute serosal inflammation with edema and neutrophil exudation.

HYPERPLASTIC POLYP

Biology of Disease

- Two thirds of cases occur in women.
- Hyperplastic polyps have no neoplastic potential and are not associated with disease in the rest of the colon.

Clinical Features

- The lesion is usually diagnosed coincidentally during appendectomy for another indication.

Gross Pathology

- In many cases, there are no gross abnormalities.
- A mucocele (a dilated appendix filled with mucus) may be present.

Microscopic Pathology

- The histologic appearance is basically similar to that of a hyperplastic polyp elsewhere in the large bowel.
- Polyps may appear as flattened, button-shaped lesions.
- Hyperplastic changes may be widespread and replace the entire mucosa of the appendix. This pattern is often associated with mucocele formation. The mucosa may become flattened rather than polypoid.
- The mucosa has a characteristic serrated growth pattern.
- The cells may contain cytoplasmic mucus, but goblet cells are less common than in normal mucosa.
- The nuclei are normal, and stratification is usually not prominent.
- Mitoses are present only at the base of the crypts.

Differential Diagnosis

Well-differentiated adenoma, including cystadenoma.

Adenomas are characterized by nuclear stratification, hyperchromasia, and dysplasia.

Lesions that appear to be combined hyperplastic polyps and adenomas are probably best regarded as exceedingly well-differentiated adenomas with maturation.

References

Appelman HD. Epithelial neoplasia of the appendix. In: Pathology of the Colon, Small Intestine and Anus, ed 2. Norris ET (ed). New York; Churchill-Livingstone; 1991:263–303.

Qizilbash AH. Hyperplastic (metaplastic) polyps of the appendix. Arch Pathol 1974;97:385–388.

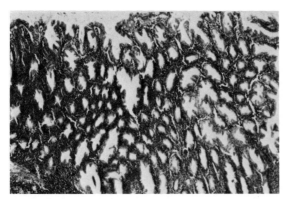

Figure 4–7. Hyperplastic polyp showing typical serrated growth pattern.

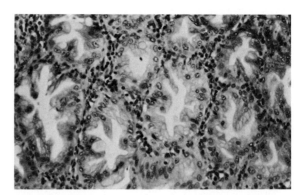

Figure 4–8. High-power view of mucosa showing absence of dysplasia.

ADENOMA

Biology of Disease

- Three major types are identified: tubular, villous, and cystadenoma. These are frequently mixed and have overlapping features.
- Tubular adenomas are rare but may be found in individuals with familial adenomatosis coli.
- Villous and cystadenomas are usually sporadic lesions, often producing a mucocele (a dilated appendix filled with mucin).
- The term *pseudomyxoma peritonei* indicates the presence of mucus in the peritoneal cavity. This may originate from any intra-abdominal organ that contains mucus-secreting epithelium. When it follows appendiceal disease, pseudomyxoma peritonei is in most cases the result of spread of an adenocarcinoma or, rarely, an adenoma. Neoplastic epithelium grows on the peritoneal surface, where it resembles and behaves like a mucinous borderline tumor of the ovary.

Clinical Features

- Adenomas are most common in women in the fifth or sixth decade of life.
- Symptomatology tends to be vague but is suggestive of mild appendicitis.
- There is an association between adenoma of the appendix and ovarian mucinous neoplasms.

Gross Pathology

- When a villous adenoma is present, the mucosal fronds may be visible on the cut surface.
- In mucoceles, the wall of the appendix is attenuated, and the dilated lumen is filled with mucus that may be solid or exceedingly viscous.

Microscopic Pathology

- The majority of mucoceles are the result of an exceedingly well-differentiated adenoma. The features of ade-

nomatous growth (nuclear stratification, hyperchromasia, and dysplasia) are best seen at the bases of the crypts. Epithelium covering the fronds may be exceedingly well differentiated and resemble a hyperplastic polyp.
- Mucoceles are usually unilocular. Large mucoceles may have very attenuated mucosa or even be ulcerated. In these instances, it is difficult to determine the basic cause of the lesion.
- A large mucocele often has an attenuated wall with fibrotic obliteration of the muscularis propria.
- Low-grade villous adenomas may produce mucoceles. Higher grade tumors may have cytoplasm that is only sparsely mucus secreting, and the tumor may resemble villous adenomas of the remainder of the large bowel.

Differential Diagnosis

Hyperplastic polyp, adenocarcinoma.

By definition, adenocarcinomas invade the underlying stroma and adenomas do not. A similar criterion may be applied to serosal deposits of these neoplasms.

Adenomatous glands are usually rounded and do not have a cribriform pattern. Carcinomatous glands may have an irregular outline and contain irregularly piled up epithelium.

Adenomas are accompanied by normal lamina propria. Carcinomas either have no stroma or fibrotic stroma.

Hyperplastic polyps are characterized by an absence of nuclear stratification, hyperchromasia, and dysplasia. Adenomas of the appendix may be well differentiated with superficial crypts having a serrated appearance.

References

Hiega E, Rosai J, Pizzimbono CA, Wise L. Mucosal hyperplasia, mucinous cystadenoma and mucinous cystadenocarcinoma of the appendix. Cancer 1973;32:1525–1541.

Gibbs NM. Mucinous cystadenoma and cystadenocarcinoma of the vermiform appendix with particular reference to mucocele and pseudomyxoma peritonei. J Clin Pathol 1973;26:413–421.

Wolff M, Ahmed N. Epithelial neoplasms of the vermiform appendix (exclusive of carcinoid). II. Cystadenomas, papillary adenomas and adenomatous polyps of the appendix. Cancer 1976;37:2511–2522.

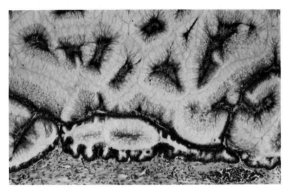

Figure 4–9. Villous adenoma of appendix.

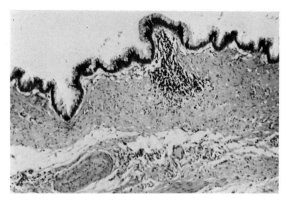

Figure 4–11. Cystadenoma of appendix.

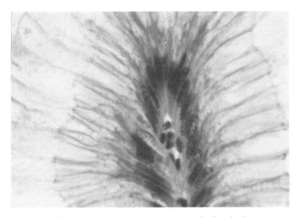

Figure 4–10. Villous adenoma showing low-grade dysplasia.

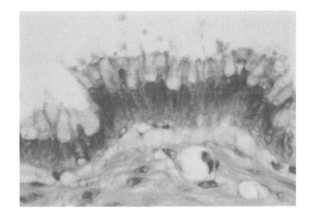

Figure 4–12. Lining epithelium of a cystadenoma.

ADENOCARCINOMA

Biology of Disease

■ It is generally accepted that most carcinomas develop in preexistent adenomas (the adenoma-carcinoma sequence).
■ Carcinomas are most likely to arise in large villous adenomas.
■ Carcinomas may or may not be accompanied by mucocele formation.
■ The 5-year survival rate is in the range of 50 to 65%.

Clinical Features

■ Adenocarcinoma is slightly more common in males than in females.
■ The peak incidence is in the fifth to seventh decades of life, with a median age at presentation of 60 years.
■ Symptoms include pain similar to that of appendicitis, a palpable mass, and bowel obstruction secondary to metastases.
■ In one quarter of cases, the carcinoma is found in an incidentally removed appendix.

Gross Pathology

■ Early lesions present only with a thickened appendiceal wall.
■ In the late stages, there is a mass of necrotic tumor and inflammation.
■ In advanced disease, the original appendix may be totally destroyed.
■ In early cases, when some residual appendix is present, the disease involves the proximal appendiceal segment in 45% of cases.
■ Twenty-five percent of cases are cystadenocarcinomas that are grossly identical with other types of mucocele.

Microscopic Pathology

■ Invasion through the muscularis mucosae is the main criterion for diagnosis.
■ As the tumor penetrates the appendiceal wall, it tends to produce large mucin-filled cysts.
■ When the tumor reaches the serosa, a large quantity of free extracellular mucin may be produced (pseudomyxoma peritonei).

- These tumors may resemble the usual type of large bowel carcinoma, but this is not common.
- Signet ring variants are distinctly unusual.

Differential Diagnosis

Adenoma, adenocarcinoma of cecum, goblet cell carcinoid.

Invasion is the key feature that distinguishes carcinomas from adenomas. Intramucosal carcinomas should be grouped with adenomas for prognostic purposes.

Cecal carcinomas may invade the base of the appendix. This possibility should always be considered when the stump of the appendix is involved by tumor.

Microglandular differentiation suggests the likelihood of a goblet cell carcinoid. A stain for endocrine granules should be performed.

References

Cerame MA. A 25-year review of adenocarcinoma of the appendix. Dis Colon Rectum 1988;31:145.

Ferro M, Anthony PP. Adenocarcinoma of the appendix. Dis Colon Rectum 1985;28:457–459.

Qizilbash AH. Primary adenocarcinoma of the appendix. A clinicopathological study of 11 cases. Arch Pathol 1975;99:556–562.

Wolff M, Ahmed N. Epithelial neoplasms of the appendix (exclusive of carcinoid). I. Adenocarcinoma of the appendix. Cancer 1976;37:2493–2510.

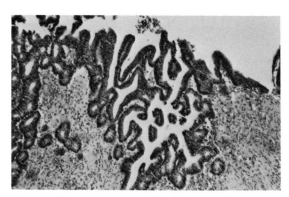

Figure 4–13. Adenocarcinoma infiltrating wall of appendix.

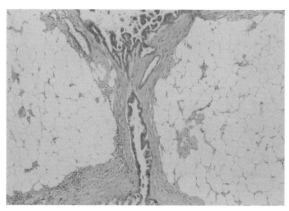

Figure 4–14. Pseudomyxoma peritonei with epithelium growing on the serosal surface.

CARCINOID

Biology of Disease

- Three types of appendiceal carcinoid tumor may be recognized, based on specific histologic and clinical features: insular, tubular, and goblet cell types.
- Goblet cell carcinoids, also referred to as *adenocarcinoids* or *crypt cell carcinoma*, probably arise from an undifferentiated stem cell and have features intermediate between those of an adenocarcinoma and an insular carcinoid.
- Carcinoids are present in 0.5 to 1.0% of all resected appendices.
- Insular and tubular carcinoids are generally benign lesions. Hemicolectomy is reserved for tumors greater than 2 cm in diameter.
- Goblet cell carcinoids have a 5-year survival rate of 80%. Hemicolectomy is recommended for all tumors that penetrate the muscularis propria or that have more than two mitoses per ten high-power fields.

Clinical Features

- The vast majority of carcinoids are discovered incidentally and are asymptomatic.

- Appendiceal carcinoids almost never result in the carcinoid syndrome.

Gross Pathology

- Three quarters of carcinoids are present at the appendiceal tip; the rest are located at the base.
- Many carcinoids are not visible grossly as tumors. Goblet cell carcinoids in particular show only an ill-defined thickening of the wall.
- The vast majority of carcinoids are 1 cm or less in diameter.

Microscopic Pathology

- Insular carcinoids consist of nests or sheets of polygonal cells, often with peripheral palisading. The nuclei are uniform with small central nucleoli and stippled chromatin. Cell borders are poorly defined and the cytoplasm is eosinophilic. Cytoplasmic granularity is sometimes evident.
- Tubular carcinoids are arranged as small, well-organized tubules and trabeculae. The lumens may contain mucus. The cells are cuboidal or columnar, with the nuclei arranged peripherally. These tumors are present in the

wall of the appendix and do not fill up the appendiceal lumen as do insular carcinoids.

■ Goblet cell carcinoids grow mainly in the submucosa, muscularis propria, and subserosa. The mucosa is generally involved only at the base of the crypts. The pattern is of small uniform nests and strands of cells. Lumina may be present but are rare. Most cells are goblet cells containing mucin. Endocrine cells are in the minority, often accounting for as little as 10% of the total. Paneth's cells may be found. Nuclei are crescent shaped and located at the periphery of the nests.

Special Techniques

■ Insular carcinoids stain positively for chromogranin, Fontana-Masson, and Diazo (argentaffin) stains. They stain negatively for carcinoembryonic antigen (CEA) and glucagon.
■ Tubular carcinoids stain strongly for CEA, glucagon, and neuron-specific enolase (NSE). They stain weakly for chromogranin and are typically argentaffin negative.
■ Goblet cell carcinoids react strongly with CEA and contain scattered argentaffin-positive cells.

Differential Diagnosis

Well-differentiated adenocarcinoma with interspersed endocrine cells.

Adenocarcinomas containing small numbers of endocrine cells look and behave like typical adenocarcinomas. They should not be diagnosed as carcinoids.

References

Burke AP, Sobin LH, Federspiel BH, Shekitka KM. Appendiceal carcinoids: correlation of histology and immunohistochemistry. Mod Pathol 1989;2:630–637.

Burke AP, Sobin LH, Federspiel BH, et al. Goblet cell carcinoids and related tumors of the appendix. Am J Clin Pathol 1990;94:27–35.

Isaacson P. Crypt cell carcinoma of the appendix (so-called adenocarcinoid tumor). Am J Surg Pathol 1981;5:213–224.

Moertel CG, Weiland LH, Nagoruney DM, Dockerty MB. Carcinoid tumor of the appendix: treatment and prognosis. N Engl J Med 1987;317:1699–1701.

Subbuswamy SG, Gibbs NM, Ross CF, Morson BC. Goblet cell carcinoid of the appendix. Cancer 1974;34:338–344.

Warkel RL, Cooper PH, Helwig EB. Adenocarcinoid, a mucin-producing carcinoid of the appendix. Cancer 1978;42:2781–2793.

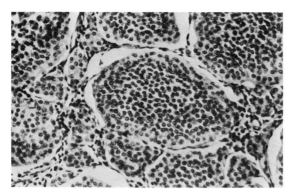

Figure 4–15. Insular carcinoid. Note islands of cells.

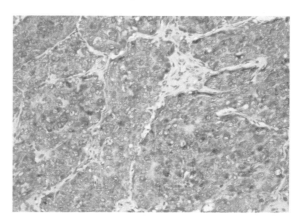

Figure 4–17. Insular carcinoid (chromogranin).

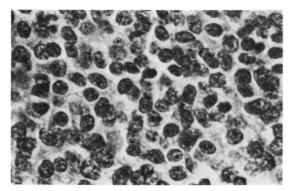

Figure 4–16. Insular carcinoid showing monotonous nuclei with small nucleoli and a stippled chromatin.

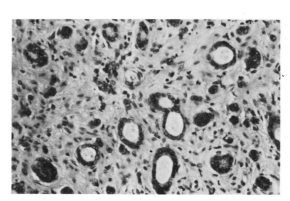

Figure 4–18. Tubular carcinoid.

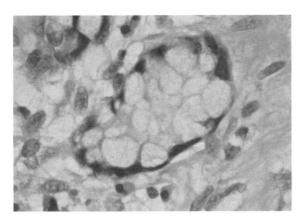

Figure 4–19. Goblet cell carcinoid.

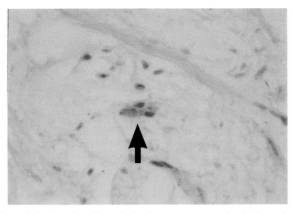

Figure 4–21. Goblet cell carcinoid showing a clump of cells (*arrow*) containing exceedingly sparse endocrine granules (Grimelius).

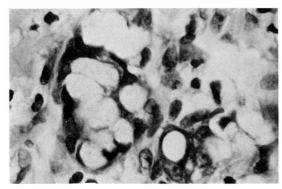

Figure 4–20. Goblet cell carcinoid.

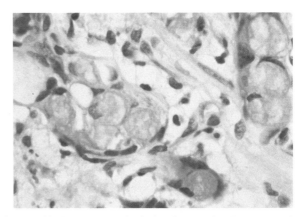

Figure 4–22. Goblet cell carcinoid showing cytoplasmic mucus production (periodic acid–Schiff).

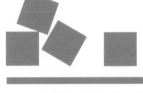

CHAPTER 5

DISEASES OF THE LARGE BOWEL

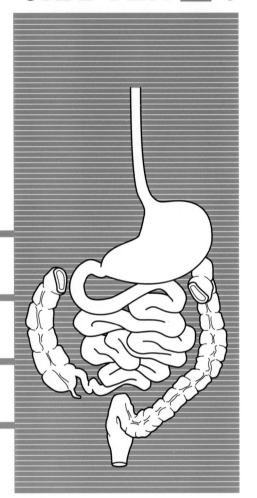

NORMAL LARGE BOWEL

Gross Anatomy

■ The *large bowel* extends from the ileocecal valve to the anus and is normally about 140 cm long in the adult. The *cecum* is the part that lies below an imaginary horizontal line drawn across the bowel at the level of the ileocecal valve. The *ascending colon* extends from this line to the hepatic flexure. The *transverse colon* reaches from the hepatic flexure to the splenic flexure. The *descending colon* stretches from the splenic flexure to the brim of the pelvis. The *sigmoid colon* runs from the pelvic brim to the rectosigmoid junction, which is opposite the promontory of the sacrum. The *rectum*, which is mainly extraperitoneal, reaches from the sacral promontory to the anus (or, by another definition, from the peritoneal reflexion to the anus).

■ The muscle coat has two layers, or coats, an outer longitudinal and an inner circular. The longitudinal coat forms three thickened bands called *teniae coli*. Contraction of the teniae coli gives the colon a sacculated appearance. The teniae are absent from the rectum.

■ The colonic mucosa displays incomplete transverse folds, the *plicae semilunares.*

■ The superior mesenteric artery supplies the ascending colon and the proximal two thirds of the transverse colon via its ileocolic, right colic, and middle colic branches. The left colic branch of the inferior mesenteric artery supplies one third of the transverse colon and the descending colon. Two or three sigmoid branches of the inferior mesenteric artery supply the sigmoid colon. An anastomotic artery, the marginal artery, runs along the medial aspect of the ascending colon, the inferior aspect of the transverse colon, and the medial aspect of the descending and sigmoid colon. This vessel interlinks the ileocolic, right colic, middle colic, left colic, sigmoid, and rectal arteries. Vasa recta extend from the marginal artery to the colonic wall. The superior rectal branch of the inferior mesenteric artery and middle rectal branches from the left and right internal iliac arteries supply the rectum. The lower rectum is supplied by left and right inferior rectal arteries from the internal pudendal arteries. The vasa recta divide at the bowel wall into subserosal arteries, which run circumferentially around the bowel wall, and penetrating arteries, which supply the submucosal and intramuscular plexuses. Veins, lymphatics, and nerves accompany arteries as they penetrate the muscle coat.

■ Lymphatics are present in the mucosal lamina propria only immediately above the muscularis mucosae. The submucosal and intramuscular lymphatic networks drain to a subserosal plexus and thence to mesocolic lymphatics, pericolic or perirectal lymph nodes close to the bowel wall, and then to lymph nodes located close to the major vessels. The upper rectum drains to pararectal nodes and then to preaortic nodes. The 10 cm of rectum above the squamocolumnar junction drains in part to inferior mesenteric nodes, in part to internal iliac lymph nodes, and in part to nodes along the inferior rectal vessels. The anal canal (inferior to the squamocolumnar junction) drains to superficial inguinal nodes.

■ The large bowel receives both parasympathetic and sympathetic nerve fibers. Both types of fiber operate through the ganglia of the myenteric (Auerbach's) or submucosal (Meissner's) plexus.

■ The colon stores feces, absorbs water and electrolytes, and ferments carbohydrate into short-chain fatty acids, which are the main energy source for colonic epithelium. The sigmoid has a sphincterlike action that controls the entry of feces into the rectum. Filling of the rectum initiates the call to stool.

Microscopic Features

■ The mucosa is composed of epithelium, lamina propria, and muscularis mucosae. The epithelium forms straight tubular crypts and has a flat surface. The lamina propria is a loose connective tissue that contains blood vessels, nerves, and immune defense cells. The muscularis mucosae is a thin muscular layer that gives the mucosa structural stability and forms its lower boundary.

■ The surface epithelium and crypts contain absorptive cells and goblet cells anchored to basement membrane. Intraepithelial lymphocytes are normally present in low numbers (about one per six epithelial nuclei). The lower portions of crypts contain endocrine cells, which are signified by their fine subnuclear eosinophilic granules. Paneth's cells are not normally present in colonic crypts. The crypt regenerative zone is in the middle third. A sheath of myofibroblasts surrounds each crypt.

■ *Innominate grooves* are infoldings in the mucosa into which several crypts open. These may give a false impression of branching (fission) of the crypts (which is usually a sign of regeneration).

■ The lamina propria contains plasma cells, lymphocytes, macrophages, eosinophils, and mast cells. The IgA immunoglobulin class of plasma cells predominates. Lymphatic vessels are present immediately above the muscularis mucosae but not in the upper half of the mucosa.

■ Lymphoid-glandular complexes are solitary lymphoid follicles located in the mucosa that are randomly scattered throughout the large bowel. The lymphoid follicles often protrude through the muscularis mucosae into the submucosa. They are a component of the mucosa-associated lymphoid tissue (MALT). The overlying epithelium includes specialized membranous enterocytes (M cells).

■ Apoptotic bodies are sometimes present in the surface epithelium but are more often seen in the lamina propria beneath the surface epithelium. Apoptosis may be the normal mode of colonic epithelial cell death (rather than shedding into the lumen). Macrophages in the lamina propria push pseudopodia through the basement membrane and engulf apoptotic bodies.

■ The submucosa is a loose connective tissue containing blood vessels and nerves. The muscle coat and myenteric plexus are similar to those in small bowel, except that the longitudinal coat is thickened into teniae coli.

References

Langman JM, Rowland R. Density of lymphoid follicles in the rectum and at the anorectal junction. J Clin Gastroenterol 1992;14:81–84.

Levine DS, Haggitt RC. Colon. In: Sternberg SS (ed). Histology for Pathologists: New York: Raven Press, 1992;573–591.

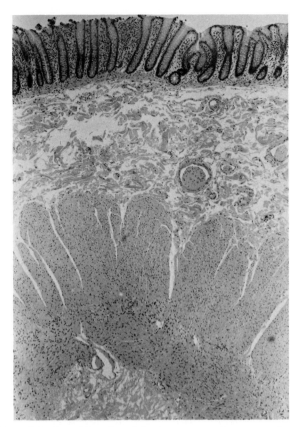

Figure 5–1. Normal large bowel showing mucosa, submucosa, and muscle coat.

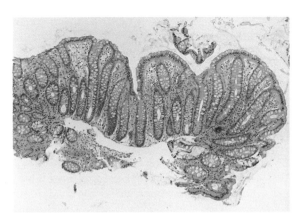

Figure 5–2. Normal colonic mucosa showing vertical crypts, columnar surface epithelium, goblet cells, and absorptive cells. In the center of the field is an innominate groove.

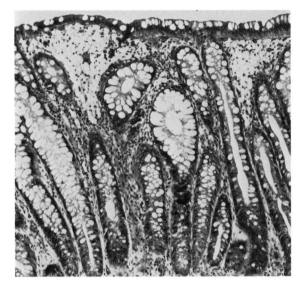

Figure 5–3. Normal colonic mucosa. Note the foamy macrophages in the lamina propria.

HIRSCHSPRUNG'S DISEASE

Biology of Disease

■ *Hirschsprung's disease* is named after its discoverer, Harald Hirschsprung (1830–1916), who was Professor of Pediatrics at the University of Copenhagen and Queen Louise Children's Hospital. This disorder is a congenital absence of autonomic ganglion cells from the rectum. The aganglionic segment is spastically contracted, fails to relax appropriately, and causes obstruction. The aganglionic segment is short and extends only to the sigmoid colon in 90% of patients. Ten percent of patients have long-segment disease.

■ Long-segment disease involves a variable length of the colon in continuity with the rectum; in the extreme, there is total colonic aganglionosis and even aganglionosis of the ileum.

■ Hirschsprung's disease affects boys more than girls in a ratio of 4:1. The male-to-female ratio is even greater among those with long-segment disease, being 28:1.

■ Hirschsprung's disease affects 1 in 5,000 livebirths. Incidence rises to 2.6% in low-birth-weight infants. Ten percent of all cases occur in Down's syndrome. Another 5% are associated with various congenital abnormalities. Siblings of index cases have an incidence of 7.2%, indicating a role for hereditary factors.

■ In the developing embryo, neuroblasts migrate cranio-caudally, reaching the rectum by 12 weeks. Arrest in migration must occur around this time.

Clinical Features

■ The infant fails to pass meconium and develops a distended abdomen and persistent vomiting within 2 to 3 days of birth. Digital examination is followed by a gush of meconium and abdominal decompression.

■ In some infants, the colon remains completely obstructed, whereas others display incomplete or recurrent obstruction. Ultimately, if the obstruction is untreated, obstructive enterocolitis or pseudomembranous colitis may develop.

■ Older infants and children may present with short-segment disease, characterized by persistent abdominal distention, fecal impaction, and constipation.

■ Barium enema displays a characteristic narrow rectal segment and dilated proximal colon.

Gross Pathology

■ The distal aganglionic segment is contracted, whereas the proximal ganglionated bowel is distended. The entire affected colon is narrow in long-segment disease.

■ Occasionally, the dilated bowel shows pseudomembranous colitis or nonspecific ulceration.

Microscopic Pathology

■ The diseased segment displays absence of ganglion cells from both submucosal and myenteric nerve plexuses. The nerve bundles in Auerbach's (myenteric) plexus are thickened.

■ There may be hypoganglionosis in the junctional area between the normal bowel and the aganglionic segment.

■ Diagnosis is made by rectal biopsy, using either a suction biopsy device or a biopsy forceps to include submucosa. Serial sections are examined, and the combination of absence of ganglion cells with increased number and size of nerve trunks establishes the diagnosis. The latter feature is consistently present in short-segment and long-segment disease but not always in total colonic aganglionosis.

Special Diagnostic Techniques

■ The biopsy specimen should be taken 2 to 3 cm above the pectinate line. An optimal specimen should include as much submucosa as mucosa. The specimen should be oriented and pinned for optimal fixation. Serial sections are cut and stained with H&E. Frozen sections may be used to determine the length of affected bowel at definitive surgery.

■ Immunoperoxidase staining of paraffin sections for neuron-specific enolase may help identify ganglia.

■ Immunostaining for S100 protein or phosphorylated neurofilament protein may demonstrate increased mucosal nerve fibers.

■ Acetylcholinesterase histochemistry on frozen sections displays increased nerve fibers in and around the muscularis mucosa.

Differential Diagnosis

Cystic fibrosis, hypothyroidism, intestinal atresia, imperforate anus, pseudo-obstruction, hypoganglionosis, zonal aganglionosis, intestinal neuronal dysplasia.

In the neonate, the differential diagnosis of constipation and colonic dilatation includes cystic fibrosis (meconium plug syndrome), hypothyroidism, intestinal atresia, small left colon syndrome (transient functional intestinal obstruction associated with maternal diabetes or use of drugs that inhibit peristalsis), and imperforate anus.

In older children or adults, and rarely in infants, intestinal pseudo-obstruction is the main differential diagnostic consideration. Rarely, visceral myopathy may mimic Hirschsprung's disease—the rectum being narrow and the colon dilated.

Hypoganglionosis is defined as the presence of only rare ganglion cells. A full-thickness biopsy is usually necessary to make the diagnosis.

Zonal aganglionosis or *skip-segment Hirschsprung's disease* is a rare condition in which a normal area of colon is interposed between aganglionic or hypoganglionic segments.

Intestinal neuronal dysplasia is a rare condition characterized by three features: (1) hyperplasia of the submucosal and myenteric plexuses with giant ganglia, (2) isolated heterotopic ganglion cells in the lamina propria and muscularis mucosae, and (3) increased acetylcholinesterase activity in the parasympathetic fibers of the lamina propria and circular muscle. Intestinal neuronal dysplasia is associated with three syndromes—multiple endocrine neoplasia type 2B, neurofibromatosis, and Hirschsprung's disease.

References

Blisard KS, Kleinman R. Hirschsprung's disease: clinical and pathological overview. Hum Pathol 1986;17:1189–1191.

Case records of the Massachusetts General Hospital. Case 52-1991. N Engl J Med 1991;325:1865–1873.

Gryboski JD. Hirschsprung's disease. In Kirsner JB, Shorter RG (eds). Diseases of the Colon, Rectum and Anal Canal. Baltimore: Williams & Wilkins, 1988;603–610.

Kapula L, Haberkorn S, Nixon HH. Chronic adynamic bowel simulating Hirschsprung's disease. J Pediatr Surg 1975;10:885–892.

Lake BD. Hirschsprung's disease and related disorders. In: Whitehead ER (ed). Gastrointestinal and Esophageal Pathology. New York: Churchill Livingstone, 1989;257–268.

Leon SH, Schuffler MD. Visceral myopathy of the colon mimicking Hirschsprung's disease: diagnosis by deep rectal biopsy. Dig Dis Sci 1986;31:1381–1386.

Yunis E, Sieber WK, Akers DR. Does zonal aganglionosis really exist? Pediatr Pathol 1983;1:33–49.

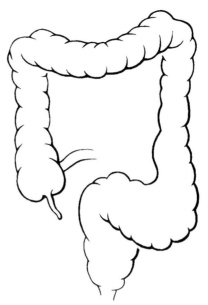

Figure 5–4. Line diagram showing the rectal narrowing and proximal dilatation as seen in Hirschsprung's disease.

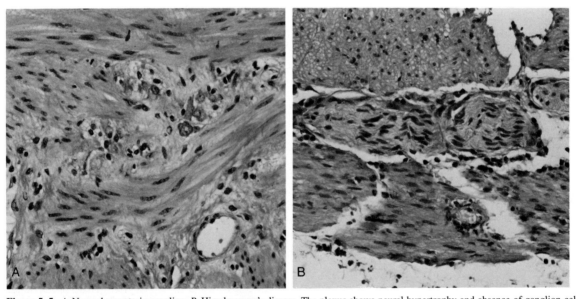

Figure 5–5. *A,* Normal myenteric ganglion. *B,* Hirschsprung's disease. The plexus shows neural hypertrophy and absence of ganglion cells.

CHRONIC GRANULOMATOUS DISEASE OF CHILDHOOD

Biology of Disease

■ Chronic granulomatous disease (CGD) was originally reported as a "syndrome of recurrent infection and infiltration of viscera by pigmented lipid histiocytes" and as "a fatal granulomatosis of childhood." It is now recognized to be a disorder of nicotinamide adenine dinucleotide phosphate (NADPH) oxidase. NADPH oxidase generates superoxide anion and other oxygen radicals that kill bacteria. A number of different molecular defects have been described.

■ The X-linked form of CGD is associated with an absence of cytochrome *b* due to a defect in the gene that encodes one of its subunits. The autosomally inherited forms of the disease are characterized by absence of one of the cytosolic oxidase component proteins.

■ CGD granulocytes can kill non–catalase-producing bacteria with the hydrogen peroxide produced by the bacteria themselves. Patients with CGD are susceptible to bacteria that produce catalase and thereby degrade their own hydrogen peroxide. The bacteria include staphylococci, *Serratia marcescens*, and gram-negative enterococci. Affected patients are also susceptible to *Aspergillus* and other fungi, because neutrophils are the main defense against the mycelial phase of fungi.

Clinical Features

- The respiratory tract bears the brunt of most infections in CGD. Gastrointestinal manifestations are uncommon and usually mimic Crohn's disease. Therefore, CGD must be considered in young patients with granulomatous colitis or enteritis in whom there is a history of recurrent respiratory infections.
- Patients may present in childhood, adolescence, or early adult life with persistent diarrhea, perianal abscesses, and granulomatous colitis mimicking Crohn's disease. Appendicitis followed by enterocutaneous fistula with granulomas and chronic gastric outlet obstruction are also described.
- Rare manifestations include esophageal candidiasis and bowel obstruction secondary to an inflammatory mass.

Gross Pathology

- The mucosa may show patchy friability, cobblestoning, small pseudopolyps, a furrowed pattern, and synechiae.

Microscopic Pathology

- The lamina propria displays an infiltrate of large, pale, foamy histiocytes containing yellow-brown pigment. These are most prominent in the small bowel villi and above the muscularis mucosae in the colon.
- Pigmented lipid histiocytes are also seen in the portal tracts of the liver and in the spleen, lymph nodes, bone marrow, and epicardium.
- Many patients display mucosal granulomas with giant cells. Granulomas may be located in lymphoid follicles or in lamina propria.

Special Diagnostic Techniques

- The nitroblue tetrazolium test performed on neutrophil leukocytes is the simplest method of confirming the diagnosis. Specific genetic testing for known defects can be performed in research laboratories.
- The yellow-brown pigment in the histiocytes is PAS positive after addition of diastase.

References

Ament ME, Hawkes HD. Gastrointestinal manifestations of granulomatous disease. N Engl J Med 1973;288:382–387.

Berendes H, Bridges RA, Good RA. A fatal granulomatosus of childhood: the clinical study of a new syndrome. Minn Med 1957;40:309–312.

Landing BH, Shirkey HS. A syndrome of recurrent infection and infiltration of viscera by pigmented lipid histiocytes. Pediatrics 1957;20:431–438.

Ochs HD, Ament ME, Davis SD. Structure and function of the gastrointestinal tract in primary immunodeficiency syndromes (IDS) and in granulocyte dysfunction. Birth Defects 1975;11:199–207.

Segal AW. Biochemistry and molecular biology of chronic granulomatous disease. J Inherited Metab Dis 1992;15:683–686.

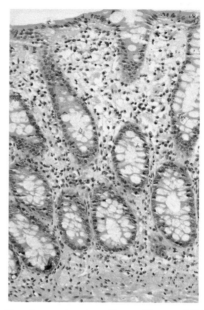

Figure 5–6. Chronic granulomatous disease. Pigmented lipid histiocytes differ from normal histiocytes by being lightly yellowish brown.

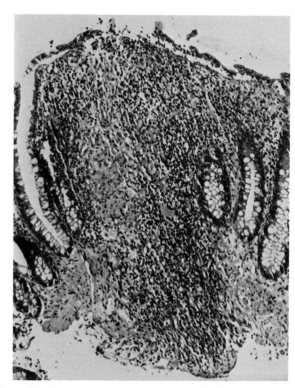

Figure 5–7. Granulomatous colitis in chronic granulomatous disease. An epithelioid granuloma is present within a lymphoid-glandular complex.

LARGE BOWEL VOLVULUS

Biology of Disease

- *Volvulus* is twisting of the bowel around its mesenteric attachment resulting in a combination of obstruction and vascular occlusion. The three main forms of large bowel volvulus are volvulus neonatorum, adult cecal volvulus, and sigmoid volvulus. Volvulus of the transverse colon is rare. In adults, the sigmoid colon is the most common site of volvulus.

- A redundant loop of sigmoid that possesses a narrow mesentery is the main cause of volvulus in high-risk areas (Africa, Eastern Europe, the Middle East). In these parts of the world, sigmoid volvulus accounts for between 30% and 50% of all intestinal obstructions (in contrast with about 5% in the United States). A diet rich in fiber is an important predisposing factor. Intertwining of an ileal loop with a sigmoid loop (ileosigmoid knotting) accounts for nearly a fifth of cases.

- In westernized countries, sigmoid volvulus, according to Hughes (1980), is "better regarded as an idiopathic megarectum extending proximally into the colon, complicated almost inadvertently by twisting as the massive loop falls down under gravity, usually only through 180 degrees or so. The mesentery is not particularly narrow at its base. The enormous hypertrophy of the colorectal musculature makes tight twisting all but impossible and the sigmoid vessels are consequently greatly enlarged and thick-walled. These changes account for the limited degree of volvulus and the chronic, intermittent nature of the attacks, as well as the rarity of gangrene and the safety of rectal deflation. This form of volvulus is called *chronic sigmoid volvulus*. Some cases seem to be akin to idiopathic colonic pseudo-obstruction.

- *Adult cecal volvulus* occurs secondary to a congenital anomaly in which the cecum is hanging free from the posterior abdominal wall on a mesentery and is capable of undergoing torsion around the ascending colon.

- Pneumatosis coli may complicate volvulus.

- *Volvulus neonatorum* is torsion leading to gangrene of the small bowel, cecum, and ascending colon. It is due to a malrotation that leaves the cecum high and free on the mesentery in continuity with the ileum. Additionally, there may be a congenital band across the duodenum around which the torsion occurs.

- Chagas's disease is an important substrate for chronic sigmoid volvulus in South America. This disorder is an infection by the flagellate protozoan *Trypanosoma cruzi* (discovered in 1909 by Carlos Chagas), which is transmitted by the feces of a blood-sucking bug that defecates as it feeds. In chronic infection, the protozoan resides in muscle and is associated with damage to autonomic nerves. Megacolon and megaesophagus often result. The internal anal sphincter fails to relax when the rectum is distended. This leads to chronic rectosigmoid distention and hypertrophy of the smooth muscle despite inefficient fecal propulsion. Sigmoid volvulus occurs as a complication of the megacolon and accounts for 20% of cases of large bowel obstruction in parts of Brazil.

Clinical Features

- Both forms of sigmoid volvulus manifest as colicky pain and rapid abdominal distention. About 80% of patients with chronic sigmoid volvulus have had previous episodes, and only 5% to 10% go on to develop gangrene. Gangrene and perforation are common sequelae of acute volvulus.

- Cecal volvulus causes acute right lower quadrant pain with abdominal distention. Plain films show a greatly dilated portion of bowel.

Gross Pathology

- In acute volvulus, the bowel shows enormous dilatation, thinning of the wall, acute congestion, and sometimes ischemia, ulceration, perforation or hemorrhagic infarction.

- Chronic sigmoid volvulus is associated with considerable thickening of the muscle coat that extends into the rectum.

Microscopic Pathology

- The microscopic appearances of acute volvulus include variable congestion, ischemia, infarction, ulceration, and inflammation with thinning of the mucosa and muscle coat.

- In chronic or recurrent sigmoid volvulus, the main finding is muscular hypertrophy. The mucosa is intact.

References

Gillon J, Holt S, Sircus W. Pneumatosis coli and sigmoid volvulus: a report of four cases. Br J Surg 1979;66:802–805.

Habr-Gama A. Chagas disease of the bowel. In: Allan RN, Keighley MRB, Alexander-Williams J, Hawkins C (eds). Inflammatory Bowel Disease. New York: Churchill-Livingstone 1983:548–555.

Hughes LE. Sigmoid volvulus. J Roy Soc Med 1980;73:78–79.

Hughes LE. The place of immediate resection in the management of sigmoid volvulus. Med J Aust 1969;1:268–273.

Shepherd JJ. The epidemiology and clinical presentation of sigmoid volvulus. Br J Surg 1969;56:353–359.

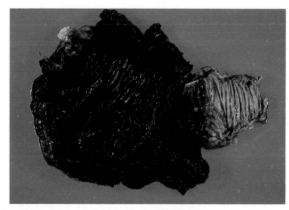

Figure 5–8. Acute cecal ischemia due to volvulus.

DIVERTICULAR DISEASE

Biology of Disease

- *Diverticula* are protrusions of the mucosa through the muscle coat. They occur mainly at points of weakness where the muscle coat is penetrated by blood vessels. Colonic diverticula are pulsion diverticula and are believed to be the result of increased intraluminal pressure.
- Low-residue diets are thought to be important in the genesis of diverticula. Vegetarians have a lower prevalence of the disease. How a low-residue diet leads to the increased intraluminal pressure required for diverticulum formation is unclear.
- Diverticulosis of the sigmoid and descending colon is extremely prevalent in affluent Western countries. It affects about 30% of people over the age of 40 years. The incidence and prevalence of diverticulosis increase with age. Women are affected more than men in a ratio of 3:2, but the incidences of complications are about equal.
- *Diverticulitis* is inflammation and ulceration of a diverticulum. It may lead to pericolic abscess, perforation, and peritonitis.
- Right-sided colonic diverticulosis is more common than left-sided in Japan and Asian countries. It also occurs in a younger age group than left-sided diverticulosis. The male-to-female ratio is 3:1.
- Uncommonly, total colonic diverticulosis occurs. The rectum is never affected.

Clinical Features

- Only 2% to 5% of all individuals with diverticulosis develop symptoms. (Only about 0.5% require surgery.)
- Uncomplicated diverticulosis may be associated with episodes of colicky left lower quadrant abdominal pain. The pain lasts from hours to days and may be worsened by eating or alleviated by passage of feces or flatus. Episodes of pain may be associated with diarrhea or constipation and may resemble the pain of irritable bowel syndrome (although there is no clear relationship between these two conditions).
- Massive hemorrhage with passage of bright red blood in an elderly person is most often due to bleeding from an ulcerated diverticulum.
- Diverticulitis manifests as left lower quadrant pain, fever, neutrophil leukocytosis, and localized tenderness or guarding. Colovesical fistula is an uncommon complication manifesting as pneumaturia, fecaluria, or urinary tract infection. Colovaginal fistula may also occur.
- Foreign bodies such as chicken bones or toothpicks may impact in a diverticulum and perforate it. The muscular narrowing of the sigmoid contributes to impaction.
- Inflammation of right-sided diverticula may mimic acute appendicitis. About four fifths of right-sided diverticula are multiple lesions.

Gross Pathology

- Prediverticular disease is characterized by thickening and contraction of teniae coli, thickening and corrugation of the circular muscle coat, narrowing of the lumen, and sacculations of the mucosa that do not protrude through the muscle coat.
- Muscle changes antedate the development of diverticula but persist throughout the course of the disease.
- Uncomplicated diverticula form two rows that protrude into the pericolic fat between the mesenteric and antimesenteric teniae. A third row of very small diverticula is sometimes seen between the two antimesenteric teniae.
- The lumen may be virtually obliterated by the combination of muscle coat contraction and redundant mucosal folds. The folds are accentuated and drawn closer together and may show polypoid projections, congestion, hemosiderin deposition, and histologic features of mucosal prolapse.
- In colectomy specimens for acute bleeding, all of the diverticula contain clot, and the site of hemorrhage is usually not identifiable.
- Diverticulitis usually affects only one diverticulum. The pathogenesis of the inflammation and ulceration is poorly understood. Diverticula often contain pellets of hard feces, which may contribute to diverticulitis through an abrasive effect or by occluding the mouth of the diverticulum.
- Specimens excised for local perforation usually display a greenish plaque of local peritonitis. A probe can often be passed through the perforated diverticulum to the peritoneum in the fresh specimen.
- In the absence of peritonitis, there may be local induration and, on the cut surface, a peridiverticular abscess. The abscess may spread longitudinally in pericolic fat for a distance of several centimeters, fistulize into the proximal colon or other viscera, or obstruct the colon. The last development may be complicated by obstructive colitis or cecitis.

Microscopic Pathology

- Diverticula are outpouchings of mucosa and muscularis mucosae through the muscularis propria. The mucosal lining of diverticula is usually normal. Lymphoid follicles may be enlarged or more numerous than normal.
- Diverticulitis is characterized by mucosal ulceration, granulation tissue, and variable inflammation. Peridiverticular abscesses contain pus and are lined by a pyogenic membrane of granulation tissue rich in plasma cells, neutrophils, and lymphocytes. Local acute peritonitis consists of a heavy neutrophil exudate.
- Segmental colitis may be seen in conjunction with diverticular disease in elderly patients. Coincidental Crohn's disease and diverticular disease may occur.

Differential Diagnosis

Intestinal pseudo-obstruction, Crohn's disease.

Wide-mouthed diverticula may be seen in chronic intestinal pseudo-obstruction.

A granulomatous response to fecal material in diverticulitis is unlikely to be misdiagnosed as Crohn's disease.

Diverticulosis is a common incidental finding in colons excised for cancer or other disorders.

References

Hughes LE. Post-mortem survey of diverticular disease of the colon. Part I: diverticulosis and diverticulitis. Gut 1969;10:336–351.

Hughes LE. Post-mortem survey of diverticular disease of the colon. Part II: the muscular abnormality in the sigmoid colon. Gut 1969;10:344–351.

Kelly JK. Polypoid prolapsing mucosal folds in diverticular disease. Am J Surg Pathol 1991;15:871–878.

Marcus R, Watt J. The prediverticular state. Br J Surg 1964;51:676–782.

Mendeloff AI. Thoughts on the epidemiology of diverticular disease. Clin Gastroenterol 1986;15:855–877.

Morson BC. Pathology of diverticular disease of the colon. Clin Gastroenterol 1975;4:37–52.

Sladen GE, Filipe MI. Is segmental colitis a complication of diverticular disease? Dis Colon Rectum 1984;27:513–514.

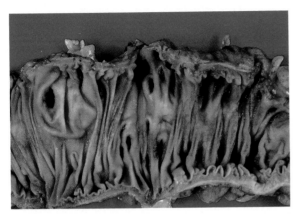

Figure 5–9. Diverticular disease of the colon. There are two rows of diverticula. The black material in the diverticula is blood—the patient presented with massive bleeding.

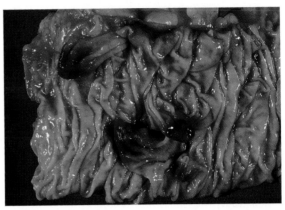

Figure 5–12. Polypoid prolapsing mucosal folds in diverticular disease. (Courtesy of Dr. Patrick Dean.)

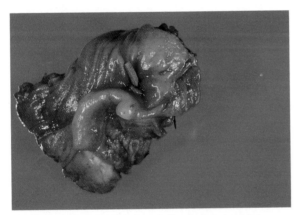

Figure 5–10. Perforated solitary cecal diverticulum (containing a green marker). The terminal ileum and ileocecal valve have been opened.

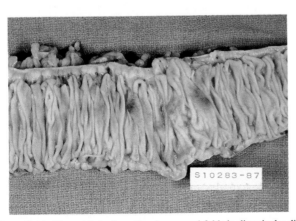

Figure 5–11. Hemosiderin deposition in mucosal folds in diverticular disease gives them a brown color. These areas are becoming polypoid.

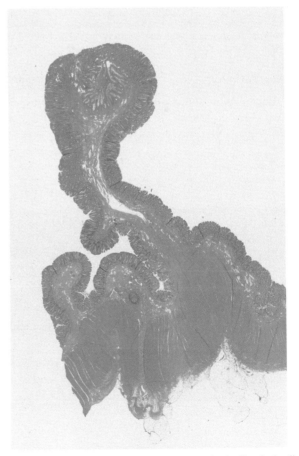

Figure 5–13. Prolapsing mucosal fold forming a polyp in diverticular disease. The mucosa shows histologic features similar to those of solitary ulcer syndrome.

MELANOSIS COLI

Biology of Disease

- Chronic uses of anthroquinone purgatives such as senna, cascara sagrada, and danthron causes an accumulation of a melanin-like lipofuscin in the macrophages of the colon. When this process is severe, the mucosa assumes a brown or black appearance to the naked eye.
- The precise mechanism by which anthroquinones induce melanosis is not understood. The pigment granules are membrane-bound, secondary lysosomes.
- Cathartic colon is associated with long-term laxative abuse due to chronic constipation. It may be an end-stage of anthroquinone-induced colonic damage, either alone or superimposed on a primary colonic pseudo-obstruction.
- Laxative abuse is a rare cause of clinically unexplained diarrhea. Where the abuse has been present for only a short time, the bowel may not appear brown on gross examination.

Clinical Features

- In mild cases, the gross appearance is normal. In severe cases, the mucosa is diffusely brown. In the most severe examples, the mucosa is black.
- The right side of the colon (including the appendix) is most affected. The lymphoid follicles stand out as tiny white spots against the dark background. Hyperplastic polyps, adenomas, and carcinomas are also free of pigment.

Gross Pathology

- Cathartic colon shows distention, thinning of the muscle coat, loss of haustra, loss of the mucosal folds, and melanosis coli.

Microscopic Pathology

- The macrophages of the lamina propria contain granules of golden-brown pigment. Those nearest to the lumen are most affected. In severe examples, pigment-laden macrophages are present throughout the mucosa and beneath the muscularis mucosae. Regional lymph nodes may contain pigmented macrophages.
- Argyrophilic neurons are decreased in number. Those remaining are shrunken and have fewer processes. Schwann's cells are increased. Most authors believe that cathartic colon is distinct from idiopathic constipation.

Special Diagnostic Techniques

- The pigment gives positive staining reactions with periodic acid–Schiff, long Ziehl-Neelsen, Nile blue sulfate, and Schmorl's stains. Reactions to iron stains are negative in the majority of cases.

Differential Diagnosis

Chronic granulomatous disease, hemosiderin.

Children or young adults with chronic granulomatous disease have pigmented lipid histiocytes in the lamina propria. The pigment is diffuse or very finely granular rather than coarsely granular as in melanosis coli.

Hemosiderin in colonic macrophages is usually a consequence of local hemorrhage and may be seen in association with diverticular disease, ischemia, or trauma or following a previous biopsy.

References

Bockus HL, Willard JH, Bank J. Melanosis coli: etiologic significance of anthracene laxatives, 41 cases. JAMA 1933;101:1–6.

Smith B. Pathologic changes in the colon produced by anthroquinone purgatives. Dis Colon Rectum 1973;16:455–458.

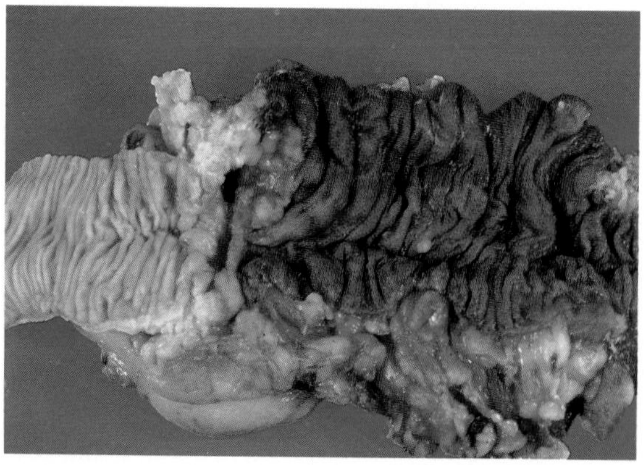

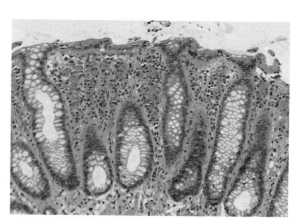

Figure 5–14. Melanosis coli contrasts with the normal ileum.

Figure 5–15. Melanosis coli. Pigmented macrophages in lamina propria.

ULCERATIVE COLITIS AND COLITIS INDETERMINATE

Biology of Disease

- *Ulcerative colitis* is a diffuse mucosal inflammatory disorder that affects a variable length of the large bowel in continuity from the anus proximally. (Inflammation confined to the rectum is called *proctitis*.)
- The disease manifests most commonly in the third decade but may do so at any time between infancy and old age.
- Sex incidences are approximately equal.
- The cause of ulcerative colitis is unknown. Genetic factors play an important role. There is higher incidence in families. Compared with the general population, the rate of ulcerative colitis among first-degree relatives of probands is increased by a factor of 9.5. Twin studies show that the genetic factor in the etiology is weaker in ulcerative colitis than in Crohn's disease. There is a higher incidence in Jews and North American whites. There are a positive association with the HLA-DR2 allele and negative associations with DR4 and DRw6.
- The risk of ulcerative colitis is reduced in smokers, and patients who smoke may have a relapse if they quit smoking.

Clinical Features

- Most patients have symptomatic episodes separated by remissions. Ten percent of patients have continuous symptoms without remission.
- Symptoms vary from mild to fulminant. About 60% of patients have mild symptoms and involvement of only the rectum or rectosigmoid. The predominant complaints are rectal bleeding and mild diarrhea. Blood loss may cause iron deficiency anemia.
- About 25% of patients have moderate symptoms consisting of four to five loose, blood-stained bowel motions per day, crampy abdominal pain, anemia, fatigue, and low-grade fever. Endoscopically, the disease extends for varying distances beyond the rectum.
- Severe or fulminant colitis may occur de novo or may punctuate the course of moderate or mild disease. The clinical manifestations of severe colitis are profuse diarrhea and rectal bleeding, tenesmus, abdominal cramps, anorexia, weight loss, weakness, fever, anemia, leukocytosis, and hypoalbuminemia. Endoscopically, the mucosa is friable, granular, and extremely congested, and may be extensively ulcerated.
- Extraintestinal manifestations of colitis include arthritis, uveitis, iritis, pyoderma gangrenosum, erythema nodosum, and thromboembolism. The last manifestation results from loss of antithrombin III in severe colitis.
- Eighty percent of all cases of primary sclerosing cholangitis occur in young men with idiopathic ulcerative colitis.
- One fifth of patients have fecal stasis and use laxatives. Diverticulosis may be present in patients with colitis.

Gross Pathology

- Extent of disease varies from a few centimeters (distal proctitis) to total colonic involvement. In the latter, the inflammation may extend into the terminal ileum (backwash ileitis).
- Endoscopic features of active disease are hyperemia, friability, granularity, and small ulcers or erosions. Resected specimens that show active disease contain blood in the lumen, and the mucosa has a granular, velvety hemorrhagic appearance. The junction between inflamed and uninflamed mucosa is usually sharp. The rectal mucosa may grossly appear less diseased than the colon, especially after steroid enemas.
- In fulminant colitis, there may be extensive ulceration, toxic dilation (diameter >5.5 cm on plain film), thinning of the muscle coat, perforation, and peritonitis.
- Specimens from chronic colitis show a shortened colon (80 to 90 cm rather than 120 to 150 cm), flat or granular mucosa, loss of mucosal folds, inflammatory polyps, focal ulceration, and variable mucosal congestion. Inflammatory polyps or sessile areas of dysplasia may be present.
- Inflammatory polyps are found clinically in 12% to 20% of cases. They follow episodes of severe disease in which ulceration, running to confluence or undermining the muscularis mucosae, leaves islands of mucosa protruding above the ulcers. When mucosa regenerates on the floors of the ulcers, the islands remain elevated and become inflammatory polyps.

Microscopic Pathology

- The mucosa shows a diffuse increase in inflammatory cells in the lamina propria, including large numbers of plasma cells, eosinophils, lymphocytes, macrophages, and neutrophils. They are distributed uniformly throughout the lamina propria, with loss of the normal superficial predominance. Basal plasmacytosis is characteristic.
- The capillary blood vessels are congested and dilated.
- The crypts display branching (fission), hyperchromatism, mucin depletion, shortening, irregularity, cystic dilatation, and villiform change (all signs of regeneration).
- Neutrophils infiltrate the surface and crypt epithelium, and crypt abscesses may form. Traditionally, neutrophil infiltration is regarded as evidence of disease activity. Ulcers begin as ruptured crypt abscesses. The inflammation spreads laterally, undermining the mucosa, which sloughs and increases the area of ulceration.
- Ulcers vary in size, shape, number, and location from case to case. In fulminant colitis, ulcers may penetrate the muscularis mucosae and spread rapidly, causing the undermined mucosa to slough or to form pseudopolyps.
- Rarely, in severe colitis treated with corticosteroids, there is superimposed cytomegalovirus infection (with inclusion bodies in endothelial, epithelial, or mesenchymal cells).
- In chronic colitis, the mucosa may have a villiform appearance owing to crypt dilatation. The mucosa may be

thinned and atrophic with crypt dropout or branching. Crypts may be shortened and may fail to reach the muscularis mucosae. Inflammation is minimal or absent. Paneth cell metaplasia, hyperplastic mucosal change, and increased numbers of enterochromaffin cells are present.

■ In chronic colitis, the muscularis mucosae is hypertrophied owing to contraction and fibrosis. Regenerated mucosa may lie directly on the muscularis propria in areas of previous deep ulceration.

■ Lymphoid follicular hyperplasia may be prominent in quiescent or active disease, particularly in the rectum (follicular proctitis).

Special Diagnostic Techniques

■ The diagnosis of idiopathic ulcerative colitis is clinicopathologic. Endoscopy, radiology, and mucosal morphology contribute to the final diagnosis.

Differential Diagnosis

Crohn's disease, infectious colitis, diversion proctitis, colitis indeterminate.

Crohn's disease (colitis) is distinguished by predominance of ulceration, patchy or discontinuous disease, ulcers separated by normal-appearing or noncongested mucosa, strictures, sinuses or fistulae, anal fistulae and tags, the presence and nature of ileal involvement, granulomas, the absence of extreme mucosal congestion, and the absence of diffuse continuous mucosal inflammation.

Prolonged shigellosis, gonorrhea, or syphilis of the rectum may histologically resemble chronic inflammatory bowel disease. In prolonged infectious colitis, the number of mucosal plasma cells increases in proportion to the time from onset of illness. Stool cultures help to establish the diagnosis. Infectious or pseudomembranous colitis

may complicate and exacerbate inflammatory bowel disease.

Diversion colitis presents with passage of mucus or blood per rectum, tenesmus, and endoscopic appearance resembling that of ulcerative proctitis. Histologic features are like those of inflammatory bowel disease or follicular proctitis.

Colitis indeterminate, a term expressing diagnostic uncertainty, is applied to severe colitis with extensive ulceration and mixed features of Crohn's disease and ulcerative colitis that make the distinction impossible. Colitis indeterminate is usually a severe pancolitis with an unremitting course from initial presentation to colectomy. It may be complicated by toxic megacolon. Acute fissures, transmural inflammation, and maintained goblet cell population may be found in cases that do not recur and are likely examples of acute ulcerative colitis. Acute fissures are accompanied by myocytolysis and capillary engorgement. The transmural inflammation is not composed of aggregated lymphocytes. If biopsy specimens from a preceding phase of low grade illness are available, they may help establish a specific diagnosis.

References

Hywel-Jones J, Lennard-Jones JE, Morson BC, et al. Numerical taxonomy and discriminant analysis applied to non-specific colitis. Q J Med 1973;62:715–732.

Lockhart-Mummery HE, Morson BC. Crohn's disease (regional enteritis) of the large intestine and its distinction from ulcerative colitis. Gut 1960;1:87–105.

Lumb GR, Protheroe RHB, Ramsay GS. Ulcerative colitis with dilatation of the colon. Br J Surg 1955;43:182–185.

Price AB. Overlap in the spectrum of non-specific inflammatory bowel disease— "colitis indeterminate." J Clin Pathol 1978;31:567–577.

Price AB, Morson BC. Inflammatory bowel disease: the surgical pathology of Crohn's disease and ulcerative colitis. Hum Pathol 1975;6:7–29.

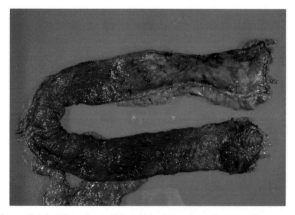

Figure 5–16. Ulcerative colitis with severe mucosal congestion, loss of mucosal folds, and a granular mucosal appearance.

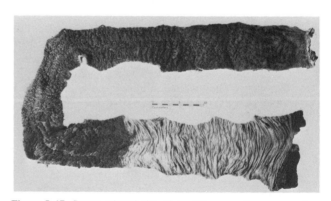

Figure 5–17. Severe subtotal ulcerative colitis spares the cecum and ascending colon. Note the skip lesion in the cecum, a feature that does not alter the diagnosis.

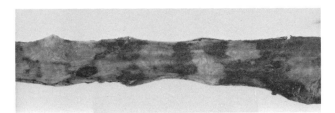

Figure 5–18. Ulcerative colitis. Patches of pale mucosa between congested patches as disease enters remission.

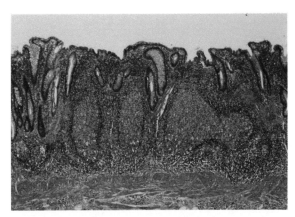

Figure 5–21. Chronic follicular proctitis. There are increased numbers of reactive lymphoid follicles in the rectal mucosa. This pattern can be seen in idiopathic ulcerative colitis, diversion colitis, and lymphogranuloma venereum.

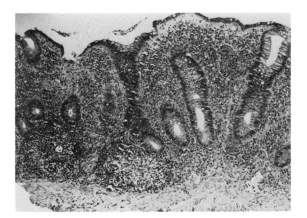

Figure 5–19. Mucosal biopsy specimen showing ulcerative colitis. Diffuse inflammation, basal plasmacytosis, and mucin depletion are noted.

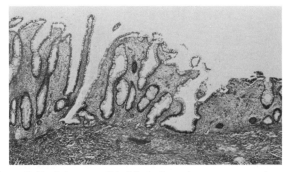

Figure 5–22. Quiescent colitis: Mucosal atrophy, crypt regeneration, and little inflammation.

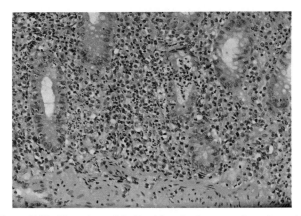

Figure 5–20. Ulcerative colitis. Basal lymphoplasmacytosis, and cryptitis are present.

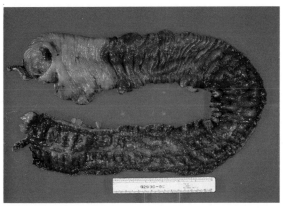

Figure 5–23. Colitis indeterminate. Severe extensive ulceration. The diffuse mucosal congestion favors ulcerative colitis.

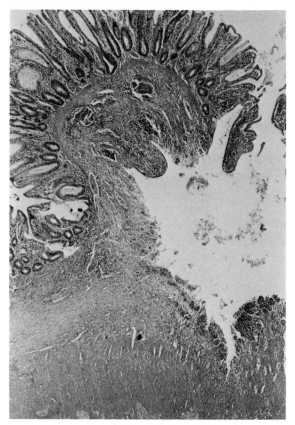

Figure 5–24. Colitis indeterminate. Ulceration undermines mucosa and penetrates into the muscle coat.

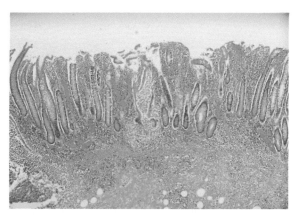

Figure 5–25. Colitis indeterminate. Mucosa at the margin of an ulcer shows diffuse inflammation and congestion. Inflammation extends into the submucosa. There is a crypt abscess in the center.

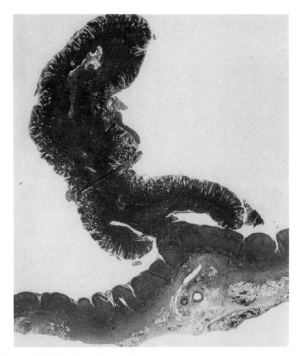

Figure 5–26. Colitis indeterminate. Undermined mucosa forms an inflammatory polyp. Note the acute fissures, which nearly traverse the muscle coat.

CROHN'S DISEASE OF THE COLON

Biology of Disease

See Chapter 3

Clinical Features

■ The extent and severity of involvement determine the clinical features. Extensive colitis is signified by chronic diarrhea, abdominal pain, weight loss, and debility. Blood loss and anemia are less prominent than in ulcerative colitis.

■ Anal disease encompasses fissures, mucosal tags, sinuses, fistulae, and perianal abscesses. Anal fistulae are usually associated with ulcers of the low rectum, above the anal sphincter. They are refractory to treatment while the rectal ulceration persists. Low ulcers tend to cause anal stenosis.

■ Complications include internal fistulae, toxic dilatation, amyloidosis (rarely), dysplasia, carcinoma, and, rarely, acute massive hemorrhage.

■ Associated diseases include ankylosing spondylitis (5%), anterior uveitis (2%), and rarely sclerosing cholangitis.

Gross Pathology

■ Crohn's colitis shows discontinuous segments of disease and asymmetric large and small ulcers separated by normal (noncongested) mucosa. Ulcers may be discrete, confluent, serpiginous, or linear. Linear longitudinal (railroad track) ulcers often overlie teniae coli. Linear longitudinal and transverse ulcers may dissect the mucosa into a cobblestone pattern. Strictures (secondary to ulcers), sinuses and fistulae, inflammatory polyps, and terminal ileal involvement are often present. Fistulae may penetrate into the duodenum, small bowel, bladder, or vagina.

Microscopic Pathology

■ Patchy inflammation and ulceration are the hallmark of Crohn's disease. Transmural inflammation consisting of lymphoid follicles is seen beneath chronic ulcers. Granulomas may be found in any layer of the bowel wall; they increase in frequency towards the anus. If the edematous skin tag at the apex of an anal fissure is removed, it often shows follicular lymphoid inflammation or granulomas. Adenocarcinoma may arise in long-standing anal fistula.

Differential Diagnosis

Idiopathic ulcerative colitis, segmental colitis, infectious and amebic colitis, diversion colitis, tuberculosis, ischemic injury, irradiation injury.

Ulcerative colitis is distinguished by diffuse mucosal inflammation in continuity from the anus, mucosal conges-tion and hemorrhage, absence of granulomas, and absence of transmural inflammation (except under deep ulcers). Although the mucosal inflammation is continuous, it may vary in severity, especially when entering remission.

Infectious colitis may present a segmental or patchy pattern endoscopically, shows mucosal edema and neutrophil infiltration, and is self-limited. Biopsies late in the course of infection may show increased plasma cells, crypt regeneration, and spotty inflammation, and the distinction from Crohn's disease may not be possible. The diagnosis of amebiasis depends on identification of amebae.

Diversion colitis may show patchy inflammation and crypt abscesses resembling Crohn's disease. The history of fecal diversion is crucial to the diagnosis.

Segmental colitis with diverticular disease is confined to the area of diverticula and shows mucosal inflammation with crypt abscesses.

Tuberculous granulomas typically show caseous necrosis. If mycobacteria are identified in tissue, diagnosis is presumptive. Culture is the definitive test.

Chronic ischemia may produce a segmental stricture. The diagnosis of ischemia is most secure when vascular occlusion is found. Irradiation injury is suggested by the history, and the mechanism of injury is ischemic.

References

Lockhart-Mummery HE, Morson BC. Crohn's disease (regional enteriris) of the large intestine and its distinction from ulcerative colitis. Gut 1960;1:87–105.
Price AB, Morson BC. Inflammatory bowel disease: the surgical pathology of Crohn's disease and ulcerative colitis. Hum Pathol 1975;6:7–29.

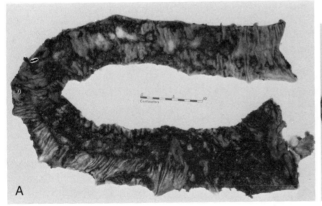
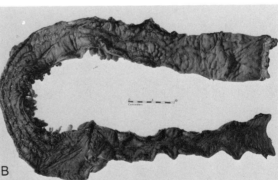

Figure 5–27. Crohn's colitis. *A,* Numerous ulcers and relatively normal intervening mucosa. *B,* "Railroad track" ulceration and typical ileal Crohn's disease.

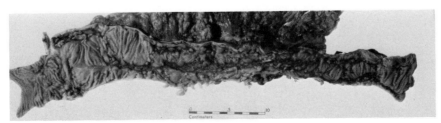

Figure 5–28. Crohn's colitis. Longitudinal ulcers with inflammatory polyps forming at the ulcer margins.

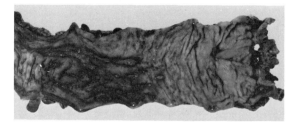

Figure 5–29. Rectal and anal Crohn's disease with rectal ulcers.

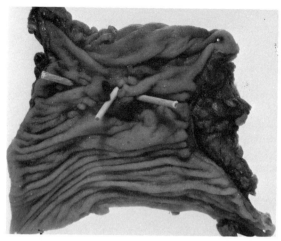

Figure 5–31. Colon: Ileocolic fistulae entering the colon. Note the small sentinel polyps.

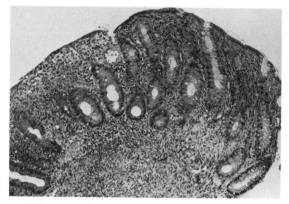

Figure 5–30. Crohn's disease, colonic biopsy. Note the granulomas in the lower half of the mucosa.

DYSPLASIA IN INFLAMMATORY BOWEL DISEASE

Biology of Disease

■ *Dysplasia* is a precancerous change that precedes the majority of colorectal cancers which complicate ulcerative colitis and Crohn's disease. Patients with chronic ulcerative colitis have a tenfold greater risk of colorectal carcinoma than does the general population. Carcinoma complicating ulcerative colitis accounts for about 1% of all large bowel cancers. The risk of colonic and ileal adenocarcinoma is increased in Crohn's disease. The severity of disease is not a risk factor, and many carcinomas arise in patients with quiescent colitis.

■ The two principal risk factors for colorectal carcinoma are the extent and duration of colitis. The risk of dysplasia begins after 10 years of disease and increases progressively thereafter. Patients with proctitis are at no greater risk for carcinoma than the general population. (Patients with total colitis are at highest risk, and patients with intermediate extent of disease have a corresponding increase in risk.) The cumulative risk of developing carcinoma or high-grade dysplasia was 4% in 15 years, 7% in 20 years, and 13% in 25 years (at St. Mark's Hospital, London). Low-grade dysplasia is an indication for more frequent colonoscopy than the standard of once every 2 years used at St. Mark's Hospital.

■ Point mutations and inactivation of the p53 protein are commonly found in dysplasias and cancers.

Clinical Features

■ Dysplasia is an asymptomatic condition. Carcinoma may present in a patient with obstruction, perforation, blood loss, or metastases.

■ Surveillance colonoscopy aims to reduce the incidence of cancer by detecting and treating premalignant dysplasia. It is highly successful except for patients who opt out (about 15% of patients). Compliance with surveillance diminishes when disease is asymptomatic. This increases the risk for patients with low-grade disease.

■ The histologic diagnosis of dysplasia is frequently very difficult and the changes may be hard to distinguish from regeneration. In these cases, biopsy may be repeated. A diagnosis of dysplasia should be confirmed by a second pathologist before colectomy is performed.

Gross Pathology

■ Dysplasia is usually an elevated plaque or nodule that may have a velvety appearance. In some instances, dysplastic mucosa is indistinguishable from the adjacent mucosa on endoscopic or gross inspection. Plaques or nodules vary in size and are often poorly circumscribed. Dysplasia-associated lesions and masses must always be excised, because a third to a half of them contain carcinoma.

■ Carcinoma in ulcerative colitis is flat, ill defined, and infiltrating. In 25% of cases, there is more than one primary tumor.

Microscopic Pathology

■ Biopsies from surveillance colonoscopies are classified either as negative, indefinite, or positive for dysplasia. The last category is divided into low-grade and high-grade dysplasia.

■ Most often, dysplasia resembles villous adenoma. Dysplastic epithelium shows nuclear stratification and hyperchromatism, increased numbers of mitoses, mitoses high in the crypts, and failure of maturation. Mucin content is diminished or confined to the apical portions of the cells. Low-grade dysplasia manifests nuclei confined to the lower half of the epithelium. The nuclei are elongated, hyperchromatic, and mildly pleomorphic. Rarely, large numbers of endocrine cells or Paneth's cells are present. The nuclei in high-grade dysplasia extend into the upper half of the epithelium and may reach the surface. They are stratified, pleomorphic, and hyperchromatic, and they may show clearing of the nucleoplasm and nucleoli. Variants of dysplasia are: incomplete maturation with a single cell layer containing nuclei that are large and hyperchromatic, dysplasia with nonmucin clear cell change, and dystrophic goblet cells. The goblet cells are located near the basement membrane and do not reach the lumen. They are disoriented, and the nucleus may be on the luminal aspect of the goblet.

■ Desmoplasia with severe dysplasia establishes the diagnosis of carcinoma; so does invasion, which can occasionally occur without desmoplasia. The presence of mucin lakes also makes carcinoma more likely.

■ Carcinomas arising in colitis are more frequently high-grade or colloid carcinomas than sporadic large bowel cancer. The prognosis for cancer in colitis is similar to that for sporadic colonic cancer, stage for stage.

■ Biopsies are classified as indefinite for dysplasia if they show unusual patterns that are neither definitely positive nor negative, as inflammatory atypia, regenerative change, and hyperplastic polyp–like change.

Special Diagnostic Techniques

■ DNA aneuploidy detected by flow cytometry on endoscopic biopsies precedes histologic dysplasia and may identify a subset of patients without dysplasia who are more likely to develop it and who might benefit from increased frequency of colonoscopy. Histology remains the gold standard for diagnosis of dysplasia.

Differential Diagnosis

Regenerative mucosa, hyperplastic mucosa, incidental adenoma.

Regenerative or inflamed mucosa may show nuclei occupying half of the cell height with stratified or large, open nuclei. Usually, some degree of surface maturation is retained.

Hyperplastic polyp–like change is serrated mucosa resembling gastric pits with interspersed goblet cells. The nuclei may occupy up to half the cell height. This change is graded as indefinite for dysplasia.

Pedunculated dysplastic lesions in patients with ulcerative colitis are best regarded as adenomas arising coincidentally with colitis. This diagnosis is obvious when a pedunculated adenoma arises in the right side of a colon with left-sided colitis. Dysplasia rarely arises in an inflammatory polyp.

References

Langholz E, Munkholm P, Davidsen M, Binder V. Colorectal cancer risk and mortality in patients with ulcerative colitis. Gastroenterology 1992;103:1444–1451.

Lennard-Jones JE, Melville DM, Morson BC, et al. Precancer and cancer in extensive ulcerative colitis: findings among 407 patients over 22 years. Gut 1990;31:800–806.

Lofberg R, Brostrom O, Karlen P, et al. DNA aneuploidy in ulcerative colitis: reproducibility, topographic distribution, and relation to dysplasia. Gastroenterology 1992;102:1149–1154.

Riddell RH, Goldman H, Ranshoff DF, et al. Dysplasia in inflammatory bowel disease: standardized classification with provisional clinical applications. Hum Pathol 1983;14:931–968.

Rubin CE, Haggitt RC, Burmer GC, et al. DNA aneuploidy in colonic biopsies predicts future development of dysplasia in ulcerative colitis. Gastroenterology 1992;103:1611–1620.

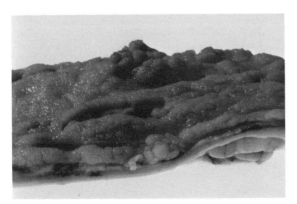

Figure 5–32. Dysplasia in chronic ulcerative colitis presenting as an elevated multinodular mass.

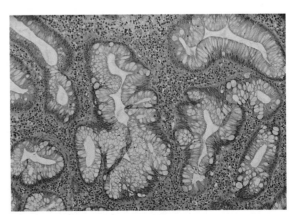

Figure 5–33. Hyperplastic change indefinite for dysplasia in chronic ulcerative colitis.

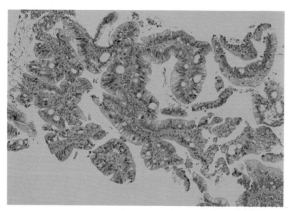

Figure 5–34. Mucosal biopsy shows dysplasia in chronic ulcerative colitis.

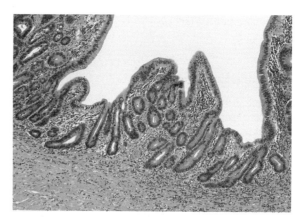

Figure 5–36. Ileal dysplasia in Crohn's disease. (Courtesy of Dr. Steve Rasmussen.)

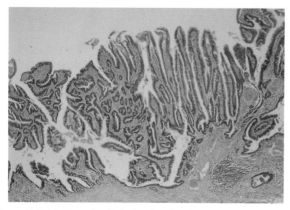

Figure 5–35. Villous dysplasia in chronic ulcerative colitis. Note the crowded hyperchromatic nuclei.

COLLAGENOUS COLITIS

Biology of Disease

- *Collagenous colitis* is a clinicopathologic syndrome of chronic watery diarrhea, normal endoscopic appearance, inflamed colonic mucosa, normal crypt architecture, increased epithelial lymphocytes, and thickened collagen table beneath the surface epithelium.
- The etiology is unknown. Immunologic factors may play a role, because some patients have celiac, thyroid, or rheumatoid disease.

Clinical Features

- Eighty percent of patients with collagenous colitis are middle-aged or elderly women.
- The typical symptom is chronic watery (nonbloody) diarrhea that has been present for months to years before presentation. There may be mild abdominal pain or flatulence.
- A history of using nonsteroidal anti-inflammatory drugs (NSAIDs) is often present.

Gross Pathology

- Endoscopically, the colon may appear normal or minimally erythematous with mucosal hemorrhage.

Microscopic Pathology

- The subepithelial collagen band is thickened (more than 10 μm).
- The crypt architecture is normal.
- The quantity of mononuclear cells in the lamina propria is increased, although the normal superficial weighting is retained.
- The number of epithelial lymphocytes is increased.
- The surface epithelium may show flattening, cuboidalization, intraepithelial eosinophils, and occasional neutrophils. It is easily removed by the trauma of the biopsy procedure.
- The abnormalities are usually diffuse throughout the large bowel, but the collagenization is variable, and the rectum may be spared. Therefore, the colon should be sampled at several sites when endoscopy is performed in cases of chronic watery diarrhea.

Differential Diagnosis

Lymphocytic colitis, ischemia, amyloidosis, ulcerative colitis, infectious colitis, artifacts of sectioning.

Lymphocytic (microscopic) colitis is distinguished by the absence of thickening of subepithelial collagen.

Ischemia may show hyalinization of the superficial lamina propria but no increase in chronic inflammatory cells or epithelial lymphocytes.

Amyloid displays apple-green birefringence after Congo red staining and is not deposited solely beneath the surface epithelium.

Ulcerative colitis shows crypt destructive and regenerative changes and diffuse mucosal inflammation with basal plasmacytosis.

Infectious colitis shows edema, capillary congestion, and neutrophil infiltration of lamina propria and crypts. Increased epithelial lymphocytes and collagenous thickening are absent.

Tangential sectioning of the normal subepithelial collagen layer may give a false appearance of thickening.

When surface epithelial nuclei are in the center of the cell, an eosinophilic basal cytoplasmic zone beneath the nuclei may be mistaken for a thickened subepithelial collagen band.

References

Gledhill A, Cole FM. Significance of basement membrane thickening in the human colon. Gut 1984;25:1085–1088.

Jessurun J, Yardley JG, Giardiello FM, et al. Chronic colitis with thickening of the subepithelial collagen layer (collagenous colitis): histopathologic findings in fifteen patients. Hum Pathol 1987;18:839–848.

Lazenby AJ, Yardley JH, Giardiello FM, Bayless TM. Pitfalls in the diagnosis of collagenous colitis. Hum Pathol 1990;21:905–910.

Lee E, Schiller LR, Vendrell D, et al. Subepithelial collagen table thickness in colon specimens from patients with microscopic colitis and collagenous colitis. Gastroenterology 1992;103:1790–1796.

Lindstrom CG. Collagenous colitis with watery diarrhea—a new entity? Pathol Eur 1976;11:87–89.

Sylwestrowicz T, Kelly JK, Hwang WS, Shaffer EA. Collagenous colitis and microscopic colitis: the watery diarrhea–colitis syndrome. Am J Gastroenterol 1989;84:763–768.

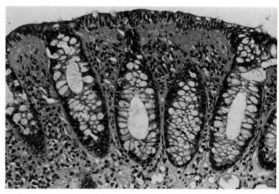

Figure 5–37. Collagenous colitis. Features include normal crypt architecture, thick subepithelial collagen layer, and mild increase in chronic inflammatory cells in the upper half of the mucosa.

LYMPHOCYTIC COLITIS

Biology of Disease

■ *Lymphocytic (microscopic) colitis* is an idiopathic clinicopathologic entity characterized by watery diarrhea, normal endoscopic appearance, normal crypt architecture, mild diffuse inflammation of the lamina propria, and increased numbers of epithelial lymphocytes. This condition differs from collagenous colitis in (1) the absence of a subepithelial collagenous band, (2) equal sex incidences and (3) an association with HLA A1.

Clinical Features

■ Patients are typically middle-aged or elderly. The sex ratio is about 1:1.
■ Diarrhea is typically watery and chronic with an average of eight to ten low-volume motions per day.
■ Lymphocytic colitis may be associated with celiac disease.

Gross Pathology

■ The endoscopic appearances are normal.

Microscopic Pathology

■ Under low magnification, the lamina propria appears hypercellular, but the inflammation does not have the basal weighting of idiopathic inflammatory bowel disease.
■ There is a marked increase in epithelial lymphocytes. Occasional neutrophils or eosinophils may be present in the surface epithelium. Crypt architecture and goblet cells are normal.
■ The condition is diffuse throughout the large bowel.

Differential Diagnosis

Collagenous colitis, idiopathic ulcerative colitis, Crohn's disease, infectious colitis, chronic amebic colitis, segmental colitis, drug-induced colitis.

Collagenous colitis shows a thickened subepithelial collagen band throughout the colon. Rectal biopsy specimens may not show the collagenous thickening, and the appearance may be confused with that of lymphocytic colitis.

Idiopathic ulcerative colitis is distinguished not only by its clinical and endoscopic features but by the intensity of the inflammation, basal plasmacytosis, crypt regeneration, neutrophil infiltration, and capillary dilatation. A marked increase in epithelial lymphocytes is not a feature of idiopathic ulcerative colitis.

Crohn's disease is characterized by multifocal deep mucosal inflammation and ulceration, not by diffuse inflammation or a marked increase in epithelial lymphocytes.

Acute infectious colitis is characterized by edema, capillary dilatation, and neutrophil infiltration. The immunocytes in the lamina propria are not increased in early infections but may be considerably increased late in the course of disease.

Chronic amebic colitis is characterized by watery diarrhea with mucus and low numbers of amebae in the stool. Diagnosis is by recognition of the organisms in either stools or biopsy specimens.

Segmental colitis associated with diverticular disease is confined to the sigmoid, spares the rectum, and resembles inflammatory bowel disease or infectious colitis.

Drug-induced colitis should be considered in any patient receiving medication. Nonsteroidal anti-inflammatory drugs (NSAIDs) may prove to play a role in lymphocytic colitis.

References

Bo-Linn GW, Vendrell DD, Lee E, Fordtran JS. An evaluation of the significance of microscopic colitis in patients with chronic diarrhea. J Clin Invest 1985;75:1559–1569.

Kingham GJC, Levison DA, Ball JA, Dawson AM. Microscopic colitis—a cause of chronic watery diarrhea. Br Med J 1982;285:1601–1604.

Lazenby AJ, Yardley JH, Giardiello FM, et al. Lymphocytic (microscopic) colitis: a comparative histologic study with particular reference to collagenous colitis. Hum Pathol 1989;20:18–28.

Sylwestrowicz T, Kelly JK, Hwang WS, Shaffer EA. Collagenous colitis and microscopic colitis: the watery diarrhea colitis syndrome. Am J Gastroenterol 1989;84:763–768.

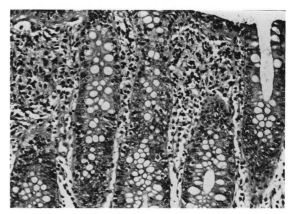

Figure 5–38. Lymphocytic colitis displays increased epithelial lymphocytes and normal crypt architecture.

DIVERSION PROCTITIS AND COLITIS

Biology of Disease

■ *Diversion (or bypass) colitis* is an inflammatory process in a portion of large bowel that is excluded from the fecal stream. Diversion colitis resolves after reanastomosis and appears to be caused by absence of the fecal stream. Short-chain fatty acids, the preferred metabolic substrate of colonic epithelial cells, may be lacking in diversion colitis, and this lack may contribute to the inflammation.

■ Diversion colitis was originally described in patients without prior inflammatory bowel disease who had undergone bypass for various indications. In patients who have had prior inflammatory bowel disease, distinguishing between diversion effect and inflammatory bowel disease may be extremely difficult.

Clinical Features

■ Diversion proctitis or colitis is usually asymptomatic. Passage of blood or mucus, tenesmus, and abdominal pain may lead the patient to seek medical attention.

■ Diversion colitis may occur as early as 1 month after diversion or many years later.

■ Treatment by local application of short-chain fatty acids has been reported to induce a dramatic improvement in both endoscopic and histologic appearances.

Gross Pathology

■ The endoscopic appearances may be similar to those of mild ulcerative colitis, including redness, petechiae, granularity, and friability. The inflammation is mainly confined to the rectum and diminishes in severity proximally.

■ The bypassed segment shrinks and may become stenotic. In resected specimens, longitudinal mucosal ridges and diffuse mucosal nodularity have been described.

Microscopic Pathology

■ Crypt architecture is minimally distorted, but the epithelium shows reactive hyperchromatism and mucin depletion. There may be expansion of the lamina propria by plasma cells, lymphocytes, and granulocytes. Some cases display focal cryptitis, crypt abscesses, and Paneth cell hyperplasia. Diffuse lymphoid follicular hyperplasia, with tiny ulcers (aphthoid ulcers) over the follicles, is often seen. Lymphoid hyperplasia is particularly marked in infants and children who have had a bypass for Hirschsprung's disease.

■ A milder form of mucosal injury comprising mild follicular lymphoid hyperplasia, an increase in lymphoplasmacytic infiltrates with absence of neutrophils, and little epithelial injury has been termed *diversion reaction*. The reaction is associated with normal gross appearance.

Differential Diagnosis

Inflammatory bowel disease, lymphoid follicular proctitis.

Despite its resemblance to inflammatory bowel disease, the inflammatory changes in diversion colitis are likely due to diversion if the original surgery was performed for conditions other than inflammatory bowel disease.

Granulomas in the bypassed mucosa in patients with a former diagnosis of Crohn's disease nearly always indicate recurrence of that disease; however, in diversion colitis, mucin granulomas have been described in relation to ruptured crypts.

Lymphoid follicular proctitis was formerly regarded as a specific form of idiopathic ulcerative colitis but may also be a manifestation of diversion colitis. When doubt exists about the recurrence of inflammatory bowel disease, a therapeutic trial of short-chain fatty acids or reanastomosis may be justified.

References

Glotzer DJ, Glick ME, Goldman H. Proctitis and colitis following diversion of the fecal stream. Gastroenterology 1981;80:438–441.

Haque S, Eisen RN, West BA. The morphologic features of diversion colitis: studies of a pediatric population with no other disease of the intestinal mucosa. Hum Pathol 1993;24:211–219.

Komorowski RA. Histologic spectrum of diversion colitis. Am J Surg Pathol 1990;14:548–554.

Korelitz BI, Cheskin LJ, Sohn N, Sommers SC. Proctitis after fecal diversion in Crohn's disease and its elimination with reanastomosis: implications for surgical management. Gastroenterology 1984;87:710–713.

Ma CK, Gotleb C, Haas PA. Diversion colitis: a clinicopathologic study of 21 cases. Hum Pathol 1990;21:429–436.

Yeong ML, Bethwaite PB, Prasad J, Isbister WH. Lymphoid follicular hyperplasia—a distinctive feature of diversion colitis. Histopathology 1991;19:55–61.

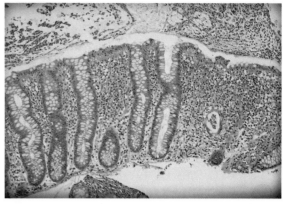

Figure 5–39. Diversion colitis shows focal inflammation and a crypt abscess.

OBSTRUCTIVE COLITIS

Biology of Disease

■ *Obstructive colitis* is the name given to nonspecific ulceration proximal to obstruction. The obstructing lesions are usually carcinoma or diverticular disease. The obstruction is often partial or incomplete.

■ The pathogenesis is poorly understood. Ischemia has been invoked on the basis of the tension in the wall and Laplace's law (the tension in the wall of a cylinder increases with the intraluminal pressure and the diameter). Altered bowel microbial flora may play a role. Pseudomembranous colitis has occurred in this context.

■ In severe cases, there may be extreme thinning of the wall and transmural necrosis with perforation and peritonitis.

Clinical Features

■ The clinical features are those of obstruction except in cases of perforation.

■ The patients are predominantly elderly women who often have hypertension, diabetes, or other preexisting illness.

Gross Pathology

■ The ulcerations are either small, shallow, and well-defined lesions measuring up to 2 cm in diameter, or confluent, circumferential lesions up to 25 cm in length. Small pseudopolyps are sometimes present. The affected areas are separated from the obstructing lesion by a segment of normal colon. Lesions occur in moderately distended colon and are not uncommonly in the cecum.

Microscopic Pathology

■ The ulcers are nonspecific, composed of granulation tissue and inflammatory cells replacing the mucosa. They extend into the submucosa or muscle coat in some instances, leading to perforation. Acute fissures can be present.

References

Glotzer DJ, Roth SI, Welch CE. Colonic ulceration proximal to obstructing carcinoma. Surgery 1964;56:950–956.

Reeders JW, Rosenbusch G, Tytgat GN. Ischaemic colitis associated with carcinoma of the colon. Eur J Radiol 1982;2:41–47.

Toner M, Condell D, O'Briain DS. Obstructive colitis: ulceroinflammatory lesions occurring proximal to colonic obstruction. Am J Surg Pathol 1990;14:719–728.

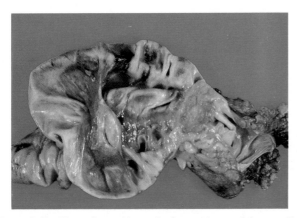

Figure 5–40. Obstructive cecitis proximal to carcinoma of the ascending colon. Note the cecal ulceration.

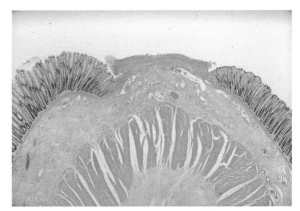

Figure 5–41. Obstructive colitis. Ulceration proximal to an obstructing carcinoma.

BACTERIAL (INFECTIOUS, SELF-LIMITED) COLITIS

Biology of Disease

■ Infectious colitis is primarily caused by *Campylobacter jejuni, Escherichia coli, Salmonella, Shigella,* and *Yersinia enterocolitica. Aeromonas* spp and *Pleisiomonas* spp may also produce diarrhea. Viruses (see Chapter 3) and specific protozoa are dealt with elsewhere.

■ Most bacteria that cause colitis colonize the bowel or invade the mucosa and produce toxins or factors that resist host defenses. Adherence or colonization factors allow bacteria to adhere to epithelium or mucus, proliferate, and resist clearance by the flow of bowel contents. These mechanisms are varied and are currently the subject of investigation. Adherence is mediated through surface fimbriae (pili). In some strains of *E. coli* (enteropathogenic and enterohemorrhagic), initial adherence is followed by formation of an extremely close attachment of bacterial and epithelial surface membranes with effacement of microvilli. This mode of adherence is called *attachment-effacement.*

■ There are two main classes of toxin—enterotoxins and cytotoxins. *Enterotoxins* cause diarrhea by promoting fluid secretion by crypt epithelium (studied experimentally in rabbit ileal loops). For example, cholera toxin and related heat-labile toxins stimulate cyclic AMP, which in turn evokes fluid secretion. *Cytotoxins* damage or kill cells. Shiga toxin, the toxin of *Shigella dysenteriae* 1 and of enterohemorrhagic *E. coli,* inhibits protein synthesis thereby causing cell death.

■ Proctitis due to *Neisseria gonorrhoeae, Treponema pallidum, Chlamydia trachomatis* (lymphogranuloma venereum (LGV) and non-LGV serotypes), herpes simplex, and cytomegalovirus may be transmitted sexually.

■ Antibiotic-induced diarrhea with colitis is a form of infectious colitis related to selective bacterial overgrowth.

■ *Acute self-limited colitis* is a term that describes an episode of acute self-limited diarrhea of infectious type. On culture, only 50% of such cases yield a bacterial pathogen.

Clinical Features

■ Two major clinical presentations are acute watery diarrhea and dysentery (acute or chronic diarrhea with blood). Classically, dysentery is caused by *Shigella* spp but may be due to verotoxin-producing *E. coli,* enteroinvasive *E. coli, Salmonella* spp, *Campylobacter jejuni,* and *Entamoeba histolytica.*

■ Other symptoms are tenesmus, fever, malaise, and abdominal cramps.

■ Acute infectious colitis is usually self-limited and requires only supportive care and fluids.

Gross Pathology

■ Endoscopically, generalized or patchy erythema can mimic inflammatory bowel disease. Aphthoid ulcers are characteristic of *Yersinia* but are also seen in salmonellosis or shigellosis. Extensive ulceration is uncommon but may be a feature of severe dysentery or enterohemorrhagic *E. coli* infection.

Microscopic Pathology

■ Infectious colitis is characterized by edema, neutrophil infiltration (including cryptitis and crypt abscesses), preservation of crypt architecture, capillary congestion, minimal increase in mononuclear cells, superficial predominance of inflammation, and absence of plasmacytosis at the base of the mucosa.

Special Techniques

■ Stool culture is the main diagnostic modality. Specific media and culture techniques are used for specific organisms.

Differential Diagnosis

Ulcerative colitis, Crohn's disease, segmental colitis, diversion colitis.

Idiopathic ulcerative colitis is distinguished by its clinical chronicity, crypt architectural changes, Paneth cell metaplasia, crypt atrophy, basal plasmacytosis, and diffuse disease.

Crohn's colitis is differentiated by clinical chronicity, the focal or patchy nature of the inflammatory process, predominance of inflammation in the lower half of the mucosa, ulceration, and granuloma formation.

Segmental colitis associated with diverticular disease is not histologically distinctive but must be considered when there is inflammation of the mucosa of the sigmoid.

The diagnosis of diversion colitis relies heavily on the history. It may resemble infection or inflammatory bowel disease.

References

Day DW, Mandal BK, Morson BC. The rectal biopsy appearances in *Salmonella* colitis. Histopathology 1978;2:117–131.

Farthing MJG, Keusch GT. Enteric Infection. Mechanisms, manifestations and management. London: Chapman and Hall, 1989.

Kumar NB, Nostrant TT, Appelman HD. The histopathologic spectrum of acute self-limited colitis (acute infectious-type colitis). Am J Surg Pathol 1982;6:523–529.

Lambert PE, Schofield PF, Ironside AG, Mandal BK. Campylobacter colitis. Br Med J 1979;1:857–859.

Loss RW, Mangla JC, Perera M. *Campylobacter* colitis presenting as inflammatory bowel disease with segmental colonic ulcerations. Gastroenterology 1980;79:138–140.

McGovern VJ, Slavutin LJ. Pathology of *Salmonella* colitis. Am J Surg Pathol 1979;2:483–490.

Shigellosis

Biology of Disease

■ Shigellae are nonmotile, gram-negative rods that are closely related to E. coli but do not ferment lactose. The genus *Shigella* contains four species: *S. dysenteriae, S. flexneri, S. boydii, and S. sonnei*. The predominant species are now *S. flexneri and S. sonnei. Shigella dysenteriae* type 1 has declined in importance since the early part of the century for unknown reasons but is still a significant pathogen in some underdeveloped countries. *Shigella boydii* is mainly encountered in India and Bangladesh. Shigellosis is endemic in tropical and subtropical underdeveloped parts of Africa, Southern Asia, and Central America, which lack water treatment and sanitation. Seasonal outbreaks and periodic regional epidemics are associated with significant morbidity and mortality.

■ Shigellae invade epithelial cells and produce a potent cytotoxin, Shiga's toxin. *Shigella dysenteriae* type 1 produces a thousandfold more Shiga's toxin than other species. The toxin is composed of one enzymatic A subunit and five receptor-binding B subunits. The intestinal receptor is the glycolipid Gb_3. After binding, the A subunit is internalized, inhibits protein synthesis, and causes cell death. Absorbed toxin circulates in the blood stream and is the likely cause of the hemolytic uremic syndrome (HUS, consisting of microangiopathic hemolytic anemia, thrombocytopenia, and renal failure).

Clinical Features

■ The majority of cases of shigellosis occur in children under 5 years of age. Breastfed infants under 6 months of age are spared because of immunity from breast milk antibodies.

■ *Shigella* is transmitted by the fecal-oral route, and clinical infection may result from very small numbers of bacteria. Water, food, and person-to-person contact are the vehicles of transmission. Though acid sensitive in vitro, *Shigella* appears resistant to gastric acid in vivo and hypochlorhydric patients do not have increased susceptibility.

■ *Shigella dysenteriae* type 1 is a virulent bacterium that causes severe dysentery with considerable mortality. *Shigella flexneri* is less virulent and may cause diarrhea or dysentery. *Shigella sonnei* infection is usually a self-limited watery diarrhea with fever lasting 48 to 72 hours. The diarrhea is mainly due to an absorption defect in the colon.

■ Classic dysentery (from *S. dysenteriae type* 1) begins with fever, abdominal cramps, and watery diarrhea. Within hours, the stools become frequent, low volume, bloody, and mucoid. Defecation is accompanied by intense abdominal pain and tenesmus, and straining at stool may cause rectal prolapse. Fever may reach 39°C or higher and is unresponsive to antipyretic agents.

■ Complications include a fulminant course and HUS. In shigellosis that runs a fulminant course with extensive ulceration and toxic megacolon, spontaneous perforation results in fecal peritonitis and 50% mortality. Either HUS or thrombotic thrombocytopenic purpura (TTP; HUS with fever and seizures or other neurologic manifestations) occurs almost exclusively with *S. dysenteriae* type 1 infection; it is a self-limited condition if the patient survives the acute renal failure.

■ Malnourished children fail to develop fever and, despite antibiotic therapy, may develop chronic colitis lasting weeks or months with persistently positive stool cultures. This chronic infection may exacerbate malnutrition and is life-threatening. The terminal event is often secondary bacteremia or pneumonia.

■ The cornerstone of treatment is antibiotic therapy with either ampicillin or trimethoprim-sulfamethoxazole. Bacterial resistance is a major problem. Nalidixic acid is effective in most resistant cases. In infants, supportive care consists mainly of maintaining nutrition, because dehydration is not a major problem.

Gross Pathology

■ The extent of involvement of the colon is variable in *S. dysenteriae* type 1 infection. The rectum is affected in 90% of cases. The rectosigmoid alone is affected in some cases. Some cases involve the entire colon and terminal ileum. Subtotal involvement is most common. In the initial stage, the disease is continuous. It becomes patchy with intervening normal mucosa during recovery. The endoscopic appearances of *S. dysenteriae* type 1 infection vary with the duration from onset of illness. The earliest abnormality is mucosal edema, appearing as swollen pale mucosa with loss of vascular pattern, sometimes sufficient to compromise the lumen. Ulceration and mucosal friability develop next. The ulcers are small, discrete, starshaped or serpiginous, and uncommonly linear or aphthoid. Punctate discrete mucosal hemorrhages are seen in all patients throughout the course of the disease. Pseudomembranes were present in 20% of fatal cases in Bangladesh. Other species of *Shigella* produce milder disease.

Microscopic Pathology

■ Biopsy findings in *S. dysenteriae* type 1 infection include edema, congestion, focal hemorrhages, crypt hyperplasia, goblet cell depletion, polymorphonuclear cell infiltration, and micro-ulcers. Marginating neutrophils, crypt abscesses, and capillary thrombi are sometimes seen. Micro-ulcers with associated inflammatory exudate are sometimes present. Abnormalities of crypt architecture comprising crypt dilatation and branching (simulating idiopathic ulcerative colitis) are present in a high proportion of cases. Increased mononuclear cells may be seen in prolonged cases.

References

Anand BS, Malnotra V, Bhattacharya SK, et al. Rectal histology in acute bacillary dysentery. Gastroenterology 1986;90:654–660.

Butler T, Dunn D, Dahus B, Islam M. Causes of death and the histopathologic findings in fatal shigellosis. Pediatr Infect Dis 1989;8:767–772.

Kelber M, Ament ME. *Shigella dysenteriae* 1: a forgotten cause of pseudomembranous colitis. J Pediatr 1976;89:595–596.

Khuroo MS, Mahajan R, Zargar SA, et al. The colon in shigellosis: serial colonoscopic appearances in *Shigella dysenteriae 1*. Endoscopy 1990; 22:35–38.

McElfatrick RA, Wurtzbach LR. Collar-button ulcers of the colon in a case of shigellosis. Gastroenterology 1973;65:303–307.

Speelman P, Kabir I, Moyenal I. Distribution and spread of colonic lesions in shigellosis: a colonoscopic study. J Infect Dis 1984;150:899–903.

Enterohemorrhagic *Escherichia coli*

Biology of Disease

■ *E. coli* O157:H7 and several other serotypes produce large amounts of Shiga's toxin or Shiga-like toxin (verotoxins) and cause outbreaks of hemorrhagic diarrhea with colitis. These strains have been called enterohemorrhagic *E. coli* (EHEC) and verotoxin-producing *E. coli* (VTEC). *E. coli* serotype O157:H7 accounts for 90% of cases.

■ EHEC is the major cause of sporadic HUS and also causes some cases of TTP. Human and experimental studies support the notion that systemic Shiga's toxemia may mediate HUS or TTP and that the endothelial cells are the targets of the toxin.

■ The bacteria are transmitted by ground beef and by contaminated water or food.

■ Outbreaks of infection may derive from restaurants, daycare centers, or nursing homes for the handicapped or elderly. Institutional outbreaks have had mortality rates of up to 26%.

Clinical features

■ *E. coli* O157:H7 produces a spectrum of effect, from asymptomatic infection through mild diarrhea to hemorrhagic colitis complicated by fatal HUS.

■ Crampy abdominal pain is followed shortly by watery diarrhea. Within 48 hours, the diarrhea becomes grossly bloody, and the bloody diarrhea lasts 3 to 4 days. Then the diarrhea gradually wanes. Fever is uncommon and never high.

■ In well-documented outbreaks, bloody diarrhea occurs in one third to two thirds of all patients.

Gross Pathology

■ The main lesions are located in the right side of the colon. The main finding on radiography is thumbprinting. Endoscopic findings are erythema, edema, hemorrhage, erosions, ulcers, and pseudomembranes.

■ Resected colons may show patchy shallow ulcers in cecum and ascending colon or a severe diffuse colitis with extensive ulceration, pseudomembranes, mucosal and submucosal hemorrhage, and submucosal edema that may cause luminal narrowing or obliteration.

Microscopic Pathology

■ The spectrum of changes in colonoscopic biopsies include normal areas, neutrophil infiltrates and edema resembling those in any infectious colitis, appearances similar to ischemia, and pseudomembranous colitis similar to that seen with *Clostridium difficile*.

■ Ischemic changes consist of mucosal epithelial loss or attenuation, hyalinization of lamina propria, and paucity of inflammatory cells. Reported cases of "transient ischemic colitis" in young patients were likely examples of EHEC infection.

Special Techniques

■ *E. coli* O157:H7 is selected by culture on sorbitol-MacConkey agar and identified by serotyping in a reference laboratory. Toxins can be sought by nucleic acid probes. The older toxin neutralization test (testing the effect of toxin on cultured cells) is not widely used.

Differential Diagnosis

Infectious colitis, pseudomembranous colitis, ischemic colitis, and idiopathic inflammatory bowel disease.

Other causes of infectious colitis are indistinguishable if the biopsy shows only neutrophil infiltration, edema, congestion, and normal crypt architecture.

Distinction of the pseudomembranous lesions caused by shigellae or *E. coli* from those caused by *C. difficile* is impossible. Infection with *C. difficile* follows antibiotic treatment, however, and is not associated with bloody diarrhea.

Ischemia may be impossible to distinguish histologically from EHEC unless some of the biopsy specimens show features of infectious colitis.

Idiopathic inflammatory bowel disease shows abnormal crypt architecture, increased chronic inflammatory cells, and basal preponderance of the inflammation.

References

Eidus LB, Guindi M, Drouin J, et al. Colitis caused by *Escherichia coli* O157:H7: a study of six cases. Can J Gastroenterol 1990;4:141–146.

Griffin PM, Olmstead LC, Petras RE. *Escherichia coli* O157:H7–associated colitis: a clinical and histological study of 11 cases. Gastroenterology 1990;99:142–149.

Karmali MA, Petric M, Lim C, et al. The association between idiopathic hemolytic uremic syndrome and infection by verotoxin-producing *Escherichia coli* O157:H7. J Infect Dis 1985;151:775–782.

Kelly JK, Oryshak A, Wenetsek M, et al. The colonic pathology of *Escherichia coli* O157:H7 infection. Am J Surg Pathol 1990;14:87–92.

Pai CH, Ahmed N, Lior H, et al. Epidemiology of sporadic diarrhea due to verocytotoxin-producing *Escherichia coli* (VTEC): a two-year prospective study. J Infect Dis 1988;157:1054–1057.

Richardson SE, Karmali MA, Becker LE, Smith CR. The histopathology of the hemolytic uremic syndrome associated with verocytotoxin-producing *Escherichia coli* infections. Hum Pathol 1988;19:1102–1108.

Riley LW, Remis RS, Helgerson SD, et al. Outbreaks of hemorrhagic colitis associated with a rare *E. coli* serotype. N Engl J Med 1983;308:681–685.

Salmonella Infection

Biology of Disease

■ Human salmonellosis may be associated with four distinct clinical syndromes—an asymptomatic carrier state, enterocolitis, enteric fever, and septicemia with metastatic suppurative foci. Typhoid (enteric) fever may be caused by *S. typhi* and *S. enteritidis*, serotypes paratyphi A or B (see Chapter 3).

■ Nontyphoid *Salmonella* are transmitted from domestic animals, particularly poultry, in eggs, milk, or meat, or by shellfish. Patients with sickle cell disease, other hemolytic diseases, and hypochlorhydria have greater susceptibility to infection.

Clinical Features

■ Nontyphoid *Salmonella* cause nausea, vomiting, fever, abdominal pain, and diarrhea within 8 to 36 hours of ingestion of contaminated food. Diarrhea is usually watery, although it may be bloody. *Salmonella* infection is a common cause of infectious enterocolitis in healthy individuals and in patients with inflammatory bowel disease. Rectal endoscopic appearances may resemble those of idiopathic ulcerative colitis.

■ Fluids and electrolytes are the mainstays of treatment, and antibiotic treatment is not beneficial in the absence of septicemia or persistent symptoms.

Gross Pathology and Microscopic Pathology

■ These are similar to those of other infectious colitides.

References

Candy DCA, Stephen J. *Salmonella*. In: Farthing MJG, Keusch GT (eds). Enteric Infection: Mechanisms, Manifestations and Management. London: Chapman and Hall, 1989;289–298.

Day DW, Mandal BK, Morson BC. The rectal biopsy appearances in *Salmonella* colitis. Histopathology 1978;2:117–131.

Lindeman RJ, Weinstein L, Levitan R, Patterson JF. Ulcerative colitis and intestinal salmonellosis. Am J Med Sci 1967;254:855–861.

McGovern VJ, Slavutin LJ. Pathology of *Salmonella* colitis. Am J Surg Pathol 1979;2:483–490.

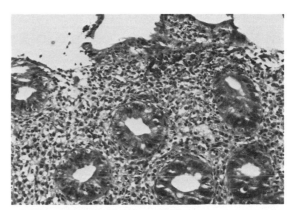

Figure 5–42. Infectious colitis. Normal crypt architecture, minimal increase in mononuclear cells, edema, and superficial neutrophil infiltrate with cryptitis.

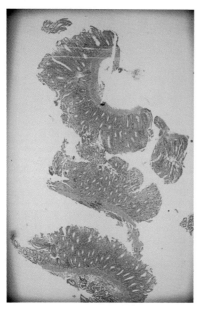

Figure 5–43. *Shigella flexneri* infection. The mucosa appears hypercellular, there is superficial mucosal damage, and the crypt architecture is preserved.

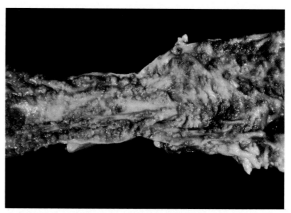

Figure 5–46. *Escherichia coli* O157:H7 colitis with a pseudomembranous pattern. (Courtesy of Dr Cynthia Trevenen.)

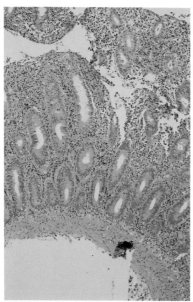

Figure 5–44. *Shigella flexneri* infection. The surface is ulcerated and the crypt architecture is preserved.

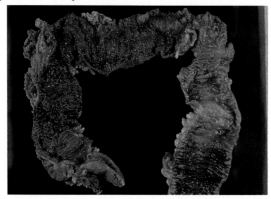

Figure 5–45. *Escherichia coli* O157:H7 infection causing hemorrhagic colitis with skip lesions. (Courtesy of Dr. Leslie Eidus.)

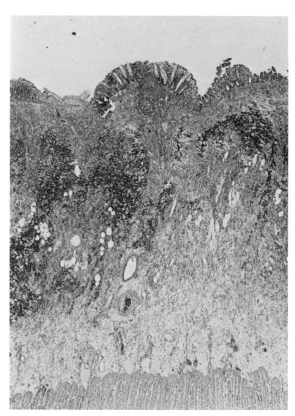

Figure 5–47. *Escherichia coli* O157:H7 infection. There is ulceration, but the most notable feature is extreme submucosal edema and hemorrhage (black material).

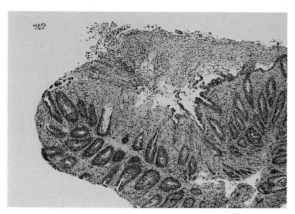

Figure 5–48. *Escherichia coli* O157:H7 colitis. Biopsy specimen displays pseudomembranous colitis.

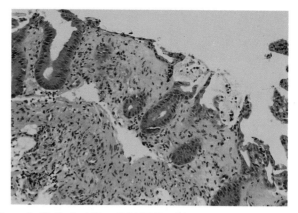

Figure 5–49. *Escherichia coli* O157:H7 colitis. Biopsy specimen displays an ischemic pattern with hyalinization of lamina propria.

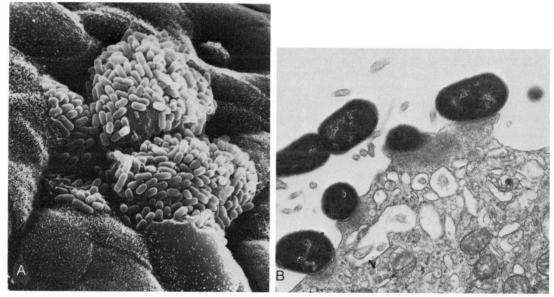

Figure 5–50. *Escherichia coli* O157:H7 infection. *A,* Bacteria adhere to surface epithelium. *B,* Transmission electron micrograph showing attachment-effacement in rabbit cecum.

PSEUDOMEMBRANOUS COLITIS

Biology of Disease

- Pseudomembranous colitis (PMC) is a form of colitis in which plaques of inflammatory exudate form a pseudomembrane on the mucosal surface.
- The principal cause is *Clostridium difficile*; others are verotoxin-producing (enterohemorrhagic) *Escherichia coli, Shigella dysenteriae,* other clostridia, and occasionally ischemia.
- The great majority of *C. difficile*–associated PMC follows the use of antibiotics, particularly clindamycin, ampicillin, and the cephalosporins. Nosocomial outbreaks due

to transmission of the organism between patients account for most cases. Sporadic cases also occur.
- *Clostridium difficile* produces two main toxins, toxin A and toxin B. Toxin A is thought to mediate the PMC. Many strains of *C. difficile* are nontoxigenic and do not produce PMC.

Clinical Features

- Patients present with watery diarrhea, intermittent fever, and abdominal pain that is sometimes colicky and severe. The diarrhea may be rich in mucus and protein, causing hypokalemia and hypoalbuminemia. Disease usually lasts for days but may persist up to 2 months.

- Severe cases may also be complicated by blood loss and anemia.
- Fulminant disease (toxic dilatation, perforation, or severe bleeding) is uncommon.

Gross Pathology

- The colon displays multiple, elevated, yellowish white plaques against a background of normal mucosa. Plaques vary from pinpoint size to 3 cm.
- The right side of the colon is most severely affected. The rectosigmoid may be spared completely or may show smaller, less numerous lesions. The terminal ileum is rarely involved.
- Sometimes abundant mucus is adherent to the surface.
- On sectioning, the bowel shows extreme submucosal edema, and if the patient has thrombocytopenia or a hemorrhagic diathesis, hemorrhage may be present. Hemorrhage is not a feature of most cases.

Microscopic Pathology

- The earliest pseudomembranous lesion follows destruction of the surface epithelium between adjacent crypts. An eruptive exudate, composed of fibrin and mucin with files of neutrophils, arises from the ulcerated surface. The exudate remains firmly attached to the mucosa. More advanced lesions show confluent surface exudate, increasing crypt dilatation, and destruction of the crypt epithelium. In the most severe lesions, the mucosa underlying the pseudomembrane is completely necrotic. The crypts are distended with mucus.
- Mucosal capillaries are markedly congested and contain marginating neutrophils. Occasional capillary thrombi are noted.
- The submucosa shows marked edema and infiltration by immunoblasts and plasma cells. Occasionally, capillary thrombi, fibrin-rich exudate, and hemorrhage are present.
- The mucosa outside the pseudomembranes may have the features of infectious colitis—edema, capillary congestion, and neutrophil infiltration.

Special Diagnostic Techniques

- Stool filtrates are assayed for the toxins of *C. difficile* either by latex fixation tests or by cytotoxicity test. Stool culture for *C. difficile* may also be performed.

Differential Diagnosis

Ischemia, enterohemorrhagic *E. coli*, prolapsing mucosa, amebiasis, cytomegalovirus infection.

Ischemic pseudomembranes are usually diffuse sheets confined to the area of ischemia, not the multiple scattered plaques seen in PMC.

Shigella dysenteriae, *E. coli* O157: H7, and other enterohemorrhagic *E. coli* form Shiga's toxin or Shiga-like toxins (verotoxins) and may cause pseudomembranes identical to those produced by *C. difficile*. More often, infections with the former show features of infectious or ischemic colitis. *Escherichia coli* O157: H7 grows on Sorbitol-MacConkey agar, is virtually always toxin producing and causes hemorrhagic diarrhea, unlike the watery diarrhea seen in PMC.

Prolapsing mucosa or solitary rectal ulcer syndrome may show surface ulceration and exudation resembling pseudomembranes, but the associated villiform change, muscularization of the lamina propria, and history of isolated rectal lesions should void any confusion with PMC.

Amebiasis and cytomegalovirus infection produce surface ulceration and exudate that lacks the explosive character of PMC.

Heavy metal poisoning, staphyloccal infection, uremia, and leukemia have been associated with PMC.

References

Bartlett JG, Moon N, Chang TW, et al. Role of *Clostridium difficile* in antibiotic-associated pseudomembranous colitis. Gastroenterology 1978;75:778–782.

Goulston SJM, McGovern VJ. Pseudomembranous colitis. Gut 1965;6:207–212.

Price AB, Davies DR. Pseudomembranous colitis. J Clin Pathol 1977;30:1–7.

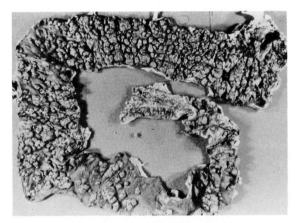

Figure 5–51. Pseudomembranous colitis due to *Clostridium difficile* in a patient taking clindamycin. Each yellow plaque is a pseudomembrane.

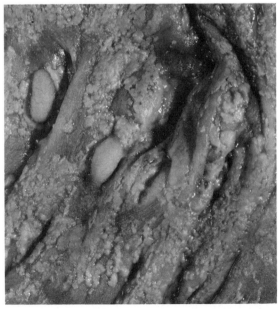

Figure 5–52. Pseudomembranous colitis due to *Clostridium difficile*.

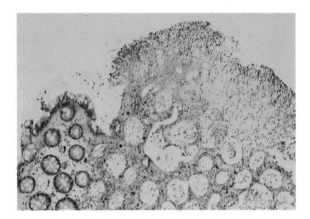

Figure 5–53. Pseudomembranous colitis in an endoscopic biopsy. The pseudomembrane (*right*) covers ulcerated mucosa and dilated crypts.

AMEBIASIS

Biology of Disease

- *Amebiasis* is caused by the protozoan parasite *Entamoeba histolytica*, which is transmitted by the fecal-oral route.
- The World Health Organization (WHO) estimates that in 1990, amebiasis caused 40,000 to 60,000 deaths worldwide. In 1981, WHO estimated that 480 million people carried amebiasis worldwide and that about 36 million of them had significant colitis.
- Though worldwide in distribution, amebiasis is most prevalent in the tropics and subtropics, where sanitation is lacking.
- In developed countries, most new infections are found among foreign travelers, recent immigrants, and homosexual men.
- *E. histolytica* may cause acute colitis, chronic colitis, or an asymptomatic carrier state. Blood-borne dissemination may result in amebic abscesses in liver or other organs.
- Not all *E. histolytica* are pathogenic: Specific enzyme patterns known as zymodemes have been used to identify pathogenic strains.

Clinical Features

- Acute amebic colitis manifests as low-volume diarrhea, hematochezia, mucus, crampy abdominal pain, and, if there is rectal involvement, tenesmus. The symptoms may resemble those of bacillary dysentery or inflammatory bowel disease.
- In chronic cases, there may be episodic attacks of diarrhea with occasional hematochezia, abdominal pain, general malaise, anorexia, and anemia. These can also masquerade as inflammatory bowel disease.
- A localized ameboma (tumorlike inflammatory mass) may cause colonic obstruction or intussusception.
- The organism may disseminate from the colon, resulting in liver abscesses. Less commonly, abscesses in lung, brain, pericardium, and other tissues can occur. Corticosteroid therapy predisposes to colonic invasion and dissemination.

- Rarely, in southern Africa, or South America, fulminant colitis with ileus occurs; it has a very high mortality.

Gross Pathology

- Endoscopically, the mucosa has a friable, erythematous, granular appearance that resembles that of idiopathic inflammatory bowel disease. There may be small, shallow, discrete ulcers or larger undermined ulcers separated by normal mucosa.
- Amebic ulcers may be limited to one part of the colon or dispersed throughout the colon. The most commonly involved site is the cecum. The ileum is rarely involved.
- Sometimes, the colon may display multiple discrete, raised, shaggy plaques of exudate. In addition, there is undermining ulceration, best seen on cross-section (collar-stud ulcers). Fistula is a rare complication.
- An ameboma or amebic pseudotumor is an uncommon localized, inflammatory, tumorlike lesion that may cause an annular constriction of the cecum or colon that resembles carcinoma both radiologically and grossly.
- First-line treatment consists of metronidazole and diloxanide furoate. If dysentery is severe, emetine hydrochloride and tetracycline are given.

Microscopic Pathology

- Endoscopic biopsies show neutrophil infiltrates in the epithelium and lamina propria, congested capillaries with marginated neutrophils, and surface intercrypt ulcers and exudate that may resemble the features of PMC.
- Amebae may be found only in surface exudate or mucus. Therefore, every fragment of mucus received with colonic biopsy specimens should be processed histologically.
- In resected specimens, classic flask-shaped ulcers extend through the muscularis mucosae and undermine the mucosa. The ulcer base displays a thin zone of "dirty" necrosis separating the amebae, which sit in the ulcer cavity, from viable tissue. Amebae may occasionally be found beneath the zone of necrosis within the tissue.
- The inflammatory response includes abundant plasma cells. Eosinophils are generally not prominent.

- Histologically, amebomas display florid granulation tissue with fibrosis and sinuses containing clusters of trophozoites.
- Two forms of *E. histolytica* are identified—trophozoites and cysts. Only trophozoites are seen in tissue. They usually measure 15 to 25 μm in diameter. The transmissible cyst passed in the stool is a multinucleate form that, in its fully developed stage, contains four nuclei and measures 10 to 20 μm in diameter. An immature cyst may contain two or three nuclei.
- In tissues, *E. histolytica* is definitively identified because it contains phagocytosed erythrocytes.

Special Diagnostic Techniques

- *E. histolytica* stains positively with periodic acid–Schiff (PAS) stain.
- Antiamebic antibodies are of limited value in intestinal disease but are nearly always present in high titer in amebic liver abscess.

Differential Diagnosis

Entamoeba coli infection, macrophages, *Balantidium coli* infection.

Nonpathogenic *E. coli* do not phagocytose blood cells.

Macrophages may be difficult to distinguish from amebae and may also ingest red blood cells. Macrophages may be PAS positive and diastase resistant, whereas amebae are glycogen rich.

Balantidium coli is much larger than *E. histolytica* and, with its homogeneous hyperchromatic macronucleus, is highly distinctive.

References

Connor DH, Neafie RC, Meyers WM. Amoebiasis. In: Binford CH, Connor DH (eds). Pathology of Tropical and Extraordinary Disease. Washington, DC: Armed Forces Institute of Pathology, 1976;308–316.

Pittman FE, El-Hashimi WK, Pittman JC. Studies of human amoebiasis. Gastroenterology 1973;65:588–603

Prathap K, Gilman R. The histopathology of acute intestinal amoebiasis. Am J Pathol 1970;60:229–245.

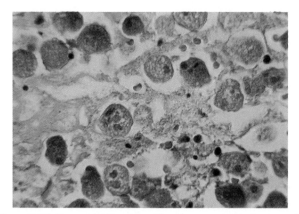

Figure 5–54. *Entamoeba histolytica*. Note that several organisms contain red cells.

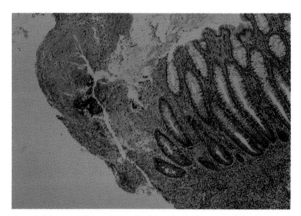

Figure 5–56. Amebic colitis. Focal mucosal necrosis with necrotic debris.

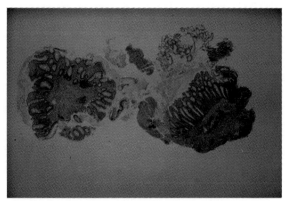

Figure 5–55. Amebic colitis. Focal necrosis at *right*.

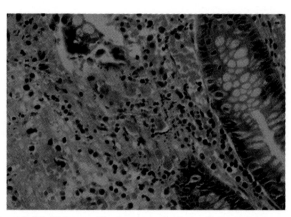

Figure 5–57. High magnification shows amebae at the base of the necrotic lesion.

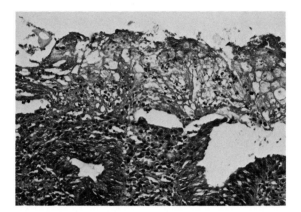

Figure 5–58. Amebic colitis mimicking pseudomembranous colitis.

LYMPHOGRANULOMA VENEREUM

Biology of Disease

- *Lymphogranuloma venereum* (LGV) is a sexually transmitted disease caused by serovars D through K of the obligate intracellular organism *Chlamydia trachomatis*. It affects the rectum following anal intercourse. Non-LGV strains of chlamydia can also produce proctitis, particularly in homosexual men.
- A 3-week course of tetracycline is usually effective treatment for chlamydial proctitis.

Clinical Features

- Patients present with anal pain, tenesmus, and blood-stained discharge.

Gross Pathology

- Endoscopically, the mucosa may be erythematous, friable, nodular, or ulcerated.
- Untreated rectal LGV causes chronic ulceration, thickening of the wall, and severe stenosis. Burnt-out lesions show a smooth, intact mucosa. The anus may be scarred and stenotic with bridging of the perianal skin.
- Squamous cell carcinoma of the anus may arise in long-standing strictures.

Microscopic Pathology

- Rectal biopsy specimens from acute chlamydial proctitis show active chronic inflammation with crypt abscesses and granulomas, a picture that closely resembles that of Crohn's disease. Following treatment, the mucosa shows regenerative features.

Special Diagnostic Techniques

- Culture of rectal swabs or biopsy specimens for chlamydia is the gold standard for diagnosis. Enzyme-linked immunosorbent assay (ELISA) for chlamydial antigens is also widely used.

Differential Diagnosis

Crohn's disease.

Crohn's disease is distinguished by involvement of other parts of the bowel, negative chlamydial cultures, and absence of a history of anal intercourse.

References

Levin I, Romano S, Steinberg M, Welsh RA. Lymphogranuloma venereum: rectal stricture and carcinoma. Dis Colon Rectum 1974;7:129–134.
Levine JS, Smith PD, Brudge WR. Chronic proctitis in male homosexuals due to lymphogranuloma venereum. Gastroenterology 1980;79:563–565.
Quinn TC, Goodell SE, Mkrtichian E, et al. Chlamydia trachomatis proctitis. N Engl J Med 1981;305:195–200.

Balantidium coli INFECTION

Biology of Disease

- *Balantidium coli* is a ciliated protozoan capable of causing a colitis or appendicitis similar to amebiasis. It is more commonly an asymptomatic parasite than a pathogen.
- In the tropics, *Balantidium* is a common parasite of pigs and primates.
- The mode of transmission is believed to be fecal-oral.
- The infection is treated by tetracycline. Alternative treatments are metronidazole and di-iodohydroxyquin.

Clinical Features

- Three states of infection are recognized—an asymptomatic carrier state, a chronic diarrheal disorder, and a severe colitic form.

■ Asymptomatic carriers may spread the infection within institutions.
■ The chronic diarrheal stage is characterized by watery or mucous bowel motions with few organisms.
■ In the severe colitic type of disease, diarrhea with mucus and blood, abdominal pain, nausea, weight loss, dehydration, tenesmus, and fever are seen. Rarely, the illness may be fulminant with extraintestinal dissemination to the peritoneum, urinary tract, vagina, liver, lung, or pleura.

Gross Pathology

■ The appearances may be similar to those in amebiasis, with multiple ulcers of varying sizes showing undermined edges. The ulcers are separated by congested mucosa.

Microscopic Pathology

■ *Balantidium coli* is an oval organism measuring between 15 and 100 μm in its long axis. It displays a large, dense, variably shaped macronucleus, cytoplasmic vacuoles and granules, and, on occasion, a small micronucleus.
■ Balantidia cluster at the bases of crypts. They are capable of penetrating through intact mucosa and muscularis mucosae to reach the submucosa. They may also be seen in the bases of ulcers and in the tissues near the margins of ulcers.
■ The inflammatory response consists predominantly of lymphocytes and plasma cells, but eosinophils may be present in large numbers.
■ The organisms tend to be found in clusters. Sometimes they are within blood vessels or lymphatics. They may migrate to lymph nodes.

Differential Diagnosis

Amebiasis.
   Entamoeba histolytica is much smaller than *B. coli*, does not have a macronucleus, and may contain ingested red blood cells.

References

Arean VM, Koppisch E. Balantidiasis, a review and report of cases. Am J Pathol 1956;32:1089–1109.
Baskerville L, Ahmed Y, Ramchand S. Balantidium colitis: report of a case. Am J Dig Dis 1970;15:722–731.
Castro J, Vazquez-Iglesias JL, Arnal-Monreal F. Dysentery caused by *Balantidium coli*—report of two cases. Endoscopy 1983;15:272–274.
Dorfman S, Rangel O, Bravo LG. Balantidiasis: report of a fatal case with appendicular and pulmonary involvement. Trans R Soc Trop Med Hyg 1984;78:833–834.
Neafie RC. Balantidiasis. In: Binford CH, Connor DH (eds). Pathology of Tropical and Extraordinary Diseases, Vol 1. Washington, DC: Armed Forces Institute of Pathology, 1976;325–327.
Walzer PD, Judson FN, Murphy KB, et al. Balantidiasis: outbreak in Truk. Am J Trop Hyg 1973;22:33–41.

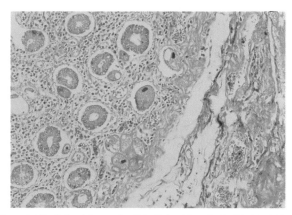

Figure 5–59. *Balantidium coli* colitis. Balantidium is signified by its large size and macronucleus.

SPIROCHETOSIS

Biology of Disease

■ *Intestinal spirochetosis* is an asymptomatic condition in which, rectal, colonic, or appendiceal surface epithelium is colonized by spiral bacteria. No inflammatory response is evoked.
■ Intestinal spirochetosis is caused by several different organisms. Some are related to the nonpathogenic spirochetes normally found in pigs.
■ The prevalence of spirochetosis appears to be diminishing in affluent Western countries, where prevalence rates vary between 1.5% and 7% in the general population. In promiscuous homosexual men, however, the rate is approximately 30% to 35%; a similar rate is reported in the general population in southern India, suggesting fecal-oral transmission.
■ Luminal antibiotics eradicate the organisms. Therefore, spirochetosis is rarely seen in resection specimens.

Clinical Features

■ Intestinal spirochetosis is an incidental finding in otherwise normal colorectal biopsy specimens or appendices.

Microscopic Pathology

■ Spirochetosis is identified on H&E-stained sections as a hematoxiphilic zone resembling an exaggerated brush border on the surface epithelium and upper portions of

the crypts. The bacteria attach at right angles to the surface epithelium.
■ Silver stains and electron microscopy confirm the diagnosis.

Special Diagnostic Techniques

■ The surface bacterial layer is periodic acid–Schiff positive and wider than normal.
■ Warthin-Starry, Steiner, and other silver stains display the individual spirochetes.

■ Electron microscopy demonstrates the organisms inserted at right angles in the epithelial surface between the microvilli.

References

MacMillan A, Lee FD. Sigmoidoscopic and microscopic appearance of the rectal mucosa in homosexual men. Gut 1984;93:1035–1041.
Parr LW. Intestinal spirochetes. J Infect Dis 1923;33:369–383.
Ruane PJ, Nakata MM, Reinhardt JF, George WL. Spirochete-like organisms in the human gastrointestinal tract. Rev Infect Dis 1989;11:184–196.

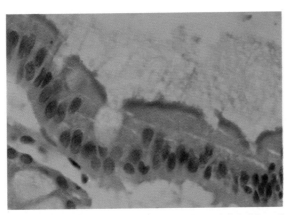

Figure 5–60. Rectal spirochetosis. The surface has a dark and fuzzy border.

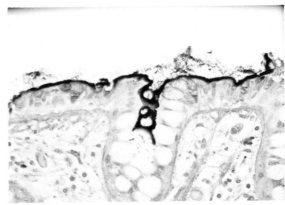

Figure 5–61. Rectal spirochetosis stained black by a silver stain (Steiner).

BEHÇET'S SYNDROME

Biology of Disease

■ Behçet's syndrome is a systemic disorder characterized by genital and oral ulcerations and a variety of other lesions—iritis or uveitis, thrombophlebitis, arthritis, and ulcerations of the gastrointestinal tract.

Clinical Features

■ Involvement of the gastrointestinal tract is a poor prognostic feature, and although there may be a response to corticosteroids, there is a high relapse rate.
■ The main sites of gastrointestinal involvement are the esophagus, colon and terminal ileum.
■ Gastrointestinal involvement may manifest as abdominal pain, bloody diarrhea, perforation, peritonitis, or anal ulceration.

Gross Pathology

■ The principal feature is ulceration of the mucosa. The ulcers vary in size from small (aphthoid) ulcers to larger discrete or confluent, serpiginous ulcers. Endoscopically, grossly, and microscopically, the morphology may be indistinguishable from that of Crohn's disease.

Microscopic Pathology

■ The ulcers have no specific morphologic features and may penetrate deep into the muscle coat. There may be an associated vasculitis of arteries or veins. Multiple sections of the vessels should be examined.
■ The intestinal lesions may be indistinguishable from those of Crohn's disease, and noncaseating granulomas may be present.

Differential Diagnosis

Crohn's disease, idiopathic ulcerative colitis, cytomegalovirus, idiopathic ulcerative jejunoileitis, Reiter's syndrome.

Crohn's disease does not have the clinical manifestations of Behçet's syndrome, particularly oral and genital ulcerations and vasculitis. In tissue specimens, the distinction may be impossible.

Idiopathic ulcerative colitis shows hemorrhagic rectocolitis, not the discrete ulcers seen in Behçet's syndrome.

Cytomegalovirus-associated ulcers show the viral inclusions in endothelial, mesenchymal, and epithelial cells.

Idiopathic ulcerative jejunoileitis does not involve the colon, is not associated with the systemic manifestations of Behçet's syndrome, and is associated with jejunal enteropathy.

Reiter's syndrome is a reactive seronegative polyarthritis that may follow dysentery or venereally acquired urethritis. Many affected patients possess the HLA-B27 antigen and have microscopic ileocolitis resembling Crohn's disease.

References

Baba S, Maruta M, Ando K, et al. Intestinal Behçet's disease: report of five cases. Dis Colon Rectum 1976;19: 428–440.

Chong SK, Wright VM, Nishigame T, et al. Infantile colitis: a manifestation of intestinal Behçet's syndrome. J Pediatr Gastrol Nutr 1988;7:622–627.

Kasahara Y, Tanaka S, Nishino N, et al. Intestinal involvement in Behçet's disease: review of 136 surgical cases in the Japanese literature. Dis Colon Rectum 1981;24:1103–1106.

Lakhanpal S, Tani K, Lie JT, et al. Pathological features of Behçet's syndrome: a review of Japanese autopsy data registry. Hum Pathol 1985;16:790–795.

Lee RG. The colitis of Behçet's syndrome. Am J Surg Pathol 1986;10:888–893.

Matsumoto T, Uekusa T, Fukuda Y. Vasculo-Behçet's disease: A pathologic study of eight cases. Hum Pathol 1991;22:45–51.

O'Connell DJ, Courtney JF, Riddell RH. Colitis of Behçet's Syndrome: radiological and pathologic features. Gastrointest Radiol 1980;5:173–179.

STERCORAL ULCERS

Biology of Disease

■ Stercoral ulcers are ulcers of the rectum or colon, secondary to the pressure of impacted feces.

Clinical Features

■ Most patients are elderly, bedridden, and constipated.
■ The principal complications are bleeding and perforation. Perforation may result in pericolic abscess and localized or generalized peritonitis.
■ Patients with paraplegia, cathartic colon, or chronic colonic pseudo-obstruction are subject to fecal impaction and stercoral ulceration.

Gross Pathology

■ The ulcers may be single or multiple and may conform to the shape of the distending mass of feces. The bowel wall may show stretching and thinning.
■ Perforation tends to occur in the central portions of ulcers, where there is maximal thinning of the wall. Fissurelike splits may also perforate.
■ Dilatation and perforation of the cecum can occur proximal to impacted feces, as can perforation of a diverticulum.

Microscopic Pathology

■ Stercoral ulcers show nonspecific features such as mucosal necrosis, granulation tissue, and bacterial colonies on the surface.
■ The inflammatory response is usually mild and confined to the ulcerated surface. Perforation may lead to perirectal abscess or localized peritonitis.

Differential Diagnosis

Localized ischemia.
Ischemic bowel usually shows infarction not just ulceration. Vasculitis or atheroembolism may cause multiple ulcers and are diagnosed by the characteristic vascular pathology.

The diagnosis of stercoral ulceration depends on the presence of impacted feces. In its absence, diagnosis is presumptive only.

References

Berardi RS, Lee S. Stercoraceous perforation of the colon: report of a case. Dis Colon Rectum 1983;26:283–286.

Grinvalsky HT, Bowerman CI. Stercoraceous ulcer of the colon: relatively neglected medical and surgical problem. JAMA 1959;171:1941–1946.

Wrenn K. Fecal impaction. N Engl J Med 1989;321:658–662.

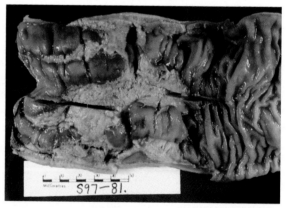

Figure 5–62. Stercoral ulceration adjacent to normal mucosa.

SOLITARY RECTAL ULCER SYNDROME

Biology of Disease

- *Solitary rectal ulcer syndrome* (SRUS) is local mucosal prolapse of the rectum that becomes secondarily ulcerated and indurated. SRUS is probably a result of incongruous contraction of the puborectalis on straining at stool. It is primarily a disease of young adult women. The prolapsing mucosa is usually on the anterior rectal wall (rarely lateral or posterior) and does not involve the entire rectal circumference.
- Mucosal prolapse is followed by venous congestion, ischemia, and mechanical trauma causing surface ulceration, regeneration, hemorrhage, hemosiderin deposition, and muscularization of the lamina propria with minimal inflammation.
- *Proctitis* (localized colitis) *cystica profunda* is a manifestation of SRUS in which crypts have been misplaced into the submucosa.
- *Inflammatory cloacogenic polyp* is a polypoid mucosal prolapse at the anorectal junction with histologic features similar to those of SRUS. Prolapsing internal hemorrhoid is similar but includes dilated submucosal veins.

Clinical Features

- Patients are young healthy adults of either sex in their 20s or 30s.
- Rectal bleeding is the most common symptom. The amounts of blood are slight in most cases.
- Mucus in the stool, anorectal discomfort, and tenesmus are commonly present.
- Patients may have a sense of anal blockage and may use digital manipulation to assist defecation.

Gross Pathology

- Rectal examination reveals an area of thickening on the anterior wall at 6 to 10 cm above the anal verge.
- At endoscopy, the anterior rectal mucosa is indurated, pale, or congested and may show one or more ulcers. The area often has a distinctly nodular appearance and may be confused with carcinoma.

Microscopic Pathology

- The crypts are elongated, branched, and dilated, imparting a villiform appearance. The tops of the villiform projections may be ulcerated and covered by pseudomembranous exudate. Focally, hyperplastic and serrated crypts resembling hyperplastic polyps may be present.
- The lamina propria is muscularized and depleted of mononuclear cells. Muscle fibers grow up into the lamina propria from the hypertrophied muscularis mucosae. The capillaries are congested. There may be hemosiderin deposition in the mucosa or submucosa.
- Crypts may be displaced into the submucosa, a condition known as colitis (or proctitis) cystica profunda.

Differential Diagnosis

Adenoma, pseudomembranous colitis, radiation proctitis, ischemia, inflammatory cloacogenic polyp, rectal prolapse, prolapsing internal hemorrhoid.

The hyperchromatic regenerating crypts in SRUS may simulate tubular or villous adenoma, but adenomas do not have muscularized lamina propria. Prominent smooth muscle bundles associated with hyperchromatic glands may be mistaken for carcinoma, but the severe epithelial dysplasia and desmoplastic reaction of carcinoma are missing.

The surface exudate of SRUS may simulate exudate seen in pseudomembranous colitis. The villiform mucosa, muscularized lamina propria, and paucity of neutrophils distinguish SRUS.

Radiation proctitis is characterized by a thinned mucosa with capillary telangiectasia and hyalinization of capillary walls.

Ischemia rarely affects the rectum. Ischemic mucosa is thinned, and the lamina propria is hyalinized rather than muscularized.

Inflammatory cloacogenic polyp is prolapse of mucosa at the anorectal junction and is identical in appearance to solitary ulcer syndrome except for admixture of squamous mucosa. Internal hemorrhoids may also show features of mucosal prolapse and admixture of squamous mucosa.

Rectal prolapse shows histologic features similar to those of solitary rectal ulcer syndrome.

References

Franzin G, Dina R, Scarpa A, Fratton A. The evolution of the solitary ulcer of the rectum— an endoscopic and histopathologic study. Endoscopy 1982;14:131–134.

Madigan MR, Morson BC. Solitary ulcer of the rectum. Gut 1969;10:871–881.

Rutter KRP, Riddell RH. The solitary ulcer syndrome of the rectum. Clin Gastrointerol 1975;4:505–530.

Saul SH. Inflammatory cloacogenic polyp: relationship to solitary rectal ulcer syndrome/mucosal prolapse and other bowel disorders. Hum Pathol 1987;18:1120–1125.

Womack NR, Williams NS, Holmfield JHM, Morrison JFB. Pressure and prolapse, the cause of the solitary rectal ulcer syndrome. Gut 1987;28:1228–1233.

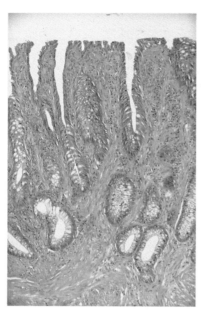

Figure 5–63. Solitary rectal ulcer syndrome. Features include muscularization of the lamina propria, a villiform appearance, and intermingling of crypts with muscularis mucosa.

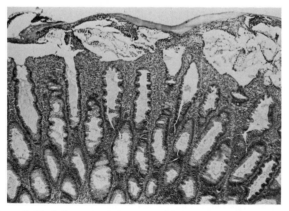

Figure 5–64. Solitary rectal ulcer syndrome. There is focal ulceration of surface intercrypt epithelium. The lamina propria is muscularized, crypts show reactive change, and capillaries are dilated.

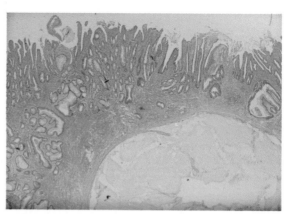

Figure 5–65. Solitary rectal ulcer syndrome with localized colitis cystica profunda forming a mucinous cyst in the submucosa. Note the villiform appearance and surface ulceration.

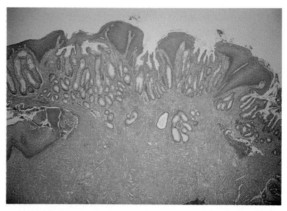

Figure 5–66. Prolapsing mucosa at the anal rectal junction may represent an internal hemorrhoid or spontaneous prolapsing mucosa, which has been designated "cloacogenic polyp." It includes an intimate admixture of squamous mucosa with columnar mucosa showing features of mucosal prolapse similar to those seen in solitary ulcer syndrome.

PNEUMATOSIS COLI

Biology of Disease

■ *Pneumatosis coli* and *pneumatosis cystoides intestinalis* of the small bowel are conditions in which multiple gas-filled cysts are present in the wall of the intestine without evidence of infection.
■ The gas within the cysts is similar to flatus, comprising atmospheric air with added hydrogen and methane. Bacterial cultures of gas cysts are usually sterile.
■ The theory that raised intraluminal pressure forces luminal gas into the bowel wall through mucosal defects is widely accepted.

■ A large number of intestinal disorders have been associated with pneumatosis, including peptic ulcer disease, intestinal obstruction, collagen vascular disorders, bowel surgery, ischemia, chronic inflammatory disorders, trauma, and virtually all ulcerating conditions. Chronic obstructive airways disease is also associated.

Clinical Features

■ Patients present with a variety of symptoms, such as crampy abdominal pain, diarrhea, constipation, and abdominal distention. Pneumatosis is usually discovered on radiologic examination, during endoscopy, or at laparatomy.

Gross Pathology

■ In resected specimens, gas cysts are present in mucosa, submucosa, mesentery, and serosa. Crepitus is noticed on handling the specimen. Cysts are generally less than 2 cm in diameter but may measure up to several centimeters.

■ On the mucosal surface, the cysts may give a multinodular appearance.

Microscopic Pathology

■ Gas cysts of chronic pneumatosis are lined by macrophages, including macrophage giant cells. Some cysts may be lined by endothelial-type cells of lymphatic origin. The cysts of recent-onset pneumatosis may have no lining other than connective tissue.

■ Gas insufflated during endoscopy (insufflation pneumatosis) appears as numerous tiny cystic spaces within the lamina propria, particularly near lymphoid-glandular complexes.

Differential Diagnosis

Emphysematous gastroenteritis, pseudolipomatosis.

Secondary pneumatosis in the bowel wall may be caused by infections by gas-forming organisms.

Insufflation of gas at endoscopy may force gas into the mucosa, giving a microcystic appearance on histology that has been called pseudolipomatosis.

References

Ghahremani GG, Port RB, Beachey MC. Pneumatosis coli in Crohn's disease. Am J Dig Dis 1974;19:315–323.

Haboubi NY, Honan RP, Haselton PS, et al. Pneumatosis coli: a case report with ultrastructural study. Histopathology 1984;8:145–155.

Kozarek RA, Ernest DL, Silverstein ME, Smith RG. Air pressure induced colon injury during diagnostic colonoscopy. Gastroenterology 1980;78:7–14.

Snover DC, Sandstad J, Hutton S. Mucosal pseudolipomatosis of the colon. Am J Clin Pathol 1985;84:575–579.

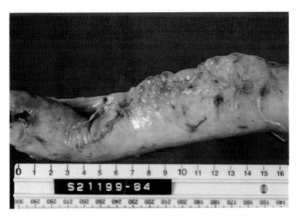

Figure 5–67. Pneumatosis intestinalis. Note gas cysts on the mesenteric border of ileum.

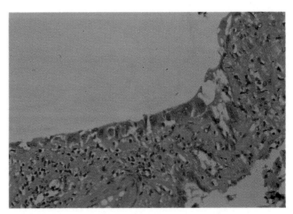

Figure 5–69. Cyst of chronic pneumatosis lined by macrophages.

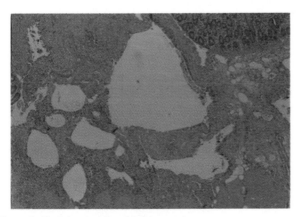

Figure 5–68. Submucosal cystic pneumatosis.

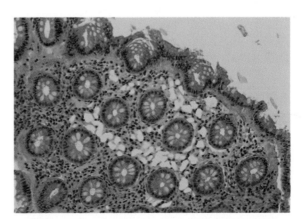

Figure 5–70. Insufflation pneumatosis caused by inflation of the bowel at endoscopy, mimicking lipomatosis.

HYPERPLASTIC (METAPLASTIC) POLYPS

Biology of Disease

■ *Hyperplastic polyps*, or benign epithelial lesions of the large bowel, are the most common polyps of the large bowel. They are found in up to 85% of adults in affluent Western countries, but in only 2% to 3% of adults in underdeveloped countries.

■ The prevalence and number of hyperplastic polyps increase with age. Hyperplastic polyps are present in the rectum in up to 90% of cases of rectal carcinoma.

■ More than 90% of rectal polyps less than 3 mm in diameter are hyperplastic.

Clinical Features

■ Hyperplastic polyps are usually incidental findings at endoscopy or in resected specimens. They rarely produce independent clinical manifestations.

Gross Pathology

■ Hyperplastic polyps are small, sessile, mucosal elevations, usually less than 5 mm in diameter. They are slightly paler than the background mucosa and are nonpigmented in melanosis coli.

Microscopic Pathology

■ Hyperplastic polyps show a characteristic serrated appearance in the upper halves of the crypts. Goblet cell numbers are diminished, and the cells in between the goblet cells resemble gastric surface epithelial cells more than normal absorptive cells.

■ The basal halves of the crypts have a hyperplastic appearance.

■ Paneth's cells are occasionally present.

■ Inverted hyperplastic polyps penetrate through the muscularis mucosae and may resemble invasion histologically.

Differential Diagnosis

Adenoma, serrated adenoma, adenocarcinoma, hyperplastic change.

Obliquely cut hyperplastic polyps may be misdiagnosed as adenomas. Correct diagnosis depends on identifying the serrated superficial component. In obliquely cut specimens, the basal crypts may be intermingled with fibers of the muscularis mucosae, giving an appearance that may be misinterpreted as carcinoma. The absence of desmoplasia and the presence of hemosiderin should suggest pseudoinvasion.

Rarely, features of both adenoma and hyperplastic polyp are present in the same lesion. The components may be side by side or may consist of adenoma with serrated tubules. These lesions are called either mixed hyperplastic-adenomatous polyps or serrated adenomas.

Hyperplastic polyp–like change may be seen focally in chronic ulcerative colitis, inflammatory polyps, juvenile polyps, and prolapsing mucosa.

References

Gebbers J-O, Laissue JA. Mixed hyperplastic and neoplastic polyp of the colon: an immunohistological study. Virchows Arch [A] 1986;410:189–194.

Jass JR. Metaplastic polyps and polyposis of the colorectum. Histopathology 1980;4:579–581.

Lane N, Kaplan H, Pascal RR. Minute adenomatous and hyperplastic polyps of the colon: divergent patterns of epithelial growth with specific mesenchymal changes. Gastroenterology 1971;60:537–551.

Longacre TA, Fenoglio-Preiser CM. Mixed hyperplastic adenomatous polyps/serrated adenomas: a distinct form of colorectal neoplasia. Am J Surg Pathol 1990;14:524–537.

Sobin LH. Inverted hyperplastic polyps of the colon. Am J Surg Pathol 1985;9:265–272.

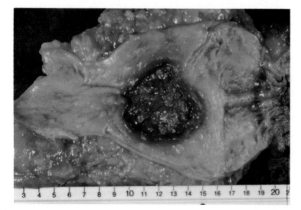

Figure 5–71. On the left of this ulcerating adenocarcinoma of the rectum there are several small pale sessile hyperplastic polyps.

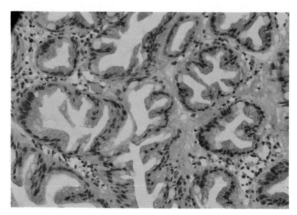

Figure 5–72. Hyperplastic polyp. Note the serrated pattern and the low number of goblet cells.

MIXED HYPERPLASTIC ADENOMATOUS POLYPS AND SERRATED ADENOMAS

Biology of Disease

■ Rarely, features of both adenoma and hyperplastic polyp are present in the same lesion. Three forms of mixed tumor are possible: (1) collision tumor (hyperplastic and adenomatous glands side by side with a sharp junction), (2) combined tumor (intermingled hyperplastic and adenomatous glands), and (3) serrated adenoma in which serrated glands with eosinophilic cytoplasm evince dysplasia (as characterized by nuclear stratification, nuclear atypia, increased nucleocytoplasmic ratio, and mitotic figures extending into the upper zone of the crypts).

Clinical Features

■ These mixed polyps constitute about 0.5% of all colonic polyps. The male-to-female ratio is approximately 3:2, and the mean age is 63.4 years (range 15 to 88 years). Only 3.1% of patients are under 40 years of age. Half of the polyps are in the rectosigmoid, and the remainder are distributed evenly throughout the colon.

Gross Pathology

■ They range in diameter from 0.2 to 7.5 cm, 20% being more than 1 cm in diameter.
■ Twelve percent are pedunculated, and the others are sessile.

Microscopic Pathology

■ Hyperplastic polyps show serrated crypt outlines, increased numbers of nongoblet cells, mature overdistended goblet cells, and expanded proliferative zones. Adenomas display crowded tubules composed of incompletely differentiated columnar cells, crowding of cells, nuclear hyperchromatism, immaturity of goblet cells, and mitoses throughout the length of the crypt.
■ Serrated adenomas have features of both adenoma and hyperplastic polyp in the same lesion. Hyperplastic and adenomatous glands may be intimately intermingled as metaplastic areas in adenomas or may merely abut one another as in collision tumors. Serrated adenomas display serrated glands with eosinophilic cytoplasm and cytologic dysplasia: nuclear stratification, increased nucleocytoplasmic ratio, and expanded proliferative zone.
■ High-grade dysplasia or intramucosal carcinoma is seen in 10% of mixed polyps.

Differential Diagnosis

Hyperplastic polyp, goblet cell–rich adenoma.

The distinction from hyperplastic polyp is based on the presence of dysplasia, particularly near the surface of the lesion, in serrated adenoma.

Goblet cell–rich adenoma is not serrated and generally shows a much greater number and proportion of goblet cells than does hyperplastic polyp or serrated adenoma.

References

Gebbers J-O, Laissue JA. Mixed hyperplastic and neoplastic polyp of the colon: an immunohistological study. Virchows Arch [A] 1986;410:189–194.

Longacre TA, Fenoglio-Preiser CM. Mixed hyperplastic adenomatous polyps/serrated adenomas. A distinct form of colorectal neoplasia. Am J Surg Pathol 1990;14:524–537.

Sumner HW, Wasserman NF, McClain CJ. Giant hyperplastic polyposis of the colon. Dig Dis Sci 1981;26:85–89.

Urbanksi SJ, Marcon N, Kossakowska AE, Bruce WB. Mixed hyperplastic adenomatous polyps — an underdiagnosed entity: report of a case of adenocarcinoma arising within a mixed hyperplastic adenomatous polyp. Am J Surg Pathol 1984;8:551–556.

Williams GT, Arthur JF, Bussey HJR, Morson BC. Metaplastic polyps and polyposis of the colorectum. Histopathology 1980;4:155–170.

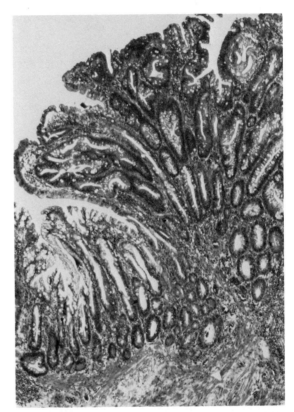

Figure 5–73. Hyperplastic polyp (*left*) adjacent to serrated adenoma (*right*).

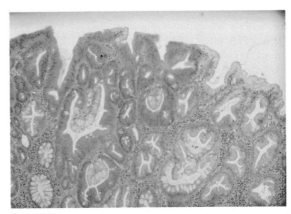

Figure 5–74. Serrated adenoma. Part of the lesion is common hyperplastic polyp, and part is unequivocally dysplastic.

JUVENILE POLYPS

Biology of Disease

■ *Juvenile polyps* are solitary rectal polyps composed of cystically dilated crypts and an excess of lamina propria. Multiple juvenile polyposis is a rare syndrome inherited as an autosomal dominant trait. The pathogenesis of juvenile polyps is poorly understood.

Clinical Features

■ Juvenile polyps usually manifest as rectal bleeding. Polyps on a long stalk may rarely prolapse during defecation.

■ Approximately 75% of all juvenile polyps are found in the rectum.

■ They are rare in the first year of life, most common between the ages of 1 to 7 years, and may manifest well into adult life.

Gross Pathology

■ Most juvenile polyps are single, pedunculated, and smooth-surfaced with multiple tiny gelatinous cysts on cut surface.

■ These polyps range in height from 3 mm to 2 cm.

Microscopic Pathology

■ Juvenile polyps display surface ulceration, granulation tissue, and excess lamina propria at the expense of glands. The lamina propria contains large numbers of plasma cells, eosinophils, and lymphocytes. The crypts are distended by mucin and may show branching and hyperchromatism, particularly near the ulcerated surface.

■ There may be considerable neutrophil infiltration at the ulcerated surface.

■ Focally, the epithelium may have a serrated hyperplastic appearance.

■ There are rare case reports of dysplasia or carcinoma occurring in solitary juvenile polyps.

■ Dysplasia and adenocarcinoma are well-recognized complications of multiple juvenile polyposis.

Differential Diagnosis

Inflammatory polyps, hyperplastic polyp, adenoma, Peutz-Jeghers polyp, granulation tissue polyp.

Inflammatory polyps arise from inflammatory bowel disease. They display a core of muscularis mucosae and show mucosal regeneration, inflammation, and ulceration but do not usually show widespread glandular dilatation or excess of lamina propria. They are almost always multiple.

Hyperplastic polyps are distinguished by their characteristic microscopic morphology. Hyperplastic change in juvenile polyps is usually a focal phenomenon.

Tubular adenomas may display ulceration and focal glandular dilatation, but the glands are dysplastic and the volume of lamina propria is diminished.

Peutz-Jeghers polyps display a branching core of mus-

cularis mucosae surmounted by essentially normal mucosa.

Granulation tissue polyps are composed almost entirely of granulation tissue and are usually seen in inflammatory bowel disease. It has been suggested that some juvenile polyps may arise from granulation tissue polyps through a process of progressive epithelialization.

References

Dajani YF, Kamel MF. Colorectal juvenile polyps: an epidemiological and histopathological study of 144 cases in Jordanians. Histopathology 1984;8:765–779.

Goodman ZD, Yardley JH, Milligan FD. Pathogenesis of colonic polyps in multiple juvenile polyposis: report of a case associated with gastric polyps and carcinoma of the rectum. Cancer 1979;43:1906–1913.

Haggitt RC, Pittcock JA. Familial juvenile polyposis of the colon. Cancer 1970;26:1232–1238.

Jass JR, Williams CB, Bussey HJR, Morson BC. Juvenile polyposis—a precancerous condition. Histopathology 1988;13:619–630.

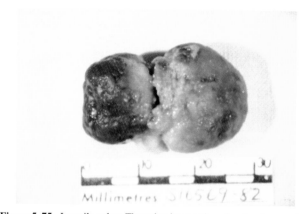

Figure 5–75. Juvenile polyp. The polyp is smooth surfaced and congested.

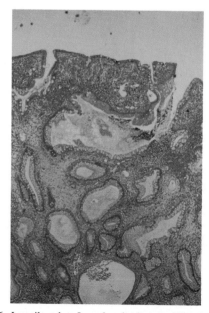

Figure 5–76. Juvenile polyp. Irregular glands, some dilated. Focal excess of lamina propria.

INFLAMMATORY POLYPS

Biology of Disease

- *Inflammatory polyps*, composed of mucosa and muscularis mucosa, follow episodes of severe inflammatory bowel disease. They begin as pseudopolyps—mucosal islands and undermined mucosal tags in a sea of ulceration. When mucosa regenerates across the ulcers, the islands of original mucosa protrude above the regenerated mucosa as inflammatory polyps. With time, these polyps may be progressively elongated by the propulsive action of the gut.
- In clinical series, inflammatory polyps are found in approximately 15% of patients with ulcerative colitis, but 60% of resected specimens of ulcerative colitis and 40% of specimens of Crohn's disease of the colon show inflammatory polyp(s).
- Secondary changes in inflammatory polyps include traumatization and ulceration.

Clinical Features

- The clinical features of inflammatory bowel disease dominate most cases. The polyps are incidental findings.
- Large inflammatory polyps may give rise to abdominal pain and anemia due to blood loss.

Gross Pathology

- Inflammatory polyps vary in size and shape. Some are short and stubby, others long and threadlike, still others bulbous. They range from a few millimeters to more than 5 cm in height. The diameter of bulbous polyps may reach 2 cm.

Microscopic Pathology

- The mucosa constitutes the major portion of the polyp and may display branching or dilated crypts, inflammation, dilatation of capillaries, surface ulceration, granulation tissue, and focal hyperplastic-metaplastic change. Inflammatory polyps usually include a core of muscularis mucosae, submucosa, and dilated blood vessels. This core may not be visible in obliquely cut polyps.
- Hemosiderin deposition may be present.
- The mucosa adjacent to inflammatory polyps shows regenerative features. The muscularis mucosae is scarred, hypertrophied, or fused with the muscularis propria. These features indicate repair following ulceration.
- The presence of inflammatory bowel disease adjacent to polyps may be important in the diagnosis of inflammatory polyps.
- Rarely, small sessile polyps are formed entirely of granulation tissue and may resemble pyogenic granuloma. Bizarre mesenchymal cells showing enlarged hyperchromatic nuclei and abundant cytoplasm are occasionally present. They have been designated *pseudomalignant* or *pseudosarcomatous*, and indeed they do raise the question of malignancy. These cells show positive immunostaining for the mesenchymal intermediate filament vimentin, and sometimes also for actin, suggesting that they are myofibroblastic. Results of cytokeratin stains are negative.

Differential Diagnosis

Juvenile polyps, adenomas, hyperplastic polyps.

Inflammatory polyps do not have an excess of lamina propria and glandular dilatation as juvenile polyps do. Juvenile polyps do not have a core of muscularis mucosae.

Adenomatous polyps are dysplastic. Inflammatory polyps are not.

Hyperplastic change may be seen focally in inflammatory polyps but the change is not generalized, as in hyperplastic polyps.

References

Kelly JK, Gabos MD. The pathogenesis of inflammatory polyps. Dis Colon Rectum 1987;30:251–254.
Kelly JK, Langevin JM, Price LM, et al. Giant and symptomatic inflammatory polyps of the colon in idiopathic inflammatory bowel disease. Am J Surg Pathol 1986;10:420–428.

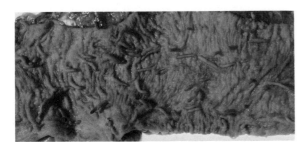

Figure 5–77. Inflammatory polyps in quiescent colonic Crohn's disease. The polyps remain after mucosa has regenerated around them.

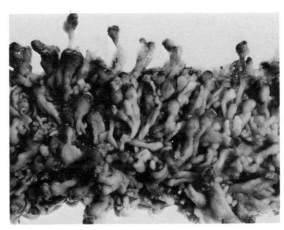

Figure 5–78. Giant inflammatory polyps which measure up to 5 cm in length. The heads of the polyps are ulcerated and congested.

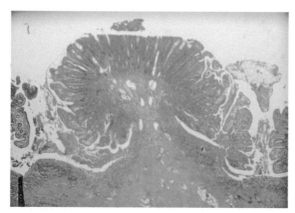

Figure 5–79. A mucosal island surrounded by ulceration is destined to become an inflammatory polyp.

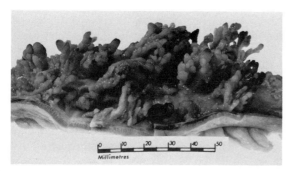

Figure 5–81. Inflammatory polyps. A cluster of giant inflammatory polyps may cause abdominal pain and blood loss.

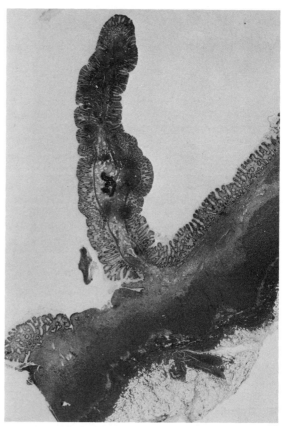

Figure 5–80. Inflammatory polyp. A central core of muscularis mucosae and dilated blood vessels is characteristic.

LIPOMAS

Biology of Disease

■ *Lipomas* are benign proliferations of mature fatty tissue that arise in the submucosa. Local excision is curative. The majority occur in adults between the fourth and seventh decades of life. Rare cases are associated with familial multiple lipomatosis.

Clinical Features

■ The majority of lipomas are asymptomatic. Lipomas are distributed throughout the colon with a slight preference for the cecum.
■ Symptomatic lipomas manifest as intussusception or hemorrhage. Rarely, a lipoma may prolapse through the anus.
■ Lipohypertrophy of the ileocecal valve is a common variant of normal.

Gross Pathology

■ Lipomas are usually sessile, smooth-surfaced, yellowish, nodules covered by intact mucosa. Pedunculated lesions are smooth surfaced but may show secondary ulceration and hemorrhage.
■ On the cut surface, lipomas are a uniform pale yellow and have the yielding consistency of fatty tissue. In cases of intussusception, hemorrhage, necrosis, and cyst formation may be present.
■ The smooth contours and absence of fixation are radiologic features that suggest a benign lesion.
■ Occasional lipomas have a dumb-bell shape, with both serosal and submucosal components.

Microscopic Pathology

■ The vast majority of lipomas are composed of mature adipose tissue.
■ Infrequently, lipomas display atypical features (particularly in association with surface ulceration). The atypical

changes include enlarged hyperchromatic nuclei, fibroblastic proliferation, and the presence of mitoses.

- Rarely, colonic lipomas contain numerous blood vessels, warranting the designation angiolipoma.

References

Ackerman NB, Chughtai SQ. Symptomatic lipomas of the gastrointestinal tract. Surg Gynecol Obstet 1975;141:565–568.

Comfort MW. Submucosal lipomata of the gastrointestinal tract: report of twenty eight cases. Surg Gynaecol Obstet 1930;52:101–118.

Haller JD, Roberts TW. Lipomas of the colon: a clinical pathologic study of 40 cases. Surgery 1964;55:773–781.

Snover DC. Atypical lipomas of the colon. Dis Colon Rectum 1984;27:485–488.

Taylor BA, Wolff BG. Colonic lipomas. Dis Colon Rectum 1987;30:888–893.

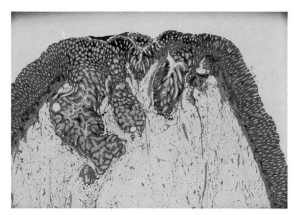

Figure 5–82. Colonic lipoma composed of mature adipose tissue and covered by intact mucosa.

ADENOMAS

Biology of Disease

- *Adenomas* are benign neoplasms of colonic epithelium. They form sessile or pedunculated masses with architectural and cytologic dysplasia. The majority of adenocarcinomas of the colon arise in adenomas.
- Statistically, adenomas are distributed evenly throughout the colon, but in individual patients, they may be clustered in a particular segment of the colon. The prevalence of adenomas is increased in families with a high rate of colorectal cancer, suggesting hereditary predisposition to adenomas, even in patients who do not have familial adenomatous polyposis (FAP).
- Adenomas are uncommon before the age of 30 years. In younger patients, adenomas are more common in the rectum and left colon, whereas in the elderly, they are more common in the right colon.
- The incidence of adenomas rises with age. In countries with a high incidence of colorectal cancer, adenomas are found at autopsy in 25% to 50% of people. In countries with a low incidence, adenomas are rare.
- A patient with one adenoma is likely to develop further adenomas.
- Beer drinking is a risk factor for colorectal adenomas in men. Whether smoking is a risk factor is controversial.
- Removal of all polyps within reach of the sigmoidoscope has been shown to dramatically reduce the incidence rate of carcinoma in that region of the bowel. This determination confirms the adenoma–carcinoma sequence.
- *Familial adenomatous polyposis (familial polyposis coli)* is an autosomal dominant condition characterized by the presence of at least 100 adenomas in the large bowel. In affected patients, the adenomas are visible by the early teenage years. Adenocarcinoma invariably develops by the fifth decade unless prophylactic colectomy is performed. *Gardner's syndrome* is familial adenomatous polyposis together with desmoid tumors, osteomas, and dental abnormalities. The extracolonic features of Gardner's syndrome are apparently the pleiotropic effect of the adenomatous polyposis coli (APC) gene (*APC*). This gene is located in region 21 of the long arm of chromosome 5 (5q 21), harbors a germ-line mutation in FAP patients. At the time of writing, 126 different *APC* mutations are recognized. These mutations are usually inactivation mutations that generate stop codons or frame shifts that truncate the protein. In an attenuated version of APC, defined as fewer than 100 polyps and delayed onset, the *APC* mutations are clustered at the beginning of the APC gene.

Clinical features

- Bleeding is the most common sign, appearing as frank blood, streaking of stool, or chronic anemia. Most adenomas are asymptomatic.

Gross Pathology

- Small adenomas are sessile nodules that may be slightly redder than the surrounding mucosa.
- Larger adenomas may be pedunculated (on a distinct stalk) or sessile (broadbased). Tubular adenomas tend to be lobulated, whereas villous adenomas are sessile and composed of delicate fronds or villi. Tubulovillous adenomas generally are multinodular or combine nodular areas with fine fronds. A small minority of adenomas are flat plaques.
- Pedunculated adenomas are particularly liable to undergo hemorrhage or ulceration.

Microscopic Pathology

- Architecturally, adenomas may be either tubular, villous, or tubulovillous. Lesions with 75% or more of tubular or villous form are called *tubular* or *villous*. Lesions with less than 75% of the dominant pattern are given the intermediate term *tubulovillous*. The tubules or villi are generally much longer than normal colonic crypts. They retain normal lamina propria.

- The great majority of adenomas are tubular. They mimic the morphology of normal crypts but are more closely packed and more complex architecturally.
- The diagnosis of adenoma depends on the presence of dysplasia. Features include epithelial hyperchromatism, mucin depletion, increased numbers of nuclei per unit length of epithelium, pseudostratification, increased mitoses, and lack of maturation. The nuclei of low-grade dysplasia are confined to the basal halves of the cells. The luminal half of the cytoplasm frequently is mucin containing. The nuclei of high grade dysplasia extend into the upper half of the epithelium and approach the surface. The nuclei are large and show clearing of the nucleoplasm and thickening of the nuclear membrane. Crypts may have secondary budding and back-to-back growth. Carcinoma in situ is regarded by most authors as synonymous with high-grade dysplasia.
- Flat adenomas are sessile tubular adenomas up to 1 cm in diameter. Flat adenomas are found in 8.5% of patients with adenomas. About half show high-grade dysplasia and aneuploid DNA content, and it is postulated that they may be the origin of so-called de novo adenocarcinomas —small carcinomas that do not contain residual adenoma.
- Torsion of pedunculated adenomas may cause displacement of crypts into the submucosa, giving a false impression of invasion. Displaced crypts are dilated, and the stroma shows hemosiderin deposition. In the majority of cases, the absence of desmoplasia and the presence of low-grade dysplasia allow easy diagnosis of displaced crypts. Displaced crypts that show high-grade dysplasia and are mingled with smooth muscle fibers may be difficult to distinguish from carcinoma.
- Carcinoma invading the stalk of an adenoma (malignant polyp) is signified by the combination of high-grade dysplasia, desmoplasia, and an infiltrative growth pattern. The former two criteria are sufficient for the diagnosis. Polypectomy alone is likely to be curative if three conditions are fulfilled: (1) the carcinoma does not extend to the cauterized line at the base of the stalk, (2) the tumor is not poorly differentiated, and (3) there is no evidence of vascular or lymphatic invasion.
- Endocrine cells are found in about 50% of adenomas. Paneth's cells are very uncommon. Rarely, melanin has been found in adenomas. Squamous metaplasia (morules)

occurs in about 1 per 200 adenomas. Mucin-negative clear cell change is a rare phenomenon that must be distinguished from metastatic renal cell carcinoma.
- Surface ulceration is the histologic basis for bleeding from adenomas.

Differential Diagnosis

Hyperplastic polyp, regenerating mucosa, adenocarcinoma.

Hyperplastic polyp may be mistaken for an adenoma if the biopsy specimen is cut obliquely so that only the crypts are visible in the section.

Regenerating mucosa following ulceration, inflammation, or rapid turnover may appear hyperchromatic and hypermitotic but does not show the tumorous growth or the architectural complexity of adenoma. Regenerating mucosa may display cuboidal or stretched cells focally and may show nuclear stratification or large, open nuclei. Usually, some degree of surface maturation is retained.

Adenocarcinoma is distinguished from adenoma by the presence of invasion and desmoplastic reaction.

References

Bansal M, Fenoglio CM, Robboy SJ, King DW. Are metaplasias in colorectal adenomas truly metaplasias? Am J Pathol 1984;115:253–265.

Correa P, Strong JP, Reif A, Johnson WD. The epidemiology of colorectal polyps: prevalence in New Orleans and international comparison. Cancer 1977;39:2258–2264.

Cottrell S, Bicknell D, Kaklamanis L, Bodmer WF. Molecular analysis of APC mutations in familial adenomatous polyposis and sporadic colon carcinomas. Lancet 1992;340:626–630.

Eide TJ. Prevalence and morphological features of adenomas of the large intestine in individuals with and without colorectal carcinoma. Histopathology 1986;10:111–118.

Eide TJ, Scheweder T. Clustering of adenomas in the large intestine. Gut 1984;25:1262–1267.

Gilbertson VA, Nelms JM. The prevention of invasive carcinoma of the rectum. Cancer 1978;41:1137–1139.

Muto T, Masaki T, Suzuki K. DNA ploidy pattern of flat adenomas of the large bowel. Dis Colon Rectum 1991;34:696–698.

O'Brien MJ, Winawer SJ, Zauber EG, et al. National polyp study: patient and polyp characteristics associated with high grade dysplasia in colorectal adenomas. Gastroenterology 1990;98:371–379.

Sobin LH. The histopathology of bleeding polyps and carcinomas of the large intestine. Cancer 1985;55:577–581.

Wolber RA, Owen DA. Flat adenomas of the colon. Hum Pathol 1991;22:70–74.

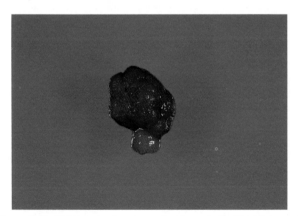

Figure 5–83. Tubular adenoma removed endoscopically. Note the smooth lobulated surface.

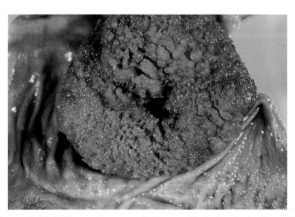

Figure 5–84. Villous adenoma of rectum. Note the finely frond-like surface.

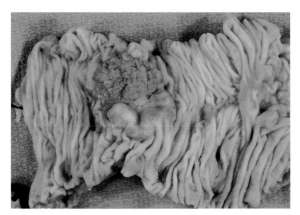

Figure 5–85. Adenocarcinoma arising in villous adenoma.

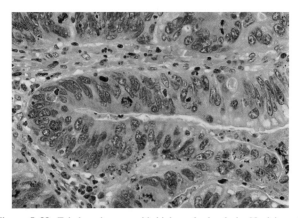

Figure 5–88. Tubular adenoma with high-grade dysplasia. Nuclei reach the surface in many areas.

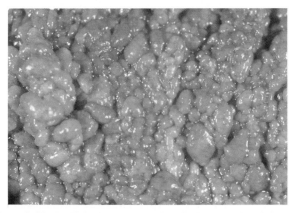

Figure 5–86. Familial adenomatous polyposis. Innumerable tubular adenomas cover the colonic mucosa.

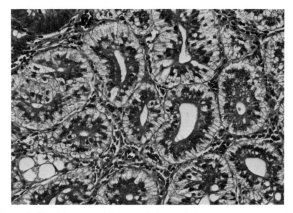

Figure 5–89. Adenoma with areas of clear cell change, an uncommon feature.

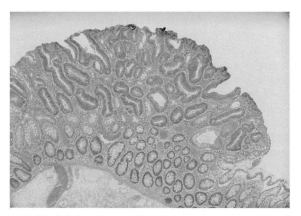

Figure 5–87. Tubular adenoma. The adenomatous crypts are hyperchromatic, and the epithelium fails to mature.

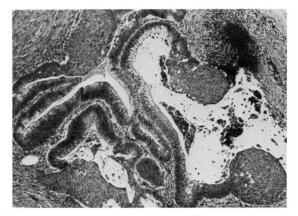

Figure 5–90. Colonic adenoma with pseudoinvasion and squamous morules. One in 200 adenomas shows squamous morules.

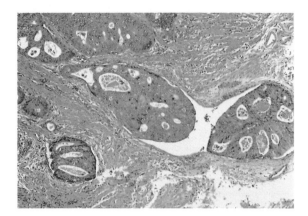

Figure 5–91. Invasion of a thin-walled vessel in the stalk of a polyp. This is an indication for surgical excision.

OTHER POLYPS

■ Other polyps include residual stalks, granular cell tumor, inflammatory "cap" polyps, Cowden's disease, polyps in schistosomiasis, polypoid mucosa in diverticular disease, Peutz-Jeghers polyps (see Chapter 3), ganglioneuromatous polyps (see Chapter 9), granulation tissue polyps with bizarre cells (see discussion of inflammatory polyps), and lymphoid polyps.

Residual Stalks

■ Residual stalks of pedunculated adenomas appear as persistent polyps at repeat endoscopy.
■ They are smooth surfaced and do not have a distinct head.
■ Histologically, there are usually a recanalizing artery in the stalk and evidence of repair at the tip.

Granular Cell Tumor

■ Granular cell tumors occur in the lamina propria or submucosa.
■ These tumors consist of sheets of large granular cells that are positive on both diastase-PAS and S100 protein stains.

Inflammatory "Cap" Polyps

■ Inflamatory "cap" polyps are distinctive inflammatory polyps of the rectosigmoid that show features of prolapsing mucosa.
■ Male and female adults of any age (17 to 82 years) are affected. There is no family history. Disease associations have included ulcerative colitis and sigmoid adenocarcinoma, but there is no strong association.
■ Symptoms such as mucous diarrhea, tenesmus, and rectal bleeding are often relieved by polypectomy, but if there are multiple polyps, rectosigmoid resection may be needed to control mucous diarrhea.
■ Grossly, the polyps may number from as few as 1 to as many as 70. They are dark red, sessile, and commonly situated on the apices of transverse mucosal folds, the intervening mucosa being normal.
■ Microscopically, inflammatory "cap" polyps consist of elongated, tortuous, and often distended crypts covered by a cap of inflammatory granulation tissue. The crypt epithelium is regular, but it is attenuated toward the luminal surface, and metaplastic-like areas are sometimes present.

Cowden's Disease

■ Numerous small bowel and colonic polyps are seen in one third of patients with Cowden's disease, an autosomal dominant disorder.
■ The polyps may resemble juvenile polyps or show fibrosis of the lamina propria or ganglioneuromatous proliferation.
■ The syndrome consists of multiple facial trichilemmomas, oral papillomas, fibrocystic disease or carcinoma of the breast, and benign or malignant lesion of the thyroid.

Schistosomiasis

■ *Schistosomiasis* is infection by flukes 1 to 2 cm long that live in veins and deposit eggs in the host tissue. The eggs elicit an inflammatory response.
■ *Schistosoma mansoni* and *Schistosoma japonicum* can both affect the colon. They are both geographically confined to intermediate host territories (Africa, Carribean, Central and South America, and Southeast Asia).
■ The colonic disorder affects mainly the descending colon and rectosigmoid and results from numerous granulomas around eggs. These can give rise to inflammatory polyps that may be secondarily ulcerated, causing diarrhea with blood and mucus.
■ Treatment with praziquantel is highly effective, and the polyps regress rapidly.
■ Diagnosis is based on the characteristic morphology of the eggs.

References

Carlson GJ, Nivatvongs S, Snover D. Colorectal polyps in Cowden's disease (multiple hamartoma syndrome). Am J Surg Pathol 1984;8:779–786.
Johnston J, Helwig EB. Granular cell tumors of the gastrointestinal tract and perianal region: a study of 74 cases. Dig Dis Sci 1981;26:807–816.
Williams GT, Bussey HJR, Morson BC. Inflammatory "cap" polyps of the large intestine. Br J Surg 1985;72(Supp):133.

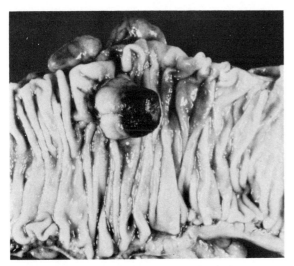

Figure 5–92. Polypoid residual stalk of pedunculated adenoma.

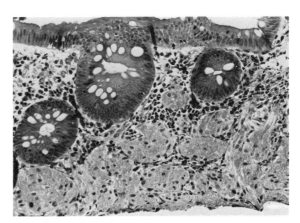

Figure 5–93. Cecal biopsy specimen showing granular cell tumor.

COLORECTAL ADENOCARCINOMA

Biology of Disease

- *Adenocarcinoma* is a malignant neoplasm of crypt epithelium. This term does not include premalignant dysplasia.
- Colorectal adenocarcinoma (CRC) is the third most common cancer in Western countries after lung and breast cancer. The incidence of CRC is rising in North America and Western Europe. The incidence is low in Asia and Africa. An estimated 156,000 patients develop CRC annually in the United States, resulting in 58,000 deaths.
- This disease is uncommon before the age of 40 years. The greatest number of cases manifest in the sixth decade. Sex distribution is about equal.
- Risk factors under investigation include antioxidants and a diet that is high in animal fat and low in vegetable fiber. Dietary alterations may have secondary effects on bacterial flora and bile acids. Following cholecystectomy, the risk of colorectal adenocarcinoma increases threefold in women. Beer drinking predisposes to adenomas and carcinomas.
- Specific syndromes and conditions that predispose to CRC include hereditary nonpolyposis colonic carcinoma (HNPCC), hereditary flat adenoma syndrome, familial adenomatous polyposis (FAP) and its variants (Gardner's syndrome, Turcot's syndrome and Oldfield's syndrome), autosomal-dominantly inherited tendency to develop occasional adenomatous polyps and CRC, Peutz-Jeghers syndrome, Muir-Torre syndrome (CRC with multiple sebaceous adenomas or carcinomas and keratoacanthomas), inflammatory bowel disease, previous irradiation, ureterosigmoidostomy, and cholecystectomy.
- HNPCC accounts for between 6% and 13% of CRCs. There are two forms, Lynch syndrome I and Lynch syndrome II. Lynch syndrome I is an autosomal dominant trait predisposing to CRC at an early age (circa 44 years), a predilection for the proximal colon, and an excess of synchronous and metachronous CRCs. Lynch syndrome II combines those features with carcinomas of the endometrium or other organs. The criteria for the diagnosis are as follows: (1) three or more relatives with histologically verified CRC, one of whom is a first-degree relative of the other two, (2) CRC involving at least two generations, and (3) one or more CRC cases diagnosed before age 50.
- Most CRCs have at least two genetic mutations and often have four or more. Tumor suppressor gene function is commonly lost by inactivation of both alleles either by chromosomal deletion or point mutation. Adenomatous polyposis coli (*APC*) mutations are acquired in some sporadic CRC cases. There is frequently loss of heterozygosity on chromosome 5 in adenomas. The "mutated in colorectal cancer" gene (MCC), which is encoded close to *APC*, is also commonly mutated in sporadic CRC. The evolution of adenomas into frank carcinomas is accompanied by inactivation-mutation of the deleted in colonic carcinoma (DCC) suppressor gene on chromosome 18 and the *p53* suppressor gene on chromosome 17. The *p53* gene is mutated in the germline of families with Li-Fraumeni syndrome, but these families do not have a predilection for colonic cancers.
- Oncogenes are dominant and require alteration of only one allele to express an effect. Sixty percent of large adenomas have a mutated, activated allele of the K-*ras* oncogene. Mutations occur at codons 12, 13, or 61. Counterintuitively (for a mutation occurring at the adenoma stage), the genotypes of K-*ras* point mutations in carcinomas may predict tumor aggressiveness! The c-*myc* oncogene encodes a nuclear phosphoprotein. In 60% to 70% of CRCs, c-*myc* RNA is elevated, but the mecha-

nism for deregulation of expression is not yet known. Transcripts of the oncogene *c-src* are also raised in 62% of cancers.

■ A novel defect was recently described in HNPCC and localized on chromosome 2. The defect results in widespread mutations in short repeated DNA sequences, suggesting that numerous replication errors had occurred during tumor development.

Clinical Features

■ Colorectal adenocarcinomas are clinically silent until they have grown to a considerable size.
■ Symptoms of anemia—fatigue, angina, or dyspnea—are common presenting complaints. Chronic low-grade blood loss in the stools ultimately leads to iron deficiency. Frank bleeding per rectum or blood admixed with stool is more common with distal lesions.
■ Bowel obstruction may present as colicky abdominal pain after meals.
■ Some patients present with disseminated disease, malaise, cachexia, jaundice, or hepatomegaly.
■ Metachronous CRC occurs at a rate of 0.35% per annum.

Gross Pathology

■ Small adenocarcinomas are most often discovered to be arising within adenomatous polyps. Polyps containing cancer may show a localized depression, expansion of the stalk, or no distinctive features. Small carcinomas may be flat, plaquelike, or depressed. A minority of small flat carcinomas apparently arise de novo, although some of these may originate in flat adenomas.
■ Most carcinomas display central ulceration and raised, rolled edges. Circumferential tumors are often stenosing. Rare diffusely infiltrating variants may show nodular and ulcerated areas and thickening of the bowel wall, simulating Crohn's disease. On cut surface, about 10% of tumors contain cysts filled with gelatinous mucus.
■ Occasionally, an inflammatory sinus penetrates a tumor and causes free perforation, inflammatory adhesion to an adjacent viscus, or fistula. Carcinomas may also directly invade and create fistulas into adjacent organs, such as small bowel, stomach, and bladder.
■ Two independent cancers are found synchronously in 5% of patients. A further 6% of patients develop a second tumor metachronously.

Microscopic Pathology

■ Eighty percent of CRCs are either well differentiated with well-formed glands lined by columnar epithelium or intermediate-grade, moderately differentiated carcinomas.
■ About 10% to 15% of colonic cancers are mucoid (colloid) carcinomas in which more than 60% of the tumor volume is mucin. Mucinous carcinomas are more common in persons under the age of 40 years and in the proximal (right side) colon. More than half of all right-sided carcinomas contain a mucinous component, compared with only a quarter of left-sided tumors. Studies that did not apply multivariate analysis concluded that mucinous tumors behave more aggressively and have a poorer prog-

nosis than nonmucinous adenocarcinomas, but more recent studies applying multivariate analysis do not confirm this. The signet-ring carcinoma subcategory that is included with mucinous carcinomas probably accounts for the perceived poorer prognosis, but also, mucinous carcinomas tend to manifest at a more advanced stage than do nonmucinous carcinomas. Whereas 15% of nonmucinous carcinomas of the rectum were classified as Dukes' stage A, only 3% of mucinous carcinomas were Dukes' stage A. The best evidence at this time is that when site, stage, and grade of tumor are adjusted for, the presence of a mucinous component does not imply a poorer prognosis unless that predominating component is of signet-ring type. Only 1% to 2% of all tumors are pure signet-ring cell carcinomas.

■ The remaining 5% to 10% of tumors are poorly differentiated and include tumor variants such as adenosquamous carcinomas, squamous carcinomas, and endocrine carcinomas. Poorly differentiated tumors display little tendency to form glands.
■ The stroma of CRC almost always displays a desmoplastic reaction consisting of a proliferation of spindle cells in a weakly hematoxiphilic stroma.
■ Depth of invasion and lymph node metastasis are major prognostic determinants. Dukes's original staging system for carcinoma of the rectum is the basis of all modern staging systems. Clinicians should learn whichever modification is in use in their institution. (In the original Dukes' classification, stage A is tumor confined to the submucosa or muscle coat, stage B is tumor that has penetrated through the entire thickness of muscle coat, and stage C is any tumor with lymph node involvement.)
■ A follicular lymphocytic response to the tumor (similar to that seen in Crohn's disease) is a favorable prognostic indicator.
■ Venous invasion outside the muscle coat is an adverse prognostic factor.
■ The presence of endocrine cells or Paneth's cells does not influence prognosis.

Special Diagnostic Techniques

■ Barium enema with air contrast examination may suggest the diagnosis. Colonoscopy allows inspection and biopsy.

Differential Diagnosis

Pseudoinvasion, carcinoids, carcinoma of prostate, metastases, endometriosis.

In pedunculated adenomas, the distinction between pseudocarcinomatous invasion and carcinoma may occasionally be difficult, because the criteria for carcinoma—invasion and desmoplasia—are both subjective.

Carcinoids of the rectum show small regular well-differentiated glands composed of monotonously regular cells.

Direct invasion of the rectum by prostatic carcinoma can occur. The morphology of prostatic cancers is usually distinctive. Well-differentiated prostatic cancers show small glands lined by regular cells with central single nucleoli. Intermediate-grade tumors may be cribriform, and higher-grade tumors form poorly differentiated cords of cells. Immunostains for prostate-specific antigen and carcinoembryonic antigen may be helpful.

Metastases from stomach or breast (especially lobular carcinoma) may mimic primary signet-ring carcinoma. Ovarian, renal, or uterine carcinomas and melanoma may have distinctive features. Metastases are often multiple and invade from the serosa.

Endometriosis may be seen beneath the mucosa in rectosigmoid biopsy specimens; it is distinguished from adenocarcinoma by its stroma, glands, hemosiderin, and location.

References

Burt RW, Groden J. The genetics and molecular diagnosis of adenomatous polyposis coli. Gastroenterology 1993;104:1211–1214.

Griffin PM, Life JM, Greenberg RS, Clark WS. Adenocarcinoma of the colon and rectum in persons under 40 years old: a population-based study. Gastroenterology 1991;100:1033–1040.

Halvorsen TB. Site distribution of colorectal adenocarcinomas: a retrospective study of 853 tumours. Scand J Gastroenterol 1986;21:973–978.

Halvorsen TB, Seim E. Degree of differentiation in colorectal adenocarcinomas: a multivariate analysis of the influence on survival. J Clin Pathol 1988;41:532–537.

Halvorsen TB, Seim E. Influence of mucinous components on survival in colorectal adenocarcinomas: a multivariate analysis. J Clin Pathol 1988;41:1068–1072.

Lynch HT, Smyrk TC, Watson P, et al. Genetics, natural history, tumor spectrum, and pathology of hereditary nonpolyposis colorectal cancer: an updated review. Gastroenterology 1993;104:1535–1549.

Muto T, Bussey HJR, Morson BC. The evolution of cancer of the colon and rectum. Cancer 1975;36:2251–2270.

Sasaki O, Atkin WS, Jass JR. Mucinous carcinoma of the rectum. Histopathology 1987;11:259–272.

Smith DM, Haggitt RC. The prevalence and prognostic significance of argyrophil cells in colorectal carcinomas. Am J Surg Pathol 1984;8:123–128.

Talbot IC, Ritchie S, Leighton M, et al. Invasion of veins by carcinoma of rectum: method of detection, histologic features and significance. Histopathology 1982;5:141–163.

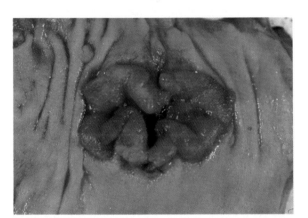

Figure 5–94. Adenocarcinoma with central ulceration and raised, rolled edges.

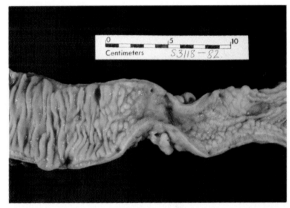

Figure 5–96. Carcinoma of sigmoid with linitis plastica-like pattern resembling Crohn's disease. This tumor was poorly differentiated histologically.

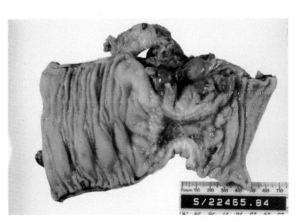

Figure 5–95. Excavated annular carcinoma which proved to be poorly differentiated histologically.

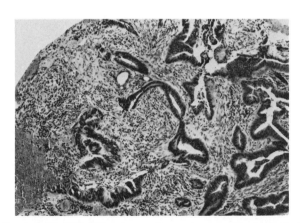

Figure 5–97. Well-differentiated adenocarcinoma with desmoplastic stroma.

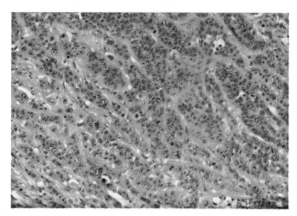

Figure 5–98. Poorly differentiated colonic carcinoma growing in cords, not forming tubules, and showing many mitoses.

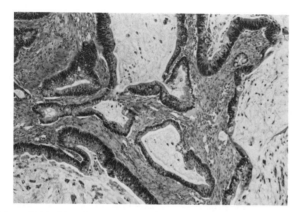

Figure 5–99. Mucoid carcinoma of colon with large amounts of extracellular mucin.

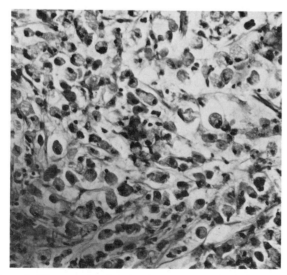

Figure 5–100. Mucoid carcinoma with signet ring cells.

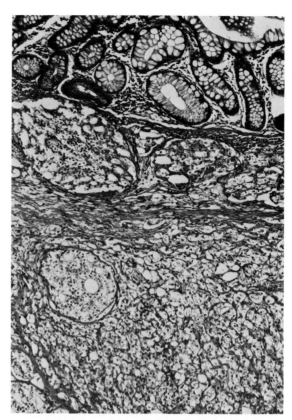

Figure 5–101. Prostatic adenocarcinoma invading the rectum. Cribriform and clear cell patterns.

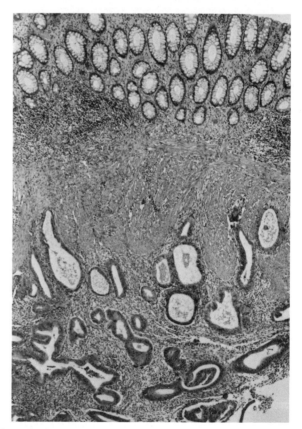

Figure 5–102. Endometriosis in a high rectal biopsy specimen must not be taken for adenocarcinoma.

SMALL CELL UNDIFFERENTIATED (NEUROENDOCRINE) CARCINOMA

Biology of Disease

- Small cell undifferentiated carcinoma of the colon resembles small cell carcinoma of the lung. The term "neuroendocrine carcinoma" emphasizes that these carcinomas may show endocrine differentiation.
- Most of these tumors are highly aggressive neoplasms. About 70% of them have metastasized to the liver at the time of diagnosis.

Clinical Features

- Small cell undifferentiated carcinomas of the colon occur most often between the sixth and eighth decades of life. The age range of patients in reported cases is 25 to 88 years.
- The clinical course is usually short, and two-thirds of patients are dead within 6 months. Some respond to chemotherapy regimens used for small cell carcinoma of the lung.

Gross Pathology

- Small cell undifferentiated carcinomas are usually large, annular, ulcerating tumors measuring between 4 and 12 cm in diameter, but some are extremely small. Some have a polypoid or fungating surface component of adenoma or well-differentiated adenocarcinoma.

Microscopic Pathology

- Forty-five percent of small cell carcinomas are associated with, and appear to arise from, adenomas or well-differentiated adenocarcinomas. There is usually a sharp junction between the two components.
- Small cell carcinomas are composed of small or intermediate-sized cells either alone or in combination.
- The cells lack distinct cytoplasm and show dark-staining, fusiform nuclei with dispersed chromatin and inconspicuous nucleoli. Intracytoplasmic mucin is absent.
- Squamous differentiation (metaplasia) is present focally in 20% of cases.
- Well-differentiated carcinoid-like areas are seen in some cases.
- Endocrine differentiation is common in small cell carcinomas if liberally defined as either argyrophilia, neuron-specific enolase, or synapatophysin immunopositivity, or as dense core granules on ultrastructural examination.
- Central necrosis, rosettelike structures and vascular invasion are often present.

Special Diagnostic Techniques

- Argyrophil stain may show positivity in some cells. Immunostaining for neuron-specific enolase, synaptophysin, and other neuroendocrine markers may be focally positive. Immunostaining for epithelial membrane antigen, melanoma markers, and lymphoma markers is negative.
- Ultrastructurally, the presence of dense core granules may help establish neuroendocrine differentiation. The granules are usually not numerous.

Differential Diagnosis

Metastatic small cell carcinoma, lymphoma, melanoma.

Uncommonly, metastatic small cell carcinoma of lung may be widely disseminated from an occult primary.

Lymphoma is signified by characteristic nuclear appearances, dyscohesive cells, immunostaining characteristics, and gene rearrangement studies.

Melanomas show sheets of cells with inclusion-like nucleoli. Immunostains for S100 protein or HMB-45 are positive. Cytokeratin and lymphocyte markers are negative.

Basaloid cloacogenic carcinoma arises from the transitional zone of the anal canal and shows a nested growth pattern with peripheral nuclear palisading and central necrosis or squamous differentiation. Ultrastructurally, they show desmosomes and lack dense core granules. Immunostaining for epithelial membrane antigen, carcinoembryonic antigen, and cytokeratins is positive.

References

Burke AB, Shekitka KM, Sobin LH. Small-cell carcinomas of the large intestine. Am J Clin Pathol 1991;95:315–321.

Cleary AP, Dockerty MC, Waugh JM. Small-cell carcinoma of the colon and rectum: a clinicopathologic study. Arch Surg 1961;83:22–30.

Gibbs NM. Undifferentiated carcinoma of the large intestine. Histopathology 1977;1:77–84.

Mills SE, Allen MS, Cohen AR. Small-cell undifferentiated carcinoma of the colon: a clinicopathologic study of five cases and their association with colonic adenomas. Am J Surg Pathol 1983;7:643–651.

Wick MR, Weatherby RP, Weiland LH. Small-cell neuroendocrine carcinoma of the colon and rectum: clinical, histologic and ultrastructural study and immunohistochemical comparison with cloacogenic carcinoma. Hum Pathol 1987;18:9–21.

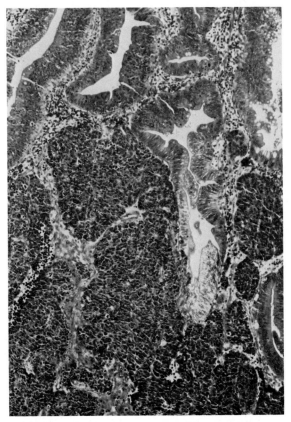

Figure 5–103. Undifferentiated small cell carcinoma arising in an adenoma.

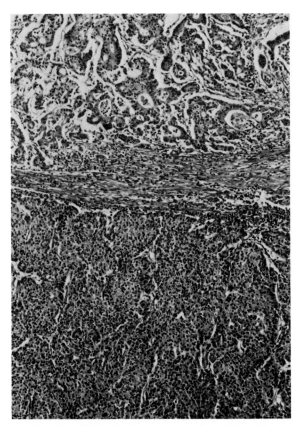

Figure 5–104. Small cell "neuroendocrine" carcinoma (*below*) arising in and abutting on moderately differentiated adenocarcinoma.

CARCINOID TUMORS

Biology of Disease

■ Carcinoids are rare in the colon but not uncommon in the rectum and sigmoid. Rectosigmoid carcinoids are usually small submucosal tumors composed of well-differentiated glands or ribbons of columnar cells. Only a minority resemble classic carcinoids of the appendix or small bowel.

■ Approximately half of rectal carcinoids stain positively with argyrophil techniques.

■ Behaviorally, carcinoids are indolent if confined above the muscularis propria, inactive mitotically, and less than 2 cm in diameter.

■ Colonic carcinoids tend to be large invasive tumors that often have metastasized at the time of diagnosis. They show a spectrum of differentiation, merging at the anaplastic end with small cell undifferentiated carcinoma.

Clinical Features

■ Half of all rectal carcinoids are discovered during digital or endoscopic rectal examination of asymptomatic patients. Most of the remainder are discovered during examination for unrelated symptoms of anorectal conditions.

■ The peak age incidence is in the fifth decade. The age range is from the third to the eighth decade.

Gross Pathology

■ Rectal carcinoids are usually firm, pale, yellow, smooth-surfaced nodules. Two thirds of rectal carcinoids are less than 0.4 cm in diameter, and the great majority are less than 2 cm in diameter.

■ Carcinoids larger than 2 cm in diameter may be ulcerated. The majority of carcinoids greater than 2 cm in diameter are malignant.

■ About 2% of cases are multiple.

Microscopic Pathology

- Carcinoids are usually located in the lamina propria and submucosa.
- The tumor may form anastomosing ribbons with a prominent vascular stroma, solid nests, tubuloacinar structures, and rosettes with central blood vessels. There may be considerable stromal fibrosis.
- The only consistently reliable criterion of malignancy is invasion of the muscularis propria. Cytologic features of malignancy such as nuclear pleomorphism, hyperchromatism, and high mitotic index are usually present.

Special Diagnostic Techniques

- Most rectal carcinoids stain positively for neuron-specific enolase and prostatic acid phosphatase. About half of all tumors stain positively for chromogranin, serotonin, and pancreatic polypeptide.

References

Burke M, Shephard N, Mann CV. Carcinoid tumors of the rectum and anus. Br J Surg 1987;74:358–361.

Federspiel BH, Burke AP, Sobin LH, Shekitka KM. Rectal and colonic carcinoids: a clinicopathologic study of 84 cases. Cancer 1990;65:135–140.

Rosenburg JM, Welch JP. Carcinoid tumors of the colon: a study of 72 patients. Am J Surg 1985;149:775–779.

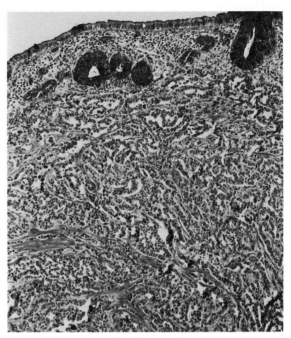

Figure 5–105. Rectal carcinoid with a glandular pattern.

ANGIODYSPLASIAS, TELANGIECTASIAS, AND HEMANGIOMAS

Biology of Disease

- *Angiodysplasias* and *telangiectasias* are acquired vascular dilatations of degenerative type. They consist of congeries of dilated capillaries and venules forming a well-defined lesion that is usually fed by a single arteriole. There is no impression of vascular proliferation (*hemangioma*).
- Telangiectasias are classically associated with Osler-Weber-Rendu disease, Turner's syndrome, systemic sclerosis (CREST syndrome), or irradiation. In most of these conditions, telangiectasias are not confined to the bowel.
- Angiodysplasias are acquired vascular ectasias that are usually multiple, and despite the name, they seem to be no more than acquired telangiectasias.
- Colonic hemangiomas are similar to those that occur elsewhere in the body. They may be associated with a variety of syndromes, but especially with the blue rubber bleb nevus syndrome.

Clinical Features

- Angiodysplasias (degenerative telangiectasias) are a common cause of recurrent acute colonic bleeding in patients older than 60 years. They can be diagnosed endoscopically and treated by cauterization. Angiography may also detect them.
- Hemangiomas manifest also as bleeding.

Gross Pathology

- Ectasias are liable to collapse after resection and may be difficult or impossible to find. In several of the published series of angiodysplasia, the authors undertook to heparinize the vessels in the operating room, to inject radiopaque contrast material, and to perform specimen radiography or corrosion casts—procedures that are too laborious for routine practice.
- Most ectasias are less than 5 mm in diameter.
- Hemangiomas may be considerably larger than telangiectasias, diffusely involving large areas of the bowel.

Microscopic Pathology

- Angiodysplasias and telangiectasias are small collections of dilated thin-walled blood vessels in the mucosa and submucosa. The vessels are intimately mixed with other, normal tissue components.
- Hemangiomas show large numbers of blood vessels, not simply dilated vessels. They may be capillary, cavernous, or mixed. The cavernous variants are most common.

References

Pounder DJ, Rowland R, Pieterse AS, et al. Angiodysplasia of the colon. J Clin Pathol 1982;35:824–829.

Vase P, Grove O. Gastrointestinal lesions in hereditary hemorrhagic telangiectasia. Gastroenterology 1986;91:1079–1083.

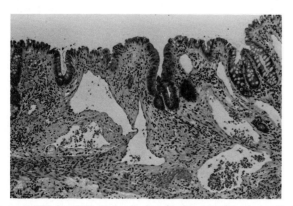

Figure 5–106. Angiodysplasia of colon showing telangiectatic vessels in mucosa and submucosa. (Courtesy of Dr. Steve Rasmussen.)

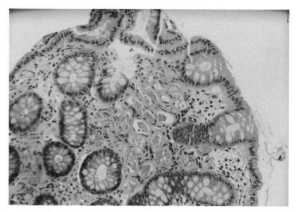

Figure 5–107. Colonic mucosa showing capillary hemangioma.

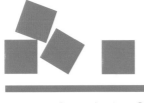

DISEASES OF
THE ANUS

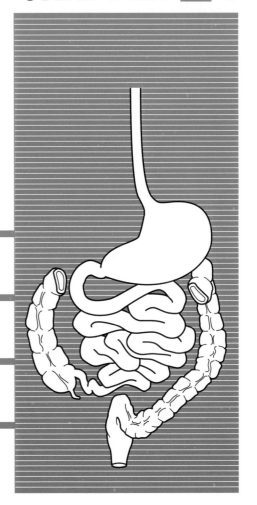

CHAPTER 6

ANATOMY AND HISTOLOGY

Gross Anatomy

■ The histologic anal canal extends from the lower margin of the rectum, which is lined by columnar epithelium, to the anal verge, where there is hair-bearing skin.

■ The only reliable grossly recognizable landmark in the anal canal is the dentate (pectinate) line. This wavy line, which runs transversely around the anus, represents the embryologic junction between the cloaca and the proctodeum.

■ Above the dentate line lies the so-called transitional zone, which is covered by nonkeratinizing squamous epithelium and/or transitional type epithelium. The junction between the transitional zone and the rectal mucosa is not recognizable macroscopically. The transitional zone is 0.5 to 1.0 cm in length.

■ Below the dentate line lies the anal margin, which is covered by non–hair-bearing squamous epithelium that is partly nonkeratinizing and partly keratinizing. The point at which this epithelium merges with skin is vague, and the junction may extend 1 to 2 cm.

■ Immediately above the dentate line are the columns of Morgagni. These consist of 6 to 10 longitudinal folds, which are joined at their bases by small semilunar valves.

■ Mucus-secreting anal glands are found in the transitional zone. Most have ducts that open immediately above the anal valves.

Microscopic Appearance

■ The anal transitional zone consists of nonkeratinizing squamous or transitional epithelium.

■ Typical transitional epithelium consists of four to nine basal layers covered by umbrella cells. It resembles urothelium.

■ The nonkeratinizing squamous epithelium may have cuboidal or polygonal cells on the surface, or there may be 1 to 2 layers of flattened cells.

■ The junction between transitional and rectal epithelium is extremely irregular, and a single section may show alternate islands of both types.

■ The anal glands are simple tubular mucous glands that empty into a duct lined by transitional epithelium. Occasional goblet cells may be present in the gland ducts.

■ Melanocytes are frequently demonstrated in the epithelium of the anal margin. The transitional zone contains occasional melanocytes.

References

Clemmensen OJ, Fenger C. Melanocytes in the anal canal epithelium. Histopathology 1991;18:237–241.

Fenger C. The anal transitional zone. Location and extent. Acta Pathol Microbiol Scand [A] 1979;87:379–386.

Fenger C. Histology of the anal canal. Am J Surg Pathol 1988;12:41–55.

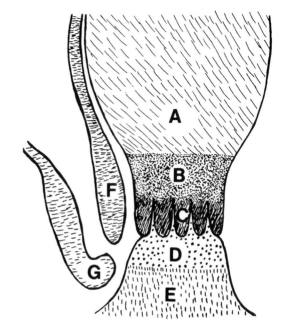

Figure 6–1. Lower rectum and anal canal, consisting of *A*, rectum; *B*, anal columnar zone; *C*, transitional zone; *D*, anal margin, *E*, perianal skin, *F*, internal sphincter, and *G*, external sphincter. The anatomical anal canal consists of zones *B*, *C*, and *D* that are covered by the internal sphincter.

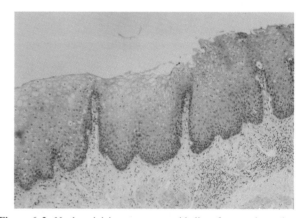

Figure 6–2. Nonkeratinizing squamous epithelium from anal margin.

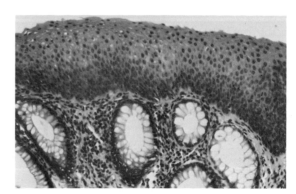

Figure 6–3. Transitional zone with nonkeratinizing squamous epithelium apparently overlying rectal mucosa.

HEMORRHOIDS

Biology of Disease

- Hemorrhoids represent a dilatation of veins in either the external or the internal venous plexuses originating either above or below the dentate line.
- They are more common in developed countries, suggesting that they may be associated with a low-residue diet and straining at stool.
- In some patients, they may be the result of an age-related degeneration of connective tissue accompanied by fibrosis.

Clinical Features

- Hemorrhoids usually present with bright red bleeding.
- Larger hemorrhoids produce a polypoid mass that prolapses down the anal canal and may require manual reduction.
- Pain can occur when hemorrhoids become infected or undergo thrombosis.

Gross Pathology

- When a hemorrhoidectomy specimen is received in the laboratory, the veins are usually collapsed and inconspicuous.
- Internal hemorrhoids are covered by columnar and transitional zone mucosa. External hemorrhoids are covered by nonkeratinizing squamous epithelium.

Microscopic Pathology

- The histology is variable but consists basically of dilated veins. They may be of variable size and have thick or thin walls.
- Between the veins is a fibromuscular stroma, which generally only shows mild inflammatory changes.
- The veins may undergo thrombosis with recanalization.

Differential Diagnosis

Histologically, hemorrhoids are characteristic and unlikely to be confused with anything else. However, it is important that all hemorrhoidectomy specimens be examined microscopically, since gross inspection alone can miss an associated carcinoma in situ, or even an invasive carcinoma.

References

Haqqani MT, Hancock BD. Internal sphincter and hemorrhoids: a pathological study. J Clin Pathol 1978;31:268–270.

Thomson WHF. The nature of hemorrhoids. Br J Surg 1975;62:542–552.

Thulesius O, Gjores JE. Arteriovenous anastomoses in the anal region with references to the pathogenesis and treatment of hemorrhoids. Acta Chir Scand 1973;139:476–479.

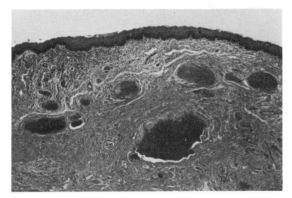

Figure 6–4. Hemorrhoids showing a polypoid appearance with thick-walled vessels.

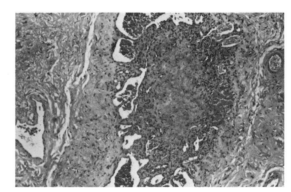

Figure 6–5. Hemorrhoids with thrombosis.

CONDYLOMA ACUMINATUM

Biology of Disease

- These venereally transmitted warts are caused by a papillomavirus.
- Virus types 6 and 11 are most regularly identified, but occasionally other types, including 16 and 18, are encountered.
- Condylomas typically affect young adults.
- Lesions are frequently multiple.
- Tetraploidy and octaploidy are almost invariably present.

Clinical Features

- Small lesions may be asymptomatic.
- Larger condylomas may cause irritation or may bleed.
- Warts may also be present on the external genitalia.

Gross Pathology

■ Condylomas are warty (cauliflower-like) growths that are often as much as several centimeters in diameter.

■ They typically arise in the epithelium of the anal margin.

Microscopic Pathology

■ Condylomas are well-defined lesions with a distinct margin.

■ Architecturally, they are squamous papillomas with well-developed fibrous cores covered by acanthotic squamous epithelium.

■ The basal layer is 1 to 5 cells thick and contains normal mitoses.

■ The malpighian layer shows orderly maturation with regular rounded, but slightly enlarged nuclei.

■ Koilocytic changes may be present in which the intermediate and superficial cells have a clear cytoplasm and a slightly pyknotic nucleus.

Special Techniques

■ Immunologic techniques, especially in situ hybridization, will demonstrate papillomavirus in up to 75% of cases.

Differential Diagnosis

Verrucous carcinoma, anal intraepithelial neoplasia.

Verrucous carcinomas (giant condylomas of Buschke and Lowenstein) are usually more than 2 cm in diameter and have prominent rete pegs that extend down into the underlying tissue. Nonirritated condylomas do not have this invasive pattern at the base.

Anal intraepithelial neoplasia is usually a flat lesion; however, it can occur in condylomas where it is identified by the presence of epithelial atypia.

References

Ferenczy A, Mitao M, Nagai N, et al. Latent papilloma virus and recurring genital warts. N Engl J Med 1985;313:784–788.

Shevchuk MM, Richart RM. DNA content of condyloma acuminatum. Cancer 1982;49:489–492.

Wells M, Griffiths S, Lewis F, et al. Identification of human papillomavirus in paraffin sections of anal condylomas and squamous carcinomas by in-situ DNA hybridization. J Pathol 1987;151:64A.

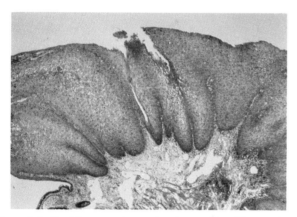

Figure 6–6. Condyloma acuminatum showing usual frondlike growth pattern.

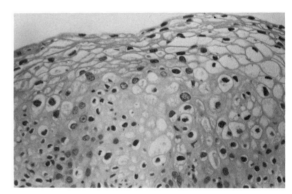

Figure 6–7. Koilocytic change.

ANAL INTRAEPITHELIAL NEOPLASIA

Biology of Disease

■ Anal intraepithelial neoplasia (AIN) may occur in flat mucosa or in condylomas.

■ As at other sites, the degree of dysplasia may vary, but it is necessary to identify only two grades: low grade and high grade. The latter category includes Bowen's disease and carcinoma in situ.

■ AIN is considered to be the result of papillomavirus infection, particularly types 16 and 18. It is more common in women and homosexual men.

Clinical Features

■ AIN may present with rectal itching or burning.

■ AIN in flat mucosa may involve the transitional zone, anal margin, or perianal skin.

■ Flat lesions may be identified grossly by the presence of hyperkeratosis or red patches.

■ The presence of AIN in condylomas is generally unrecognizable by gross inspection.

■ Ten percent of cases are discovered incidentally on examination of resected hemorrhoids.

■ Recurrence after local excision is common.

■ The subsequent development of invasive carcinoma is common and may occur in as many as 60% of cases of high-grade dysplasia.

Gross Pathology

■ The diagnosis of AIN is histologic. The disease may be present in condylomas or in flat mucosa.

Microscopic Pathology

■ AIN is characterized by the presence of dysplasia. The diagnostic features are (1) nuclear crowding (i.e., an apparent expansion of the basal layer); (2) nuclear enlargement; (3) nuclear pleomorphism with irregular nuclear outline and uneven distribution of chromatin; (4) mitotic activity above the level of the normal basal layer; (5) atypical mitoses; and (6) individual cell keratinization.

■ In low-grade dysplasia, the abnormalities occupy the lower one third to one half of the mucosal thickness. Full-thickness or virtually full-thickness changes are seen in high-grade dysplasia.

■ Keratinization may be present on the surface.

■ Koilocytic changes may be found in both flat and condylomatous AIN. Although this should be recorded in the diagnosis, it does not affect the grade of AIN or its biologic significance.

Differential Diagnosis

Epithelial hyperplasia without dysplasia, nondysplastic condyloma, invasive carcinoma, podophyllin effect.

Dysplasia must be present for the diagnosis of AIN. Sometimes this can be difficult to distinguish from reactive changes secondary to inflammation. Fortunately, such marginal cases may be safely managed by follow-up with repeat biopsy.

Early invasive carcinoma is recognized by the presence of irregular downward growth of tongues of squamous epithelium.

Podophyllin effect may produce inflammation and hyperplasia. Increased mitotic activity may be present with inflammatory atypia. There may be no reliable way to distinguish this from true dysplasia other than by the history.

References

Ehecjan GC, Idikio HA, Nayak B, Gardiner JP. Malignant transformation in an anal condyloma acuminatum. Can J Surg 1983;79:178–181.

Frazer IH, Medley G, Crapper RM, et al. Association between ano-rectal dysplasia, human papilloma virus and human immunodeficiency virus in homosexual men. Lancet 1986;2:657–660.

Marfing TE, Abel ME, Gallagher DM. Perianal Bowen's disease and associated malignancies. Results of a survey. Dis Colon Rectum 1987;30:782–785.

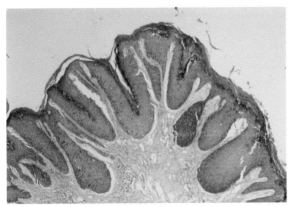

Figure 6–8. Anal intraepithelial neoplasia showing epithelial thickening and hyperkeratosis.

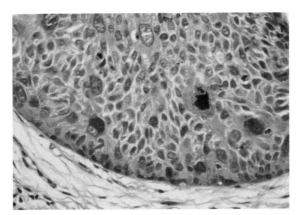

Figure 6–10. Scattered severely atypical cells. Note individual cell keratinization.

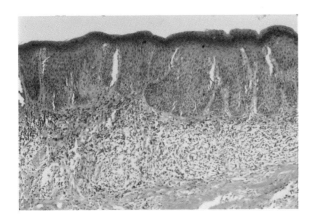

Figure 6–9. Full-thickness epithelial atypia with hyperkeratosis and a mixed chronic infiltrate in the lamina propria.

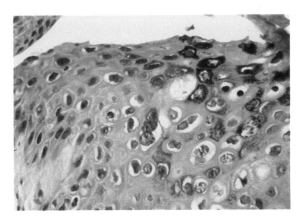

Figure 6–11. Atypia plus koilocytic change.

ANAL SQUAMOUS CARCINOMA

Biology of Disease

- These tumors may arise from the transitional zone or from the anal margin epithelium below the pectinate line.
- Tumors arising in the transitional zone comprise 75% of all anal carcinomas. They are twice as common in women as in men and behave aggressively.
- Tumors arising from the anal margin are four times more common in men than in women. They are relatively less aggressive and occur more frequently in third world countries.
- Associated and predisposing factors include anal intraepithelial neoplasia, condylomas, human papillomavirus infection, and Crohn's disease.

Clinical Features

- Patients present with rectal bleeding and pain. Sometimes a mass may be noted.
- Treatment is predominately by radiotherapy and chemotherapy, rather than by abdominoperineal excision.

Gross Pathology

- These tumors are usually indistinguishable grossly from adenocarcinomas of the rectum.
- They tend to be ulcerated with rolled edges.
- Polypoid lesions are less commonly encountered.

Microscopic Pathology

- Tumors arising in the anal margin are usually well to moderately differentiated keratinizing squamous carcinomas.
- Two thirds of transitional zone carcinomas are keratinizing squamous carcinomas. Typically, they are moderately to poorly differentiated. They resemble squamous carcinomas at other sites.
- One third of transitional zone carcinomas are cloacogenic (basaloid), consisting of basal type cells with small quantities of cytoplasm. They grow in islands with central necrosis and palisading at the edge. The mitotic rate is generally high, and focal keratinization may be present. The stroma is desmoplastic.

References

Boman B, Moertel CG, O'Connell MJ, et al. Carcinoma of the anal canal. A clinical and pathological study of 188 cases. Cancer 1984;54:114–125.

Daling JR, Weiss NS, Hislop G, et al. Sexual practices, sexually transmitted diseases, and the incidence of anal cancer. N Engl J Med 1987;317:973–977.

Greenall MJ, Quan SH, Stearns MW, et al. Epidermoid cancer of the anal margin: pathologic features, treatment and clinical results. Am J Surg 1985;149:95–101.

Palmer JG, Shepherd NA, Jass JR, et al. Human papillomavirus type 16 DNA in anal squamous carcinoma. Lancet 1987;2:42.

Papillon J, Montbaron JT. Epidermoid carcinoma of the anal canal: a series of 276 cases. Dis Colon Rectum 1987;30:324–333.

Shepherd NA, Scholefield JH, Love SB, et al. Prognostic factors in anal squamous carcinoma: a multivariate analysis of clinical, pathological and flow cytometric parameters in 235 cases. Histopathology 1990;16:545–555.

Slater G, Greenstein A, Aufses AH. Anal carcinoma in patients with Crohn's disease. Ann Surg 1984;199:348–350.

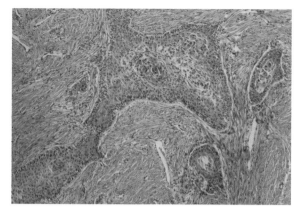

Figure 6–12. Keratinizing-type squamous carcinoma.

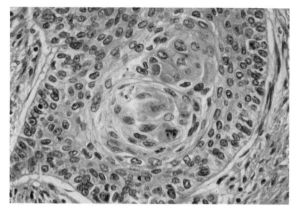

Figure 6–13. Keratinizing squamous carcinoma with cells containing abundant eosinophilic cytoplasm.

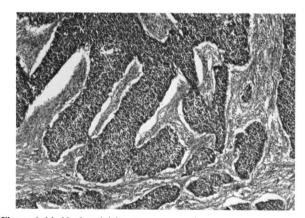

Figure 6–14. Nonkeratinizing squamous carcinoma.

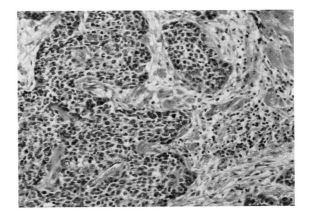

Figure 6–15. Nonkeratinizing squamous carcinoma with basaloid cells.

VERRUCOUS CARCINOMA

Biology of Disease

- This lesion, also referred to as the *giant condyloma of Buschke and Lowenstein*, occurs mainly in the anal margin mucosa.
- The lesions are large, generally over 2 cm in diameter, and extend laterally and invade underlying tissues but never metastasize unless dedifferentiation occurs.

Clinical Features

- Verrucous carcinoma presents as a large, slow-growing, cauliflower-shaped mass.
- If neglected, it can invade the underlying tissue, causing sinuses and fistulae.
- Treatment is surgical, preferably by local excision, but by abdominoperineal excision if necessary. Radiation can cause dedifferentiation of the tumor.

Gross Pathology

- Apart from their size, these tumors are indistinguishable from condylomas.

Microscopic Pathology

- Verrucous carcinomas very closely resemble simple condylomas and do not have marked cellular atypia. There may be mild basal layer atypia.
- The growth pattern is papillomatous with an arborizing fibrous stromal core.
- The base of the lesion shows invasion into the underlying connective tissue. However this may be hard to recognize, because the tumor is so well differentiated.
- Koilocytic change is usually not prominent but may be seen.

Differential Diagnosis

Condyloma acuminatum.

A high index of suspicion should be entertained for all "condylomas" in excess of 2 cm diameter.

Invasion at the base is the key distinguishing feature of carcinomas. Tongues of sharply angulated, well-differentiated squamous cells extend into the dermal collagen bundles.

References

Bogomoletz WV, Potet F, Molas G. Condylomata acuminata, giant condylomas acuminatum (Bushke-Lowenstein tumor) and verrucous squamous carcinoma of the perianal and anorectal region: a continuous precancerous spectrum? Histopathology 1985;9:155–169.

Gingrass PJ, Burbrick MP, Hitchcock CR, et al. Anorectal verrucous squamous carcinoma: report of two cases. Dis Colon Rectum 1978; 21:120–122.

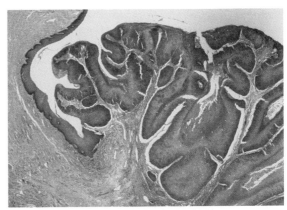

Figure 6–16. Verrucous carcinoma. Note the low-power similarity to a condyloma, although the base of the lesion extends below the level of the normal squamous epithelium.

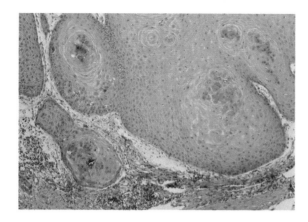

Figure 6–17. Invasion into dermal collagen at the base of the lesion.

ANAL GLAND CARCINOMA

Biology of Disease

- These tumors arise from the ducts of anal glands, rather than from the glands themselves.
- Three different histologic types are described: well-differentiated adenocarcinoma, mucinous carcinoma, and mucoepidermoid carcinoma.
- Well-differentiated carcinomas have a good prognosis. They are slow growing and easily excised locally.
- Mucinous carcinomas have a poor prognosis. They are difficult to excise locally, because of infiltration. They readily metastasize. This tumor tends to occur in elderly individuals and may complicate chronic anal fistulae in Crohn's disease.
- Mucoepidermoid carcinomas contain squamous carcinoma and areas of glandular differentiation.

Clinical Features

- All types of anal gland carcinoma may present with a perianal mass, bleeding, pain, and anal irritation.

Gross Pathology

- There are few useful gross diagnostic features. The mucinous carcinomas may appear slimy.

Microscopic Pathology

- The well-differentiated carcinomas consist of large duct-like structures lined by an exceedingly bland columnar epithelium similar to that seen in large bowel adenoma.
- Mucinous carcinomas consist of large cystlike structures filled with mucin. The lining may vary from a simple tall mucus-secreting epithelium to a more obviously malignant epithelium that resembles a colonic colloid carcinoma.
- Mucoepidermoid carcinoma is somewhat different from similar tumors of the salivary glands. It contains an intimate mixture of squamous (cloacogenic) carcinoma with mucoid differentiation.

References

Berg JW, Love F, Stearus MW. Mucoepidermoid anal cancer. Cancer 1960;13:914–916.

Jensen SL, Shokouh-Amiri MH, Hagen K, et al. Adenocarcinoma of the anal ducts. A series of 21 cases. Dis Colon Rectum 1988;31:268–272.

Prioleau PG, Allen MS, Roberts T. Perianal mucinous adenocarcinoma. Cancer 1977;39:1295–1299.

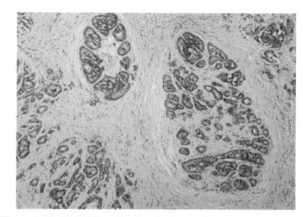

Figure 6–18. Well-differentiated anal adenocarcinoma.

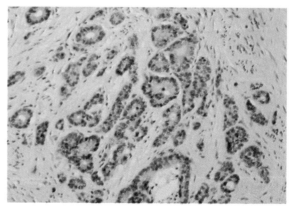

Figure 6–19. Tumor composed of distinctive, well-differentiated glandular structures.

ANAL MALIGNANT MELANOMA

Biology of Disease

- Most anal melanomas arise in the transitional zone.
- They affect adults in a variety of age groups.
- They have a poor prognosis.

Clinical Features

- Anal melanomas usually present as a bleeding mass.
- Occasionally, they may be polypoid and undergo prolapse.

Gross Pathology

- About two thirds of anal melanomas show varying degrees of pigmentation.
- The tumors average 4 cm in diameter at presentation.

Microscopic Pathology

- They resemble cutaneous melanomas and consist predominately of plump epithelioid cells with smaller numbers of spindle cells.
- Nesting may be present.
- Junctional activity may be seen at the tumor edge.

Special Techniques

- In common with other types of melanoma, they may stain positively with Fontana-Masson, Schmorl's, S100, and HMB 45 stains.

Differential Diagnosis

Poorly differentiated squamous cell carcinoma and adenocarcinoma, epithelioid leiomyosarcoma, large cell lymphoma.

Reliance must be placed on special stains to confirm the diagnosis.

Ultrastructural examination will confirm the presence of melanosomes or premelanosomes.

References

Cooper PH, Mills SE, Allen MS. Malignant melanoma of the anus. Report of 12 patients and analysis of 255 additional cases. Dis Colon Rectum 1982;25:693–670.

Mason JK, Helwig EB. Anorectal melanoma. Cancer 1966;19:39–50.

Wanebo HJ, Woodruff JM, Farr GH, Quan SH. Anorectal melanomas. Cancer 1981;57:1891–1900.

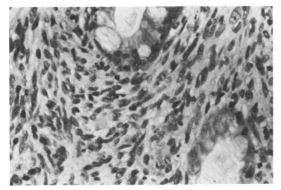

Figure 6–20. Anal canal melanoma showing a spindle cell pattern. It is infiltrating rectal mucosa.

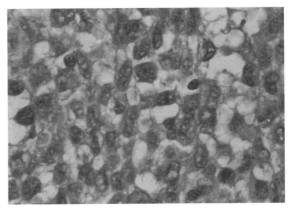

Figure 6–21. Anal melanoma showing typical plump epithelioid cells.

PAGET'S DISEASE

Biology of Disease

- Paget's disease predominately involves the perianal skin but can also occur in the anal canal.
- It consists of intraepidermal spread of adenocarcinoma as either single cells or small groups of cells.
- In many cases of Paget's disease, there is a coexistent invasive adenocarcinoma arising in perianal glands or rectal mucosa. However, in a substantial number of cases, the disease is apparently primary in the skin, and no invasive tumor develops.

Clinical Features

- Perianal Paget's disease commonly presents with pruritus.
- Reddish patches or plaques may be seen on examination.

Gross Pathology

■ There may be reddish patches or plaques that eventually ulcerate.

Microscopic Pathology

■ The squamous component of the epithelium may be inflamed and there may be excess surface keratinization. However, the squamous cells do not show features of neoplasia.
■ Paget cells are present in single cells or aggregates of cells. They generally have a clear cytoplasm and large irregular hyperchromatic nuclei.

Special Techniques

■ Mucin stains, such as Alcian blue and periodic acid-Schiff (PAS) with diastase, may be positive. Paget cells may also be immunopositive for immunostains for keratin and carcinoembryonic antigen (CEA).

Differential Diagnosis

Melanoma, squamous carcinoma in situ.

Melanoma cells may have a pagetoid appearance. They may be positive on immunostaining with S100 and/or HMB 45. They are mucin and CEA negative.

Squamous carcinoma in situ (Bowen's disease) is negative for S100, HMB 45, mucin or CEA.

References

Beck DE, Fazio VW. Perianal Paget's disease. Dis Colon Rectum 1987;30:263–266.
Kariniemi AL, Ramaekers F, Lehto VP, Virtanen I. Paget's cells express cytokeratin typical of glandular epithelia. Br J Dermatol 1985;112:179–183.
Wood WS, Culling WG. Perianal Paget's disease. Arch Pathol 1975;99:442–445.

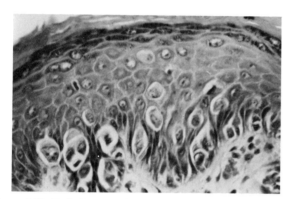

Figure 6–22. Typical Paget cells, which appear shrunken. They are surrounded by a clear halo.

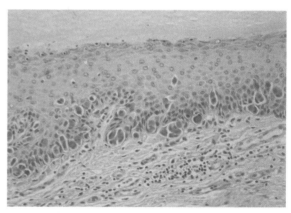

Figure 6–23. Paget cells showing cytoplasmic mucin positive with a PAS/diastase stain.

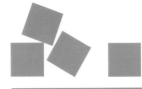

DISEASES THAT
MAY AFFECT
MULTIPLE ORGANS

CHAPTER ■ 7

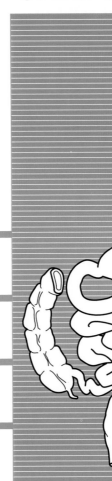

HERPES SIMPLEX

Biology of Disease

- Herpes simplex most commonly involves the squamous epithelium of the esophagus or anal canal. Distal colonic and gastric columnar epithelial involvement can occur but is much rarer.
- Most cases occur in immunosuppressed individuals, particularly AIDS patients, bone marrow transplant recipients, and leukemia patients. Herpes may also affect apparently immunocompetent persons.
- In the esophagus, most infections are due to herpes simplex type I. In the anal region, 80% are the result of herpes type II infection.

Clinical Features

- Esophageal herpes causes odynophagia and dysphagia. On examination, vesicles or aphthous ulcers may be seen, but more often there are widespread erosions resembling peptic esophagitis.
- Perianal herpes presents with severe anorectal pain, tenesmus, constipation, fever, difficulty in urinating, inguinal lymphadenopathy, and sacral parasthesia. Vesicles or ulcers are seen in the anus and in the distal 5 cm of the rectum.

Gross Pathology

- Herpes simplex ulcers are characteristically small (1 to 2 mm), shallow, and contain whitish slough with an erythematous edge. Larger ulcers may have nonspecific findings.
- Vesicles are also 1 to 2 mm in diameter and appear whitish in color.

Microscopic Pathology

- The center and base of a herpetic ulcer may show nonspecific slough and granulation tissue.
- The diagnostic morphology is the presence of basophilic "ground-glass" intranuclear inclusions (Cowdry B), or eosinophilic inclusions with a clear halo (Cowdry A).
- Multinucleated squamous cells may be present.
- Concomitant candidiasis or cytomegalovirus inclusions may be seen in immunosuppressed patients.

Special Techniques

- Immunostains for herpes are available and will positively identify the intranuclear inclusions.

References

Agha FP, Lee HH, Nostrant TT. Herpetic esophagitis: a diagnostic challenge in immunocompromised patients. Am J Gastroenterol 1986;81:246–253.

Boulton AJ, Slater DN, Hancock BW. Herpes virus colitis: a new cause of diarrhea in patients with Hodgkin's disease. Gut 1982;23:247–249.

Corey L, Spear PG. Infections with herpes simplex. N Engl J Med 1986;314:749–757.

Freiden W, Borchard F, Burrig KF, Pfitzer P. Herpes esophagitis. Light microscopical and immunohistochemical observations. Virchows Arch [A] 1984;404:1067-1076.

Goodell SE, Quinn TC, Mkrtichian E, et al. Herpes simplex virus proctitis in homosexual men. N Engl J Med 1983;308:868–871.

Howiler W, Goldberg HI. Gastroesophageal involvement in herpes simplex. Gastroenterology 1976;70:775–778.

Nash G, Ross JS. Herpetic esophagitis. A common cause of esophageal ulceration. Hum Pathol 1974;5:339–345.

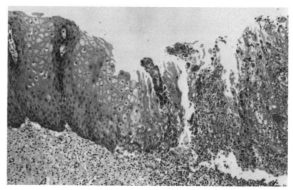

Figure 7–1. Herpetic ulceration of esophagus. Note the necrotic epithelial slough.

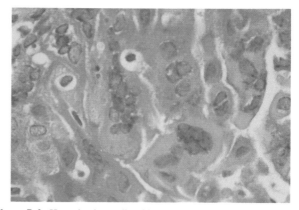

Figure 7–2. Herpetic giant cells with ground-glass nuclei.

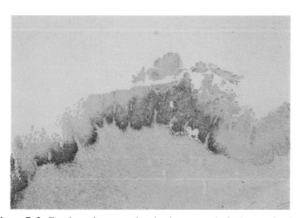

Figure 7–3. Esophageal mucosa showing immunostain for herpes simplex.

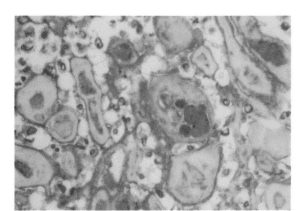

Figure 7–4. Immunostain showing positivity of the intranuclear inclusions.

CYTOMEGALOVIRUS

Biology of Disease

■ Cytomegalovirus (CMV) infection usually occurs in immunodeficient individuals, especially AIDS patients and transplant recipients.

■ In rare instances, infection can occur in immunocompetent patients (1) as a self-limited proctitis, or (2) in cases of ulcerative colitis with fulminant colitis (usually treated with corticosteroids).

■ CMV can affect any part of the gastrointestinal tract but is most common in the small and large bowel.

■ Infection is assumed to be present when CMV inclusions are seen. CMV may secondarily infect tissues damaged by another agent.

Clinical Features

■ There are no specific features. Patients often have severe diarrhea. Ulcers may cause hematochezia or perforation.

Gross Pathology

■ In early infection, the mucosa may appear virtually normal.

■ With more advanced disease, there may be mucosal erythema or edema suggestive of active inflammation.

■ Severe advanced disease is characterized by ulceration. These ulcers may be shallow or deep and can give rise to bleeding or perforation.

■ Rarely, CMV infection may produce extensive thickened mucosal folds in the gastric body.

Microscopic Pathology

■ Cytomegaly and intranuclear inclusions are the hallmarks of CMV and may be found in columnar epithelial and stromal (usually endothelial) cells.

■ Intranuclear inclusions consist of homogeneous eosinophilic masses with a clear zone separating the inclusion from the nuclear membrane.

■ Cytoplasmic inclusions are multiple, granular, and basophilic.

■ In upper gastrointestinal biopsies of nonulcerated epithelium, inclusions are most common in Brunner's glands.

■ Inclusions may occur in acute or chronically inflamed mucosa or in noninflamed mucosa.

■ In ulcers, the inclusions are most commonly found in swollen endothelial cells of granulation tissue at the ulcer base.

■ In some cases, classical inclusions are not encountered, but smudge cells may be present. These are enlarged cells with a loss of distinction between nucleus and cytoplasm. Special techniques may be necessary to identify CMV positivity.

Special Techniques

■ An immunoperoxidase method is available to demonstrate CMV antigen. This helps to distinguish small inclusions from large nucleoli or to confirm doubtful cases.

References

Cooper HS, Raffensperger EC, Jonas L, Fitts WT. Cytomegalovirus inclusions in patients with ulcerative colitis and toxic dilatation requiring colonic resection. Gastroenterology 1977;72:1253–1256.

Elta G, Turnage R, Eckhauser FE, et al. A submucosal antral mass caused by cytomegalovirus infection in a patient with acquired immunodeficiency syndrome. Am J Gastroenterol 1976;81:714–717.

Francis ND, Boylston AW, Roberts AH, et al. Cytomegalovirus infection in gastrointestinal tracts of patients infected with HIV-1 or AIDS. J Clin Pathol 1989;42:1055–1064.

Hinnant KL, Rotterdam HZ, Bell ET, Tapper ML. Cytomegalovirus infection of the alimentary tract. A clinicopathologic association. Am J Gastroenterol 1986;81:944–950.

Surawicz CM, Myerson D. Self limited cytomegalovirus colitis in immunocompetent individuals. Gastroenterology 1988;94:194–199.

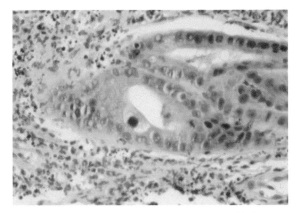

Figure 7–5. Intranuclear inclusion of CMV in gastric epithelium.

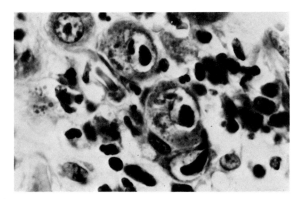

Figure 7–7. CMV in swollen endothelial cells.

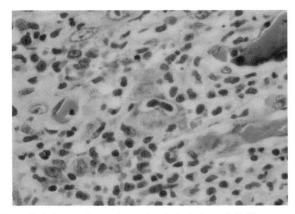

Figure 7–6. Intranuclear and cytoplasmic inclusions of CMV.

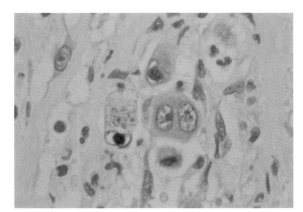

Figure 7–8. Immunostain for CMV.

FUNGAL DISEASES

Biology of Disease

- Candidiasis is by far the most frequent fungal infection of the gastrointestinal tract. Histoplasmosis, aspergillosis, phycomycosis (mucormycosis), cryptococcosis, and blastomycosis have also been described.
- Fungal diseases are distinctly more common in immunosuppressed patients.
- Candidiasis is most common in the esophagus. *Candida* infection elsewhere in the gut is usually part of systemic candidiasis.
- Traditionally, esophageal candidiasis has been divided into invasive and noninvasive forms, with invasive *Candida* considered significant and noninvasive *Candida* a surface contaminant from oral colonization. In immunosuppressed patients, however, particularly those with neutropenia, both forms are equally serious and should be treated vigorously to prevent the development of systemic candidiasis.

Clinical Features

- Esophageal candidiasis causes dysphagia and odynophagia. Sometimes it is difficult to determine to what extent the symptoms are due to *Candida* infection or to other factors.
- Histoplasmosis of the terminal ileal region may cause obstructive symptoms.
- Other fungi are usually associated with symptoms of septicemia.

Gross Pathology

- Esophageal candidiasis is characterized initially by the presence of whitish plaques. Later, there may be erosions or even deep ulceration.
- Fungemia produces shallow or deep ulcers at multiple sites.

Microscopic Pathology

■ To be considered significant in immunocompetent individuals, fungal hyphae or yeast forms must invade the epithelium and not just be present on the mucosal surface. This is particularly true in the esophagus, where hyphae may be found in swallowed saliva. In the stomach, noninvasive *Candida* may grow in slough at the base of peptic ulcers or ulcerated carcinomas. In neutropenic patients, all candidal lesions of the esophagus are considered significant.

■ To a greater or lesser extent, the esophageal epithelium in candidal infection is infiltrated by neutrophils. Where ulcers are present, the hyphae may be identified invading granulation tissue at the base.

■ In cases of fungal septicemia, widespread ulceration is present in the gastrointestinal tract, and fungal elements, most often *Aspergillus* and *Candida*, may be identified in areas of maximal inflammation.

Special Techniques

■ Special stains for fungi, especially a silver stain, such as Grocott's, methenamine silver or PAS, are strongly recommended in all cases of otherwise nonspecific inflammation or ulceration occurring in immunosuppressed patients. Hyphae may be hard to identify on routine hematoxylin and eosin sections.

References

Eras P, Goldstein MJ, Sherlock P. *Candida* infection of the gastrointestinal tract. Medicine 1972;51:367–379.
Kodsi BE, Wickremoinge PC, Kozinin PJ, et al. Candida esophagitis: a prospective study of 27 cases. Gastroenterology 1976;71:715–719.
Lyon DT, Schubert TT, Mantia AG, Kaplan MH. Phycomycosis of the gastrointestinal tract. Am J Gastroenterol 1979;72:379–394.
Pedraza MA. Mycotic infections at autopsy: a comparative study in two university hospitals. Am J Clin Pathol 1969;51:470–476.
Prescott RJ, Harris M, Banerjee SS. Fungal infections of the small and large intestine. J Clin Pathol 1992;45:806–811.

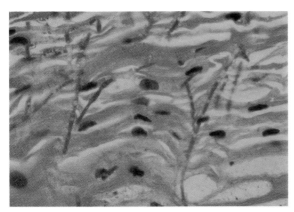

Figure 7–9. Esophagitis due to *Candida*. Note that the organisms have invaded the epithelium but there is no inflammatory response.

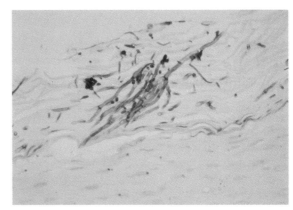

Figure 7–10. *Candida* (PAS with diastase).

GRAFT VERSUS HOST DISEASE

Biology of Disease

■ Most cases of graft versus host disease (GVHD) occur after bone marrow transplantation (BMT). The disease may rarely follow a solid organ transplant or even a blood transfusion.

■ BMT is preceded by chemoradiotherapy to ablate the recipient's original marrow. This treatment produces gastrointestinal cell necrosis and regeneration that is difficult to distinguish from GVHD. Usually these changes resolve by 21 days following transplant.

■ Acute GVHD may commence 21 days after transplant but most often presents after 28 days.

■ Acute GVHD is typically maximal in the small and large bowel. The stomach and esophagus are affected to a lesser extent.

■ Chronic GVHD may develop 80 days after transplantation, usually in patients with preceding acute GVHD.

Clinical Features

■ Symptoms of acute GVHD include an erythematous skin rash, severe diarrhea, abdominal pain, and nausea. Hemorrhage is a later complication when ulceration has occurred. Liver involvement may result in jaundice.

■ Chronic GVHD has features similar to that of systemic sclerosis and the sicca syndrome. There is a bland fibrosis involving skin and muscular layers of the esophagus and bowel. Esophageal dysmotility and strictures may result.

Gross Pathology

■ The early stages of GVHD show only mucosal erythema and friability. In the later stages, there may be mucosal sloughing and ulceration.
■ Chronic GVHD is characterized by thickening of the esophageal or bowel wall with stricture formation. Ulcers are not usually present in the bowel, although they can occur in the esophagus.

Microscopic Pathology

■ The earliest lesion of acute GVHD (grade I) is the exploding crypt cell. This is accompanied by evidence of epithelial regeneration (cells with enlarged nuclei, prominent nucleoli, and increased mitotic activity).
■ Exploding crypt cells consist of a clear vacuole containing necrotic debris (apoptotic bodies). These are present just above the basement membrane of the crypt.
■ Acute GVHD is usually not accompanied by a prominent inflammatory infiltrate, either acute or chronic, since most patients receive immunosuppressive therapy.
■ In severe cases, multiple exploding crypt cells are seen within a single crypt.
■ Grade II GVHD consists of necrotic debris within crypts, resembling crypt abscesses. Residual crypt cells are flattened, and crypts may be cystically dilated.
■ More severe or prolonged GVHD (grade III) is accompanied by crypt atrophy. The crypts are usually shortened and shrunken, as they contain fewer epithelial cells. Endocrine cells seem more resistant to GVHD than other cell types, so that eventually endocrine cell nests may survive alone deep in the lamina propria.
■ Ultimately, epithelial atrophy leads to a simplified mucosa with only a superficial layer of epithelium overlying lamina propria. At this stage, ulceration may occur (grade IV).

Special Techniques

■ No special techniques are available, but care must be taken not to miss a coexistent infection, particularly cytomegalovirus infection.

References

Epstein RK, McDonald GB, Sale GE, et al. The diagnostic accuracy of the rectal biopsy in acute graft versus host disease: a prospective study of 13 patients. Gastroenterology 1980;78:764–771.
McDonald GB, Shulman HM, Sullivan KM, Spencer GD. Intestinal and hepatic complications of human bone marrow transplantation. Gastroenterology 1986;90:460–477, 770–784.
Sale GE, Shulman HM, McDonald GB, Thomas ED. Gastrointestinal graft versus host disease in man: a clinicopathologic study of the rectal biopsy. Am J Surg Pathol 1979;3:291–299.
Snover DC, Weisdorf SA, Vercelotti GM, et al. A histologic study of gastric and intestinal graft versus host disease following allogenic bone marrow transplantation. Hum Pathol 1985;16:387–392.
Spencer GD, Shulman HM, Myerson D, et al. Diffuse intestinal ulceration after bone marrow transplantation: a clinicopathologic study of 13 patients. Hum Pathol 1986;17:621–633.

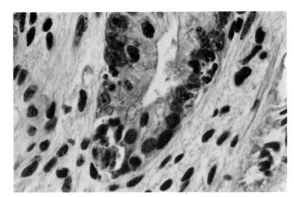

Figure 7–11. Grade I GVHD showing necrosis of individual cells at the base of a crypt.

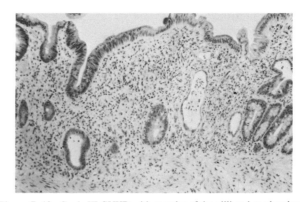

Figure 7–12. Grade III GVHD with atrophy of the villi and an abundance of edematous lamina propria.

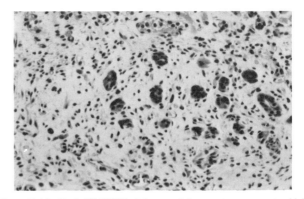

Figure 7–13. Grade III GVHD. A few surviving crypts are present, which contain mainly endocrine cells.

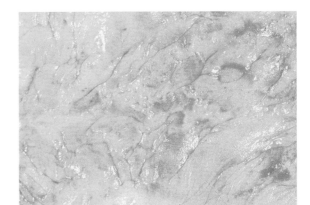

Figure 7–14. Grade IV GVHD of the large bowel with ulceration. The yellowish color of the specimen is a result of jaundice secondary to GVHD of the liver.

EOSINOPHILIC GASTROENTERITIS

Biology of Disease

- Eosinophilic infiltration of the gastrointestinal tract may be encountered in a wide variety of diseases.
- By convention, the term *eosinophilic gastroenteritis* should not be used loosely in a descriptive fashion, but should be restricted to a condition characterized by (1) the presence of gastrointestinal symptoms; (2) histologic evidence of massive eosinophil infiltration of the gastrointestinal tract; and (3) no evidence of any other condition, such as parasitic infestation, vasculitis, or systemic disease.
- The terms *eosinophilic colitis* and *allergic enterocolitis* have been used to describe the changes secondary to food allergy in young children (usually less than 2 years of age). This is probably a distinct clinical entity rather than merely a variant of adult eosinophilic gastroenteritis.
- Eosinophilic gastroenteritis has three major patterns of intestinal involvement. The most common is mucosally based, the next most frequent involves the muscularis propria, and the rarest affects the subserosa. Symptoms differ depending on which disease pattern predominates.
- Eosinophil infiltration, occurring in a bandlike fashion in the lamina propria just superficial to the muscularis mucosae, has been described in systemic sclerosis, polymyositis, and dermatomyositis.

Clinical Features

- Eosinophilic gastritis involving the mucosa may present with diarrhea and steatorrhea. There may be blood loss, leading to anemia and hypoproteinemia.
- Muscle involvement may present with features of bowel obstruction, including abdominal pain.
- Serosal disease may present with ascites and symptoms of peritonitis.
- More than 80% of patients with eosinophilic gastroenteritis have a peripheral blood eosinophilia. Usually, no food allergy can be demonstrated, but treatment with corticosteroids is generally effective.
- Eosinophilic enterocolitis in children presents with severe diarrhea, which may be blood stained. There may also be severe vomiting. Failure to thrive occurs unless treatment is instituted. In most instances, removal of milk from the diet is sufficient, although occasionally, multiple food allergies are present.

Gross Pathology

- Mucosal disease is characterized by edematous, reddened, and friable mucosa with thickened folds. Small ulcers may be present.
- Muscle disease produces inflammatory thickening of the stomach or bowel wall, which leads to luminal narrowing.
- In serosal disease, the peritoneum is thickened and opaque. Whitish or cream-colored plaques may be present.
- It is not uncommon for more than one of these patterns of disease to be present in the same patient.
- In the majority of cases, gastric or intestinal disease is localized (segmental), but diffuse involvement of the gastrointestinal tract, including the colon, is recognized also.
- The gastric antrum is affected in about 70% of patients, and about 50% have associated duodenal involvement. In about 10% of cases, only the small bowel is involved.

Microscopic Pathology

- Because the disease is patchy, the biopsy appearances may be variable. When the disease mainly involves the muscle layers, a mucosal biopsy may show only small numbers of eosinophils, although sometimes the submucosa is heavily infiltrated.
- In areas of maximal disease, the eosinophil infiltration is massive and sheetlike. Anything less than this degree of involvement should be classified as only suggestive of eosinophilic gastroenteritis.

■ In the small bowel, the villi may be either completely or partially flattened.

■ Eosinophil crypt (or pit) abscesses may be present.

■ Shallow ulcers may occur.

■ Eosinophilic enterocolitis, due to food allergy, is histologically similar to the diffuse mucosal form of eosinophilic gastroenteritis. In children, there are usually fewer eosinophils.

Differential Diagnosis

Inflammatory fibroid polyp, parasitic disease, collagen diseases, Churg-Strauss syndrome, inflammatory bowel disease, radiation changes, malignant lymphoma.

Inflammatory fibroid polyp, as the name implies, is always polypoid to a greater or lesser extent. The stroma may be infiltrated by large numbers of eosinophils, but there is usually no peripheral blood eosinophilia. Eosinophilic gastroenteritis is not characterized by the presence of polyps.

Bowel parasites that commonly result in eosinophilia include *Strongyloides*, *Trichuris,* and the herring tape worm *Eustoma rotundatum*. In addition, *Anisakis* larvae, which are ingested via raw fish, such as improperly prepared sushi, may penetrate into the stomach wall, producing an eosinophilic abscess.

In scleroderma and dermatomyositis, there may be a bandlike eosinophilic infiltrate, just superficial to the lamina propria. Obviously, the history will suggest this possibility.

The exceedingly rare Churg-Strauss syndrome is characterized by vasculitis as well as eosinophilia.

There may be considerable mucosal eosinophilia with inflammatory bowel disease, especially ulcerative colitis, particularly in the phase of resolution. However, the eosinophils are rarely sheetlike and seldom involve the muscularis propria.

Eosinophilia, often associated with enlarged hyperchromatic epithelial nuclei, may be a manifestation of early radiation enteropathy .

Certain T-cell lymphomas may be accompanied by considerable eosinophilia. However, this will not mask the basic diagnostic features of malignant lymphoma.

References

Blackshaw AJ, Levison DA. Eosinophilic infiltrates of the gastrointestinal tract. J Clin Pathol 1986;39:1–7.

Caldwell JH, Sharma HM, Hartubise PE, Colwell DL. Eosinophilic gastroenteritis—extreme allergy. Gastroenterology 1979;77:560–564.

Croese TJ. Eosinophilic enteritis: a recent North Queensland experience. Aust NZ J Med 1988;18:818–853.

De Schryver-Kecskemeti K, Clouse RE. A previously unrecognized subgroup of "eosinophilic gastroenteritis". Association with connective tissue diseases. Am J Surg Pathol 1984;8:171–180.

Goldman H, Proujansky R. Allergic proctitis and gastroenteritis in children. Clinical and mucosal biopsy features in 53 cases. Am J Surg Pathol 1986;10:75–86.

Johnstone H, Morson BC. Eosinophilic gastroenteritis. Histopathology 1978;12:348–355.

Leinbach GE, Rubin CE. Eosinophilic gastroenteritis: a simple reaction to food allergens? Gastroenterology 1970;59:874–889.

McNabb PC, Fleming CR, Higgins JA, Davis GL. Transmural eosinophilic gastroenteritis with ascites. Mayo Clin Proc 1979;54:119–122.

Sakanari JA, Loinaz HM, Deardorff TL, et al. Intestinal anisakiasis. A case diagnosed by morphologic and immunologic methods. Am J Clin Pathol 1988;90:107–113.

Shepherd NA, Blackshaw AJ, Hall PA, et al. Malignant lymphoma with eosinophilia of the gastrointestinal tract. Histopathology 1987;11:115–120.

Shimamoto C, Hirata I, Ohshiba S, et al. Churg-Strauss syndrome (allergic granulomatous angiitis) with peculiar multiple colonic ulcers. Gastroenterology 1990;85:316–319.

Talley NJ, Shorter RG, Phillips SF, Zinsmeister AR. Eosinophilic gastroenteritis: a clinicopathological study of patients with disease of the mucosa, muscle layer and subserosal tissues. Gut 1990;31:54–58.

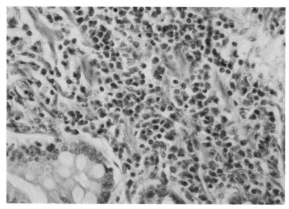

Figure 7–15. Mucosal biopsy from eosinophilic gastroenteritis. Note the sheets of eosinophils.

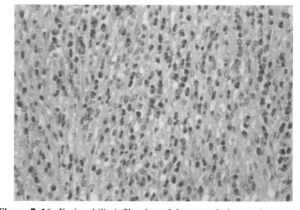

Figure 7–16. Eosinophilic infiltration of the muscularis propria.

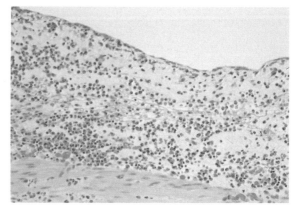

Figure 7–17. Eosinophilic serositis.

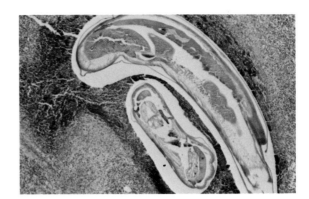

Figure 7–18. Larva of anisakine nematode in the center of an eosinophilic abscess.

ISCHEMIA

Biology of Disease

- Any part of the gastrointestinal tract may be involved, but because of the multiple arteries supplying the stomach and esophagus, ischemic damage is less common at these sites.
- A wide variety of causes of ischemia all produce basically similar lesions.
- Causes include arterial occlusion, venous occlusion, hypoperfusion as a result of hypotension, vasculitis, pancreatitis, radiation, carcinoid tumors, and cocaine abuse.
- The vast majority of arterial occlusions are the result of atherosclerosis. Often infarction is precipitated by atherosclerotic narrowing with a superimposed episode of hypoperfusion.
- Lesions may be quite variable in their extent and may be patchy.
- Emboli are much less common than atherosclerosis. Multiple atherosclerotic emboli may result in gastric ischemia secondary to occlusion of multiple vessels.
- Mesenteric venous occlusion accounts for about 13% of all intestinal infarction. Most of these cases are the result of mechanical obstruction. Other causes include accidental or surgical trauma, localized inflammation, and hypercoagulative disorders (thrombophilias).
- Ischemia may be caused by carcinoid tumors metastatic to mesenteric nodes, resulting in elastic vascular sclerosis of the arterial intima and adventia.
- An estimated 2 to 4% of patients with chronic pancreatitis have portal or mesenteric vein occlusion. Acute pancreatitis can cause damage to the arteries supplying the transverse colon.
- Fatal or transient ischemia has been described following ingestion of large quantities of cocaine. This is considered to be the result of vascular spasm.

Clinical Features

- Considerable variation in clinical findings is encountered with ischemia of different causes. There is also variation dependent on the severity and acuteness of blood supply reduction.

- The classic signs of acute intestinal ischemia due to arterial occlusion include acute abdominal pain with bloody diarrhea. If full-thickness infarction occurs, there will be peritonitis and toxic shock.
- Low-grade chronic ischemia may be characterized by intestinal angina (postprandial pain). Usually this does not give rise to fibrosis of the bowel wall.
- Acute venous insufficiency presents with gradual onset of abdominal pain (often as long as 1 week), before melena, hematemesis, or bowel perforation forces a laparotomy.
- Ischemic colitis is a clinical syndrome that mimics inflammatory bowel disease, particularly Crohn's disease. Typically, it occurs in patients over 60 years of age, who present with abdominal pain and bloody diarrhea. The ischemia is often mild and transient. In the acute stage, mucosal cobblestoning and linear ulcers may form. In the chronic stage, strictures may develop.
- Hemorrhagic enterocolitis is another, but less common, clinical syndrome that is caused by ischemia. Again, this occurs in elderly patients and is characterized by abrupt onset of a severe bloody diarrhea that is rapidly fatal. In most instances, this condition is precipitated by shock and poor intestinal perfusion. Luminal hemorrhage resulting from mucosal damage compounds the existing shock state.
- The third ischemic bowel syndrome is neonatal necrotizing enterocolitis. The pathogenesis of this condition is considered multifactorial and includes (1) ischemia precipitated by anoxia, (2) shock following sepsis (organisms such as *Escherichia coli*, *Clostridium*, and *Klebsiella* have been implicated), and (3) prematurity and poor development of the immune system. Infants develop vomiting, abdominal distension, and rectal bleeding. A characteristic finding is the presence of gas in the bowel wall, which can be identified on abdominal radiography.

Gross Pathology

- Early acute ischemia results in extreme congestion and hemorrhage of the mucosa and submucosa. This is followed by infarction and ulceration. As ischemia progresses, the muscularis propria becomes infarcted and may perforate.

- In subacute ischemia, the areas of ulceration may exude a protein-rich fluid, resulting in pseudomembrane formation.
- Chronic ischemia may produce fusiform strictures. These can be sharply delineated and are often located at the splenic flexure (watershed area between the superior and inferior mesenteric arteries). The mucosa in the strictured area may be ulcerated and replaced by granulation tissue.
- Ischemia of the stomach may produce ulcers that are indistinguishable from peptic ulcers.

Microscopic Pathology

- In the earliest stage there is mucosal and submucosal edema and hemorrhage.
- Epithelial necrosis follows. The cells first become detached from the basement membrane, and the nuclei undergo karyorrhexis, karyolysis, or pyknosis. Later, only ghost cells are present. At this stage, the entire mucosa may contain no viable nuclei. The architecture is preserved until the mucosa sloughs.
- Pseudomembranes composed of necrotic tissue, fibrin, and blood may form. These can be hard to distinguish from *Clostridium difficile*–induced pseudomembranous colitis.
- When ischemia spreads to the muscularis propria, the muscle undergoes coagulative necrosis. Nuclei are at first pyknotic but later fade. The cytoplasm is eosinophilic.
- If healing occurs, the regenerating epithelium is at first flattened and syncytial but later becomes cuboidal, then columnar. Nuclear hyperchromasia is present with multiple nucleoli.
- Hemosiderin-laden macrophages may be found within the lamina propria and submucosa.
- Fibrosis is often maximal in the submucosa but extends into the muscularis propria as many branching fibers.

Differential Diagnosis

Ulcerative colitis, Crohn's disease, pseudomembranous colitis, enterohemorrhagic *E. coli*, enteritis necroticans, neutropenic enterocolitis (typhlitis).

Acute ischemia, particularly the clinical syndrome of hemorrhagic enterocolitis, resembles acute fulminating ulcerative colitis. The key biopsy distinction is the identification of epithelial necrosis in which ghost cells and ghost crypt structures may be recognized. This occurs only in ischemia.

Distinguishing ischemic colitis or ischemic strictures of the small bowel from Crohn's disease can be difficult. Hemorrhage or hemosiderin in the mucosa and submucosa favor ischemia, as do pseudomembranes. Lymphoid aggregates in the deep submucosa and in the subserosa favor Crohn's disease. The patient's age should also be considered, although this cannot be relied on absolutely. Ischemia occurs most commonly in individuals over 60 years, whereas Crohn's disease occurs maximally in those 20 to 40 years old. Fibrous strictures are found in both conditions, but the terminal ileum is not a common location for ischemia.

The pseudomembranes of pseudomembranous colitis show a characteristic layering or streaming pattern, whereas the pseudomembranes of ischemia are more uniform and sheetlike. "Explosive" superficial crypt dilatation is most characteristic of pseudomembranous colitis.

Many cases previously referred to as "reversible ischemic colitis in young adults" are probably the result of infection by a verocytotoxin producing *E. coli*, particularly serotype O157:H7. The changes on biopsy are similar to those of ischemia, except that coagulative necrosis with preservation of the ghost outline of the mucosa is not a feature. These cases may be complicated by the hemolytic-uremic syndrome.

Enteritis necroticans is the result of bowel wall infection by *Clostridium perfringens*. It was originally described as "pig bel" and "darmbrand" in severely protein malnourished individuals who were deficient in pancreatic protease, an enzyme that deactivates the bacterial toxin. Isolated cases have been encountered in Western communities, but this is mainly a disease of the third world. As with other gastrointestinal infections, the diagnosis is best made by culture. The pathology closely mimics ischemia and knowledge of the clinical situation is required to suggest the diagnosis.

Neutropenic enterocolitis (typhlitis) is usually due to infection by *Clostridium septicum*, or less commonly *C. perfringens*, type C. The histology closely mimics that of ischemia. Thrombi may be present in superficial capillaries. Again, knowledge of the clinical situation is necessary to raise this diagnostic possibility.

References

Brophy CM, Frederick WG, Schlessel R, Barwick KW. Focal segmental ischemia of the terminal ileum mimicking Crohn's disease. J Clin Gastroenterol 1988;10:343–347.

Cherry RD, Jabbari M, Goresky CA, et al. Chronic mesenteric vascular insufficiency with gastric ulceration. Gastroenterology 1986; 91:1548–1552.

Clavien PA, Durig M, Harder F. Venous mesenteric infarction. Br J Surg 1988;75:252–255.

de Sa J. The spectrum of ischemic bowel disease in the newborn. Perspect Pediatr Pathol 1976;3:273–309.

Force T, MacDonald D, Eade OE, et al. Ischemic gastritis and duodenitis. Gastroenterology 1982;82:763–766.

Grendell JH, Ockner RK. Mesenteric venous thrombosis. Gastroenterology 1982;82:358–372.

Harvey JN, Denyer ME, Da Costa P. Intestinal infarction caused by a carcinoid associated elastic vascular sclerosis: early presentation of a small ileal carcinoid tumor. Gut 1989;30:691–694.

Kelly JK, Oryshak A, Wenetsek M, et al. The colonic pathology of Escherischia coli 0157:H7 infection. Am J Surg Pathol 1990;14:87–92.

Kosloske AM. Pathogenesis and prevention of necrotizing enterocolitis: a hypothesis based on personal observation and a review of the literature. Pediatrics 1984;74:1086–1092.

Kukora JS. Extensive colonic necrosis complicating acute pancreatitis. Surgery 1985;97:290–293.

Lindahl F, Vejlsted H, Backer OG. Lesions of the colon following acute pancreatitis. Scand J Gastroenterology 1972;7:375–378.

Ming SC. Hemorrhagic necrosis of the gastrointestinal tract and its relation to cardiovascular status. Circulation 1965;32:332–341.

Morson BC. Ischemic colitis. Postgrad J Med 1968;44:665–666.

Nalbandian H, Sheth N, Dietrich R, Georgion J. Intestinal ischemia caused by cocaine ingestion: report of two cases. Surgery 1985;97:374–376.

Severin WPJ, de la Fuente AA, Stringer MF. Clostridium perfringens type C causing necrotizing enteritis. J Clin Pathol 1984;37:942–944.

Whitehead R. The pathology of ischemia of the intestines. Pathol Ann 1976;11:1–52.

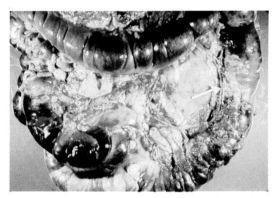

Figure 7–19. Extensive acute infarction of large bowel secondary to venous thrombosis.

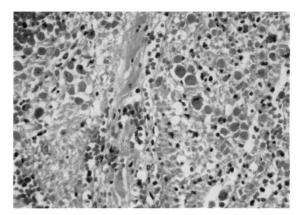

Figure 7–22. Acute infarction of muscle fibers in the bowel wall.

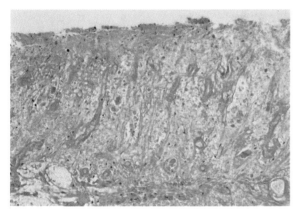

Figure 7–20. Acute infarction of large bowel. Note ghost outlines of the crypts.

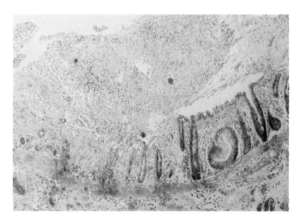

Figure 7–23. Acute infarction with pseudomembrane formation.

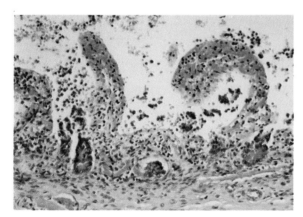

Figure 7–21. Infarction with detachment of crypt cells from the basement membrane.

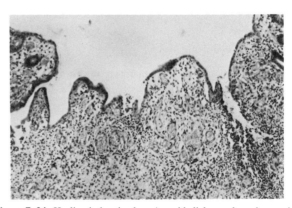

Figure 7–24. Healing ischemic ulcer. An epithelial monolayer is covering granulation tissue.

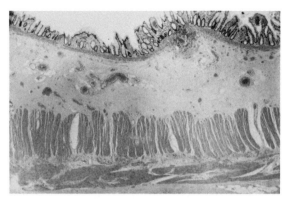

Figure 7–25. Ischemic stricture with extensive submucosal fibrosis.

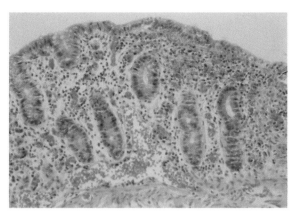

Figure 7–27. Healed ischemic colitis with abundant hemosiderin pigmentation in the lamina propria.

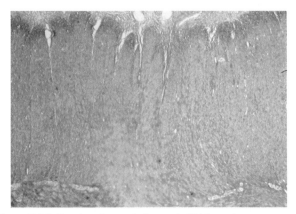

Figure 7–26. Scarring of muscularis propria (Trichrome).

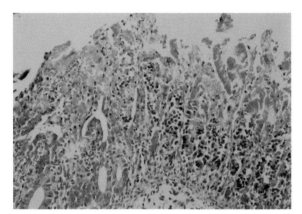

Figure 7–28. Superficial acute infarction of mucosa from a case of neonatal necrotizing enterocolitis.

RADIATION DAMAGE

Biology of Disease

■ Great individual variations in susceptibility exist. In general, severe damage does not occur at doses less than 45 Gy (4500R) although transient changes may be apparent after 12 Gy (1200R).

■ A major factor that increases susceptibility is bowel fixation due to prior surgery.

■ Radiation changes are conveniently divided into acute and chronic lesions. Acute changes do not normally persist for more than 6 months. Chronic changes generally become manifest after about 1 year.

Clinical Features

■ Acute radiation injury produces anorexia, nausea, and diarrhea. Vomiting is less common, but there may be crampy abdominal pain.

■ Chronic radiation injury produces fibrosis of the bowel with resulting diarrhea, malabsorption, and abdominal pain. Ulceration may give rise to bleeding and, in severe cases, stricture formation leading to intestinal obstruction.

Gross Pathology

■ In acute injury, the mucosa may be edematous, reddened, and friable. It may bleed when touched and superficial ulceration can be present.

■ In chronic injury, the mucosa also appears reddened. Ulcers and strictures may be present. The changes tend to be sharply circumscribed, reflecting the localized field of radiation.

Microscopic Pathology

■ Radiation changes can be quite nonspecific and difficult to distinguish from other causes of mucosal damage.

■ Acute radiation injury typically shows mucosal atrophy and thinning. In severe damage, the surface epithelium may slough, exposing the lamina propria, which contains dilated, bleeding vessels. A cryptitis, in which eosinophils are prominent, may be present and there may be karyor-rhexis of individual crypt cells (apoptotic bodies). Mitoses may be absent or reduced. In the recovery phase, regenerative changes consist of mucin loss, nuclear enlargement, hyperchromatism, prominent nucleoli, and crypt dilatation.

■ Chronic radiation damage usually results in atrophy of glandular mucosa. Within the mucosa, there may be telangiectasia and reduced numbers of inflammatory cells. The submucosa may show fibrosis with "radiation" fibroblasts (large cells with large nuclei and irregular nucleoli). The larger submucosal vessels show an obliterative angiitis. With more severe damage, there may be ulceration and/or fibrosis of the muscularis propria.

■ Intestinal metaplasia may be present in the stomach.

■ In the colon, colitis cystica profunda may be present in areas of healed ulceration.

Differential Diagnosis

Peptic ulcer, ischemic damage.

In a sense, many of the findings in chronic radiation damage are the result of ischemia following endarteritis of the submucosal vessels. It is, therefore, not surprising that these conditions are difficult to distinguish. Radiated vessels show a variety of intimal changes that are normally not encountered in simple ischemia. These include fibrinoid change and intimal fibrosis.

Peptic ulcers in the stomach and duodenum often show endarteritis of vessels at the base. Biopsies, therefore, may not help in distinguishing peptic ulcer from radiation ulcer. However, if a gastrectomy is carried out, endarteritis due to radiation may be seen in vessels distant from the ulcer base.

References

Berthrong M, Fajardo LF. Radiation injury in surgical pathology. II. Alimentary tract. Am J Surg Pathol 1981;5:153–178.

Hastleton PS, Carr N, Schofield PF. Vascular changes in radiation bowel disease. Histopathology 1985;9:517–534.

Novak JM, Collins JT, Donowitz M, et al. Effects of radiation on the human gastrointestinal tract. J Clin Gastroenterol 1979;1:9–39.

Weisbrot IM, Liber AF, Gordon BS. The effects of therapeutic radiation on colonic mucosa. Cancer 1975;36:931–940.

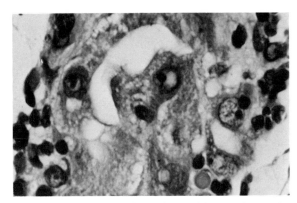

Figure 7–30. Syncytial cells with atypical nuclei but no increase in nucleus-to-cytoplasm ratio.

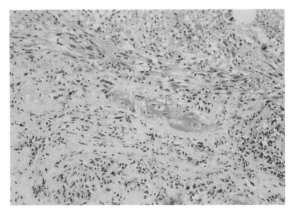

Figure 7–31. Submucosal radiation changes, including scarring and acute vascular damage (fibrinoid necrosis).

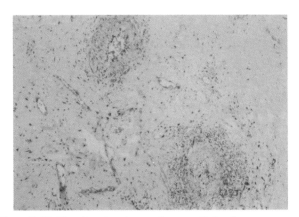

Figure 7–32. Vascular sclerosis secondary to radiation damage.

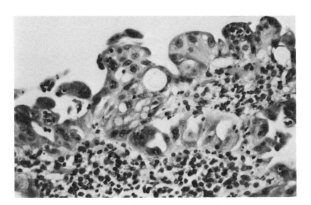

Figure 7–29. Acute radiation damage. Note vacuolization of surface epithelial cells.

EFFECTS OF CHEMOTHERAPY

Biology of Disease

■ Anticancer drugs are usually administered as combination chemotherapy, so it is extremely difficult to determine the effect of each drug in isolation. There is a marked individual variation in the effects of these drugs. For chemotherapeutic agents, such as methotrexate, the effects may be apparent within 2 hours of administration and reach a maximum in approximately 24 hours. Mitotic arrest is a common mechanism by which cell damage occurs.

■ Corticosteroids which are frequently combined with chemotherapy may cause intestinal ulceration and perforation. This can occur at any dosage level and there is often delay in treatment because steroids mask the features of peritonitis. Large and small bowel are affected as commonly as stomach and duodenum. Sigmoid diverticula are particularly prone to perforate with corticosteroid therapy.

Clinical Features

■ Following anticancer chemotherapy, patients present with nausea, vomiting, diarrhea, ileus, and hemorrhage from ulcers.

■ Generally, changes are most severe in the small bowel, since this has the highest cell turnover. Most chemotherapeutic agents affect cells when they are in the mitotic phase.

■ The syndrome of neutropenic enterocolitis (typhlitis) may partly be the result of chemotherapy. These patients often have leukemia and present with focal ulceration of the right side of the colon. Hemorrhage and shock may occur. In many cases, there is overgrowth and bowel invasion by *Clostridium septicum*.

Gross Pathology

■ Shallow or deep ulceration is a characteristic feature of gastrointestinal disease secondary to anticancer drugs. It may occur in any area of the gastrointestinal tract, including the esophagus. The ulcers are multiple in one third of cases and may be extensive.

Microscopic Pathology

■ Variation in histology may be observed between adjacent areas of mucosa. Mild damage results in the presence of isolated necrotic cells with karyorrhexic nuclei (apoptotic bodies). More severe damage may produce a variety of changes, ranging from villous atrophy through superficial epithelial necrosis and ulceration. Regenerating epithelium is typically attenuated with loss of mucin. Abundant mitoses may be present. There may be formation of cystic crypts.

■ Some chemotherapeutic agents, particularly 5-fluorouracil (5-FU), when administered by local arterial infusion, can produce extreme epithelial atypia in the stomach or duodenum with mucosal ulceration. These changes may be so bizarre that they resemble dysplasia or carci-

noma. Features that favor a diagnosis of chemotherapy associated epithelial atypia are: cytoplasmic degeneration and eosinophilia, a normal nuclear-cytoplasmic ratio, and similar bizarre changes in fibroblasts and endothelial cells.

Differential Diagnosis

Graft versus host disease (GVHD), radiotherapy.

Mucosal chemotherapy changes may be indistinguishable from radiotherapy changes. However, radiotherapy may produce obliterative changes in vessels that are not seen in chemotherapy.

The conditioning radiochemotherapy that is administered prior to a bone marrow transplant may produce mucosal changes indistinguishable from GVHD. However, these changes usually resolve by 21 days after transplant, whereas GVHD does not usually become a clinical problem prior to 28 days after transplant.

References

Kies MS, Luedke DW, Boyd JF, et al. Neutropenic enterocolitis. Cancer 1979;43:730–734.

Petras RE, Hart WR, Bukowski RM. Gastric epithelial atypia associated with hepatic arterial infusion chemotherapy: its distinction from early gastric cancer. Cancer 1985;56:745–750.

Slavin RE, Millan JC, Mullins GM. Pathology of intermittent high dose cyclophosphamide therapy. Hum Pathol 1975;6:693–709.

Trier JS. Morphologic alterations induced by methotrexate in the mucosa of the human proximal intestine. I. Serial observations by light microscopy. Gastroenterology 1962;42:295–305.

Warshaw AL, Welch JP, Ottinger LW. Acute perforation of the colon associated with chronic corticosteroid therapy. Am J Surg 1976;131:442–446.

Wiedner N, Smith JG, La Vanway JM. Peptic ulceration with marked epithelial atypia following hepatic arterial infusion chemotherapy. Am J Surg Pathol 1983;7:261–268.

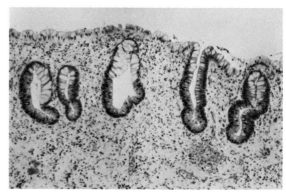

Figure 7–33. Chemotherapy changes in the large bowel. Note that normal cells are present in the upper half of the crypt. The lower half of the crypt shows regenerating cells.

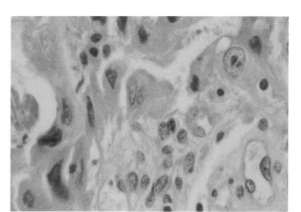

Figure 7–34. Surface epithelial changes in the small bowel after chemotherapy. The cells have atypical nuclei and syncytial cytoplasm. The nucleus-to-cytoplasm ratio is normal.

VASCULITIS

Biology of Disease

■ Almost any type of vasculitis may involve the gastrointestinal tract. Generally, the disease also affects vessels elsewhere, but occasionally vasculitis selectively targets the gut.

■ Vasculitis secondary to other diseases (rheumatoid arthritis, systemic lupus erythematosus, and dermatomyositis) may occur.

■ The major primary large vessel vasculitis is polyarteritis nodosa.

■ Primary small vessel vasculitis includes Henoch-Schönlein purpura (HSP) and Köhlmeyer-Degos syndrome.

■ The bowel may rarely be involved in Wegener's granuloma and the Churg-Strauss syndrome.

Clinical Features

■ Polyarteritis is usually a generalized disorder but can be localized to the bowel. Vascular thrombosis results in infarction, usually of the small bowel. Necrosis of the vessel wall can rarely result in intraperitoneal hemorrhage.

■ Henoch-Schönlein purpura is characterized by palpable purpura, arthritis, and abdominal pain. Bowel ischemia leads to ulceration and bleeding. This is predominantly a disease of children.

■ Köhlmeyer-Degos syndrome consists of cutaneous papules on the trunk and proximal extremities, together with a small vessel vasculitis, mainly involving the gastrointestinal tract. The gastrointestinal symptoms include abdominal pain, weight loss, and diarrhea. Intestinal infarction and perforation may result.

Gross Pathology

■ In most instances, the gross appearance is distinctive, with patchy areas of infarction and mucosal preservation produced by occlusion of multiple small vessels. Cholesterol embolism is the main differential. Rarely, the lesions are nonspecific and cannot be distinguished from ischemic disease secondary to thrombosis.

■ Occasionally in polyarteritis nodosa, the major vessels may have a beaded appearance due to the presence of small aneurysms involving segments of artery where the vasculitis has resulted in destruction of the muscle and elastic coat.

Microscopic Pathology

■ Generally, the microscopic changes present in the mucosa and bowel wall are similar to those encountered in ischemia of any cause.

■ In polyarteritis nodosa, medium to large arteries in the submucosa and subserosa are focally inflamed. The vessel walls undergo fibrinoid necrosis, which may be eccentric or concentric. Thrombosis is common. Aneurysms generally occur in healed lesions.

■ In Henoch-Schönlein purpura, the venules are mainly affected. They show a mural infiltrate of acute and chronic inflammatory cells, which may be leukocytoclastic. IgA is deposited in vessel walls, although this is usually searched for in renal, not gastrointestinal biopsy specimens.

■ In Köhlmeyer-Degos syndrome, multiple small and medium-sized arteries and veins may be affected. These show endothelial swelling and thrombosis. Vascular necrosis can occur but is unusual, and the changes tend to be confined to the intimal layer.

References

Camilleri M, Pusey CD, Chadwick VS, Rees AJ. Gastrointestinal manifestations of systemic vasculitis. Q J Med 1983;52:141–149.

Craig RD. Multiple perforations of small intestine in polyarteritis nodosa. Gastroenterology 1963;44:355–356.

Meyer GW, Lichtenstein J. Isolated polyarteritis nodosa affecting the cecum. Dig Dis Sci 1982;27:467–469.

Rodriguez-Erdmann F, Levitan R. Gastrointestinal and roentgenological manifestations of Henoch-Schönlein purpura. Gastroenterology 1968;54:260–264.

Strole WE, Clark WH, Isselbacher KJ. Progressive arterial occlusive disease (Kohlmeier-Degos). N Engl J Med 1967;276:195–201.

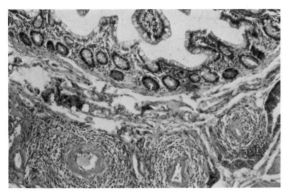

Figure 7–35. Multiple foci of polyarteritis in the small bowel.

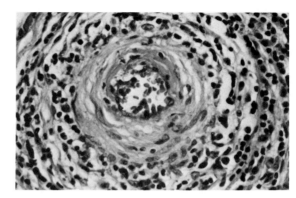

Figure 7–37. Small artery vasculitis. The adventitia contains a mixture of acute and chronic inflammatory cells.

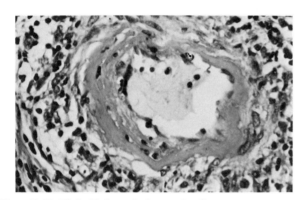

Figure 7–36. Fibrinoid change in the vessel wall.

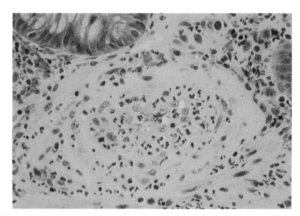

Figure 7–38. Henoch-Schönlein vasculitis. This involves a venule and is leukocytoclastic in type.

AMYLOIDOSIS

Biology of Disease

- Amyloid may be deposited in any part of the gastrointestinal tract.
- In most cases, it is present within the walls of submucosal vessels. Rarely, a localized mass (amyloid tumor) may be present. Still rarer is diffuse deposition in muscle, submucosa, and lamina propria.
- Gastrointestinal involvement is most common in primary (AL, myeloma-associated) amyloidosis, but also occurs frequently in secondary (AA, inflammation-associated) amyloidosis.

Clinical Features

- In the vast majority of cases, gastrointestinal amyloidosis is asymptomatic and is discovered by "blind" rectal biopsy.

- Rarely, massive amyloid deposition in the small and large bowel may result in motility disturbance, malabsorption, ischemia, perforation, and bleeding.

Gross Pathology

- Usually, no gross abnormalities are evident.
- Rarely, a tumorlike mass is present, or there may be diffuse thickening of mucosal folds.

Microscopic Pathology

- Amyloid is an amorphous pink-staining substance.
- In most instances, the submucosal arterioles are involved and may be narrowed. Usually, this is obvious on routine sections.
- Extravascular deposits may be found in the lamina propria (particularly in AA amyloidosis), muscularis mucosae, and submucosa (particularly AL amyloidosis).

Special Techniques

■ These are necessary to confirm that the amorphous, eosinophilic material seen on routine sections is, in fact, amyloid.

■ Congo red positivity, with characteristic apple-green birefringence, is the preferred confirmatory stain.

■ Electron microscopy will demonstrate a typical fibrillary appearance.

References

Bjornson S, Johannsson JH, Sigurjonsson F. Localized primary amyloidosis of the stomach presenting with gastric hemorrhage. Acta Med Scan 1987;221:115–119.

Glenner GG. Amyloid deposits and amyloidosis: the β-fibrilloses. N Engl J Med 1980;302:1283–1292, 1333–1343.

Kumar SS, Appavu SS, Abcarian H, Barreta T. Amyloidosis of the colon: report of a case and review of the literature. Dis Colon Rectum 1983;26:541–544.

Wald A, Kichler J, Mendelow H. Amyloidosis and chronic intestinal pseudo-obstruction. Dig Dis Sci 1981;26:462–465.

Yamada M, Hatakeyama S, Tsukagoshi H. Gastrointestinal amyloid deposition in AL (primary or myeloma associated) and AA (secondary) amyloidosis: diagnostic value of gastric biopsy. Hum Pathol 1985;16:1206–1211.

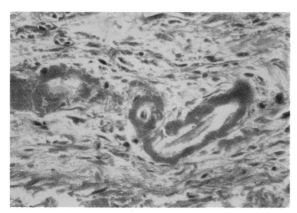

Figure 7–39. Amyloid in submucosal vessels.

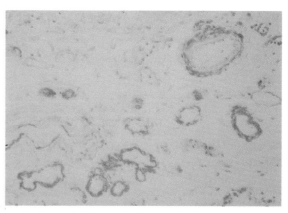

Figure 7–40. Amyloid in vessels (Congo red stain).

KAPOSI'S SARCOMA

Biology of Disease

■ Most cases of gastrointestinal Kaposi's sarcoma (KS) occur in immunosuppressed patients, particularly those with AIDS but also organ transplant recipients.

■ Most patients with gastrointestinal KS have obvious skin involvement at the time of diagnosis.

■ Co-infections, such as cytomegalovirus infection or *Mycobacterium avium-intracellulare* infection, often accompany KS.

Clinical Features

■ Fifty percent of patients with gastrointestinal KS have simultaneous involvement of the upper and lower tract. The remainder have isolated involvement of the upper tract (25%) or lower tract (25%).

■ Most gastrointestinal lesions are clinically silent, but there may be rare cases of bleeding or intestinal obstruction.

Gross Pathology

■ Endoscopically, KS lesions appear initially as foci of submucosal hemorrhage. Later, they become dome-shaped and may develop a central area of ulceration.

Microscopic Pathology

■ Early lesions are located in the submucosa. As these grow, the mucosa may become stretched over the surface.

■ Lesions consist of proliferating spindle cells with intervening vascular spaces. There may be extravasation of red cells, and hemosiderin deposition may occur. The spindle cells may be pleomorphic or relatively bland. Moderate numbers of mitotic figures are present.

Differential Diagnosis

Granulation tissue related to peptic or nonspecific ulceration.

Most granulation tissue in the gastrointestinal tract is accompanied by acute and chronic inflammation. Unless secondary ulceration is present, KS is noninflamed.

Granulation tissue contains more perfectly formed capillaries than KS, which tends to form only ill-defined slit-like spaces.

References

Blumfeld W, Egbert BM, Sagebiel RW. Differential diagnosis of Kaposi's sarcoma. Arch Pathol Lab Med 1985;109:123–127.

Friedman SL, Wright TL, Altman DF. Gastrointestinal Kaposi's sarcoma in patients with acquired immunodeficiency syndrome: endoscopic and autopsy findings. Gastroenterology 1985;89:102–108.

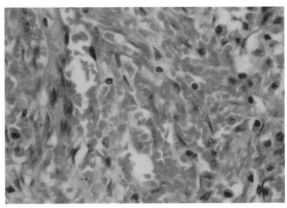

Figure 7–42. Spindle cells with slitlike spaces containing red cells.

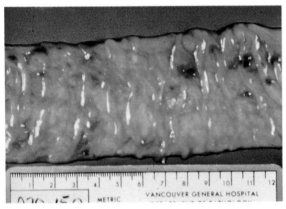

Figure 7–41. Kaposi's sarcoma of the small bowel. Note the multiple submucosal lesions. (Courtesy of Intellipath, Inc., Santa Monica, CA.)

MYCOBACTERIUM AVIUM-INTRACELLULARE (MAI)

Biology of Disease

■ Gastrointestinal infection with MAI is a common event in patients with AIDS, but is extremely rare in other types of immunosuppressed diseases.

■ The infection is usually generalized and bowel involvement occurs in association with disease in the liver, spleen, and other sites.

■ MAI commonly coexists with other gastrointestinal infections (CMV and cryptosporidiosis).

Clinical Features

■ MAI is usually identified on biopsy samples taken during investigation of diarrhea and malabsorption.

■ Generally, the contribution of MAI to symptoms is thought to be less than that for co-infecting agents.

Gross Pathology

■ The mucosa may appear normal, or there may be thickened folds, pale nodules, or shallow ulcers.

Microscopic Pathology

■ Typically, the lamina propria is expanded by a sheet-like infiltrate of macrophages. These have abundant pale or purplish staining cytoplasm.

■ Granulomas and giant cells are not usually present. Necrosis and caseation are absent.

■ Occasionally, small numbers of inconspicuous macrophages are the only biopsy finding.

■ Villi may be flattened and normal structures pushed aside, but mucosal destruction is usually not prominent.

Special Techniques

■ Normally, mycobacteria are identified in large numbers with a modified Ziehl Neelsen stain (Fite's). The organisms are generally intracellular.

■ Because some cases have only small numbers of organism-containing histiocytes, a Fite's stain is recommended in all gastrointestinal biopsies from AIDS patients.

■ Culture of tissue takes several weeks but is strongly recommended.

Differential Diagnosis

Whipple's disease, tuberculosis.

The appearances on routine section are very similar to Whipple's disease but lack the lipid droplets seen in this condition.

The organisms of Whipple's disease stain negatively with Fite's stain. Both organisms are PAS positive.

Only culture will satisfactorily distinguish MAI from other mycobacteria. In tuberculosis, organisms tend to be much less numerous.

Granulomas and necrosis may be seen in tuberculosis.

References

Klatt EC, Jensen DF, Meyer PR. Pathology of *Mycobacterium avium-intracellulare* in acquired immunodeficiency syndrome. Hum Pathol 1987;18:709-714.

Farbi DC, Mason UG, Horsburgh CR. Pathologic findings in disseminated *Mycobacterium avium-intracellulare* infection. A report of 11 cases. Am J Clin Pathol 1986;85:67-72.

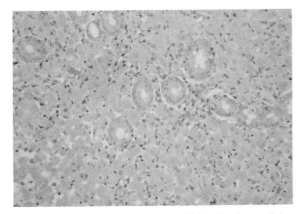

Figure 7–43. *Mycobacterium avium-intracellulare* in the small bowel. Note that the lamina propria is expanded by large numbers of histiocytes, which have a bluish-grey cytoplasm.

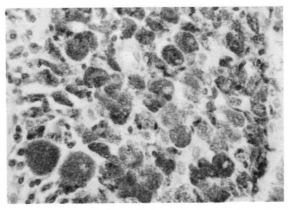

Figure 7–44. MAI-modified Ziehl-Neelsen stain. Large numbers of beaded organisms are present.

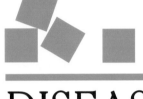

DISEASES OF
GASTROINTESTINAL
LYMPHOID TISSUE

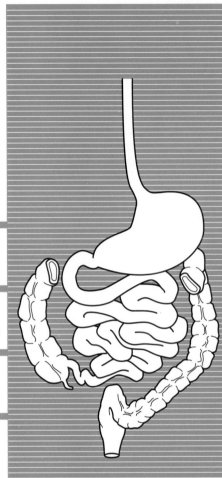

CHAPTER 8

LYMPHOID HYPERPLASIA

Biology of Disease

- Lymphoid hyperplasia can affect any part of the gastrointestinal tract. There are, however, some well-identified clinical entities, including (1) focal nodular lymphoid hyperplasia of the terminal ileum and appendix; (2) focal nodular lymphoid hyperplasia of the rectum (rectal tonsil); and (3) diffuse nodular lymphoid hyperplasia of the small or large bowel.

- The existence of tumorlike lymphoid hyperplasia (pseudolymphoma) has been reported in several areas of the gastrointestinal tract, particularly the stomach. In the past 20 years, there have been increasing reports of high-grade lymphomas arising in pseudolymphoma. More recently, the concept of low-grade lymphoma of mucosa-associated lymphoid tissue (MALToma) has been advanced. It is postulated that many cases diagnosed as pseudolymphoma were in fact low-grade MALTomas. These tumors are commonly associated with reactive lymphoid hyperplasia. It is not clear yet whether MALToma develops within a pseudolymphoma, or if all tumorlike lymphoid proliferations in the stomach are in fact MALTomas. (For more discussion on this, see the section on MALToma.)

- Lymphoid hyperplasia is common as a secondary effect of many diseases (e.g., Crohn's disease). In this section, however, only primary lymphoid hyperplasias that produce tumorlike lesions are considered.

Clinical Features

- Lymphoid hyperplasia of the terminal ileum and appendix is physiologic in children and adolescents, but is seen in older patients proximal to obstructing tumors. It is also a normal response to antigenic or bacterial challenge. The lesions may be polypoid and sometimes form the head of an intussusception.

- Lymphoid proliferation in the colon and rectum is also common in children and young adults. It may produce rectal bleeding, anemia, and anal discomfort if the lesion is located low in the rectum.

- Diffuse nodular lymphoid hyperplasia of the large bowel predominately affects children, in whom it is usually discovered incidentally on barium enema. It is rarely symptomatic. In adults, diffuse lymphoid hyperplasia may occur in association with common variable immunodeficiency (late-onset hypogammaglobulinemia), with human immunodeficiency virus infection, and idiopathically. Diffuse lymphoid hyperplasia of the small bowel not occurring in the context of common variable immunodeficiency is closely associated with low-grade lymphoma of MALT.

Gross Pathology

- Focal lymphoid hyperplasia involving the terminal ileum may predominately affect the Peyer's patches. In the colon and rectum, there are nodules with or without surface ulceration.

- Diffuse lymphoid hyperplasia is characterized by the presence of multiple sessile polyps regularly distributed throughout the affected segment of bowel. Most polyps measure 5 mm in diameter, but some may be up to 2 cm. Endoscopically, they appear as cream-colored mucosal nodules.

Microscopic Pathology

- Focal lymphoid hyperplasia at sites other than the stomach is unlikely to be confused with lymphoma, since it is more diffuse and less like a tumor. Usually these have the appearance of secondary lymphoid follicles with prominent germinal centers containing mitoses and tingible body macrophages.

- Diffuse lymphoid hyperplasia is similar histologically, whether or not hypogammaglobulinemia is present. However, in cases with immunodeficiency, there is a decrease or absence of plasma cells in the lamina propria of the adjacent bowel. The lymphoid hyperplasia consists of prominent lymphoid follicles with reactive germinal centers.

Special Techniques

- The current investigation of lymphoid lesions should include a full immunohistochemical and/or molecular analysis for cell lineage and clonality. Optimally, frozen tissue, fresh tissue, and tissue fixed in formalin and B-5 (mercury based) should be available for study.

Differential Diagnosis

Low-grade MALToma is the only significant differential diagnosis.

Generally, lymphomas are more bulky and extensive than lymphoid hyperplasia.

Generally, the infiltrate between follicles is more uniform and monotonous in lymphoma.

Reactive lymphoid follicles are present in both lesions but are found throughout the lesion in lymphoid hyperplasia.

Lymphoepithelial lesions (see section on low-grade lymphomas) are present in lymphomas, not in reactive hyperplasia.

Lymphomas may contain Dutcher bodies; lymphoid hyperplasias do not.

The interfollicular cells of a MALToma may show cytologic atypia, whereas those of pseudolymphoma do not.

Low-grade lymphoma is much more common in the stomach than at other sites and occurs in an older age group.

By immunohistochemical analysis, lymphomas show light-chain restriction; lymphoid hyperplasia does not.

Reactive germinal center cells show negative staining for bcl-2 in frozen and B-5 fixed tissues. Lymphoma cells in a follicular location may be bcl-2 positive. MALToma cells are CD20 positive and CD5 and CD10 negative.

Gene rearrangement studies are positive for a monoclonal population in lymphomas, but not in lymphoid hyperplasia.

References

Ajdukiewicz AB, Youngs GR, Bouchier IA. Nodular lymphoid hyperplasia with hypogammaglobulinemia. Gut 1972;13:589-595.

Barge J, Molar G, Potet I. Lymphoid stromal reaction in gastrointestinal lymphomas: immunohistochemical study of 14 cases. J Clin Pathol 1987;40:760–765.

Brooks JJ, Enterline HT. Gastric pseudolymphoma: its three subtypes and relation to lymphoma. Cancer 1983;51:476–486.

Burke JS, Sheibani K, Nathwani BN, et al. Monoclonal small (well-differentiated) lymphocytic proliferations of the gastrointestinal tract resembling pseudolymphoma. Hum Pathol 1987;18:1238–1245.

Charlesworth D, Fox H, Mainwaring AR. Benign lymphoid hyperplasia of the terminal ileum. Am J Gastroenterol 1970;53:579–584.

Holtz F, Schmidt LA. Lymphoid polyps (benign lymphoma) and malignant lymphoma of the rectum and anus. Surg Gynecol Obstet 1958; 106:639–642.

Ranchod M, Lewin KJ, Dorfman RF. Lymphoid hyperplasia of the gastrointestinal tract: a study of 26 cases and a review of the literature. Am J Surg Pathol 1978;2:383–400.

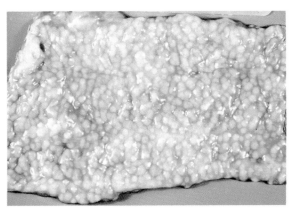

Figure 8–1. Diffuse lymphoid hyperplasia of the terminal ileum occurring in an otherwise asymptomatic child.

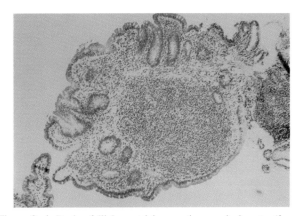

Figure 8–4. Benign follicle containing reactive germinal center (from a patient with hypogammaglobulinemia).

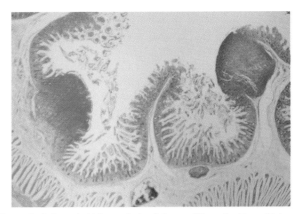

Figure 8–2. Lymphoid hyperplasia of the small bowel with multiple regularly spaced follicles.

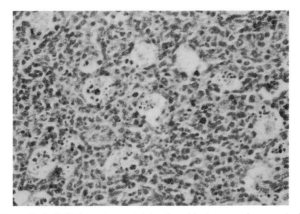

Figure 8–5. Follicle centers containing tinged body macrophages and mitotic figures.

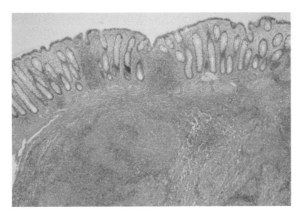

Figure 8–3. Lymphoid hyperplasia of the rectum. Note the presence of multiple submucosal follicles.

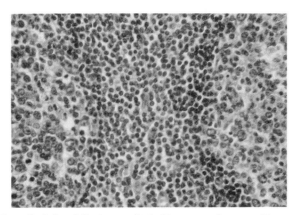

Figure 8–6. Interfollicular zone flanked by two mantle zones with mature small lymphocytes.

SMALL CELL AND FOLLICULAR LYMPHOMAS

Biology of Disease

■ The gastrointestinal tract is more commonly involved by lymphoma that is primary in the lymph nodes and becomes secondarily disseminated to the gastrointestinal tract than it is by primary gastrointestinal lymphoma. The following comments apply only to primary gastrointestinal lymphomas.

■ A primary gastrointestinal lymphoma is one in which there is no evidence of splenic, hepatic, or extramesenteric node involvement at the time of presentation. Mesenteric/omental node involvement at the time of presentation is considered the equivalent of a local "metastasis."

■ Histologically, the vast majority of small cell and follicular lymphomas fall into one of four categories: (1) MALToma; (2) mantle zone lymphoma (also called intermediate cell lymphoma, centrocytic cell lymphoma, or diffuse small cleaved cell lymphoma); (3) follicular center cell lymphoma (also called centrocytic/centroblastic lymphoma or small cleaved/large noncleaved lymphoma); and (4) Burkitt's lymphoma (small noncleaved lymphoma).

■ The majority of gastrointestinal lymphomas involve the stomach. The next most common sites are the small bowel and large bowel. Esophageal lymphomas are rare. The sex incidence is equal and most cases occur in the over-50 age group.

■ Approximately 50% of gastrointestinal lymphomas are low grade; 15% have mixed low- and high-grade components. The remainder are high grade.

■ Most lymphomas in this category are MALTomas.

■ It has recently been recognized that the majority of lesions previously referred to as *pseudolymphomas* are, in fact, low-grade MALTomas, which have run an indolent clinical course. In the early stages of MALToma, the lesions contain a large amount of benign, reactive lymphoid tissue, and it may be difficult to identify areas of tumor without specialized immunologic techniques.

■ Currently, there is controversy as to the precise nature of MALTomas. Some investigators believe they are closely related to monocytoid B-cell lymphomas.

Clinical Features

■ Gastric lymphomas may mimic peptic ulcers, with vague dyspepsia and iron deficiency anemia. Bulky tumors can result in pyloric obstruction.

■ Intestinal lymphomas may present with obstruction, hemorrhage, perforation, or occasionally intussusception.

Gross Pathology

■ Gastric low-grade lymphomas are generally solitary and most commonly resemble peptic ulcers with sharp "punched out" edges. Less commonly, they resemble adenocarcinomas and may have a rolled edge or an exophytic component. Rarely, they can be diffusely infiltrating like linitis plastica.

■ Intestinal lymphomas can present with multiple masses (usually no more than five). These masses are generally closely related anatomically.

■ Mantle zone lymphomas of the gastrointestinal tract are rare, but they characteristically present as multiple polyps. Primary intestinal follicular lymphomas are uncommon, but may be polypoid in configuration.

Microscopic Pathology

MALToma

■ Four histologic features are typical of MALToma: (1) an infiltrate of small lymphocytes and small cleaved follicle center cells (centrocyte-like, or CCL, cells); (2) reactive-appearing lymphoid follicles; (3) neoplastic plasmacytoid cells; and (4) lymphoepithelial lesions.

■ CCL cells are present in variable numbers and have a variable cytologic appearance. In most cases, they are slightly bigger than a small lymphocyte with an irregular dense nucleus and a well-defined nuclear membrane. The cytoplasm is clear. Occasionally, CCL cells are larger and resemble noncleaved small lymphocytes (lymphoblasts). In early MALTomas, CCL cells are inconspicuous and mixed with large numbers of normal-appearing small lymphocytes.

■ CCL cells are generally present in a perifollicular location, although occasionally they are encountered in an intrafollicular site.

■ Although reactive follicles are present, immunostained frozen sections demonstrate that, in some instances, the germinal centers are infiltrated by CCL cells.

■ Neoplastic plasma cells are seen in one third of cases. Because these are not bizarre or easily recognizable as malignant, immunohistochemical proof of light-chain restriction is needed to demonstrate malignancy. These plasma cells are often appear as a bandlike infiltrate immediately below the superficial epithelium.

■ Lymphoepithelial lesions consist of three or more lymphocytes present as a discrete cluster infiltrating the epithelium and displacing or partly destroying the pit lining cells.

■ The concept of MALToma is useful, but it has not yet been incorporated into the Working Formulation (or Kiel classification in Europe). Most MALTomas are classified as low-grade diffuse small cleaved cell lymphoma or well-differentiated lymphocytic lymphoma with or without plasmacytoid features.

Mantle Zone Lymphoma

■ This type of lymphoma tends to be monomorphic, and may be diffuse or nodular in pattern. Reactive lymphoid follicles may be trapped within and compressed by the tumor, and tumor cells will efface the normal mantle zone.

■ Individual lymphoma cells have a densely staining nucleus with inconspicuous nucleoli. The nuclear outline is irregular with little cytoplasm. Blast cells are not present.

■ In the Working Formulation, they are classified as a low-grade lymphoma and in the Kiel classification, as centrocytic lymphoma.

Follicular Center Cell Lymphoma

- These are true germinal center cell lymphomas. In the Kiel classification, they are centroblastic centrocytic lymphomas and in the Working Formulation, mixed cleaved and noncleaved lymphoma. The majority are nodular, although they may later become diffuse.

Burkitt's Lymphoma

- These occur primarily in children. The ileocecal region is a favored site.
- The lymphoma cells are monomorphic, medium-sized cells with regular rounded nuclei, dispersed chromatin, and several small nucleoli. Only scanty amounts of cytoplasm are present.
- A "starry sky" appearance may be seen. This is due to the presence of interspersed macrophages containing phagocytosed material.

Special Techniques

- These are extremely useful in the differential diagnosis. Frozen sections and fresh tissue may be required for some of these.
- MALTomas are usually CD5 and CD10 negative and KB61 (CDW32) positive. Gene rearrangement studies show Jh but not bcl-2 rearrangements.
- Mantle zone lymphomas are typically IgM, IgD, CD5, and CD43 positive. They are CD10 and CD23 negative.
- Follicular lymphomas have a phenotype that is IgM, IgG, and CD10 positive, but IgD, CD5, and CD43 negative.

Differential Diagnosis

Benign lymphoid hyperplasia (formerly called pseudolymphoma).

Light-chain restriction is present in lymphomas but not in hyperplasias.

Gene rearrangement is present and can be demonstrated in many lymphomas, even on biopsy material.

References

Cogliatti SB, Schmid U, Schumacher U, et al. Primary B-cell gastric lymphoma: a clinicopathologic study of 145 patients. Gastroenterology 1991;101:1159–1170.

Dragosics B, Bauer P, Radaszikiewicz T. Primary gastrointestinal non-Hodgkins lymphomas: a retrospective clinicopathologic study of 150 cases. Cancer 1985;55:1060–1073.

Hall PA, Levison DA. Malignant lymphoma in the gastrointestinal tract. Semin Diagn Pathol 1991;8:163–167.

Harris NL. Extranodal lymphoid infiltrates and mucosa-associated lymphoid tissue (MALT). A unifying concept. Am J Surg Pathol 1991;15:879–884.

Isaacson PG, Spencer J. Invited review: malignant lymphoma of mucosa-associated lymphoid tissue (MALT). Histopathology 1990;16:617-619.

Isaacson PG, Wotherspoon AC, Diss T, Langxing P. Follicular colonization in B-cell lymphoma of mucosa-associated lymphoid tissue. Am J Surg Pathol 1991;15:819–828.

Mann RB, Jaffe ES, Braylan RC, et al. Non-endemic Burkitt's lymphoma. A B-cell tumor related to germinal centers. N Engl J Med 1976; 295:685–691.

Mori N, Oka K, Nakamura K. Primary gastric mantle zone lymphoma. Arch Pathol Lab Med 1991;115:603–606.

Nizze H, Cogliatti SB, von Schilling C, et al. Monocytoid B-cell lymphoma. Morphological relationship to low-grade B-cell lymphoma of mucosa-associated lymphoid tissue. Histopathology 1991;18:404–414.

O'Briain DS, Kennedy MJ, Daly PA, et al. Multiple lymphomatous polyposis of the gastrointestinal tract. A clinicopathologically distinctive form of non-Hodgkins lymphoma of B-cell centrocytic type. Am J Surg Pathol 1989;13:691–699.

Osborne BM, Pugh WC. Practicality of molecular studies to evaluate small lymphocytic proliferations in endoscopic gastric biopsies. Am J Surg Pathol 1992;16:838–844.

Severson RK, Davis S. Increasing incidence of primary gastric lymphoma. Cancer 1990;66:1283–1287.

Sundeen JT, Longo DL, Jaffe ES. CD5 expression in B-cell small lymphocytic malignancies. Correlations with clinical presentations in sites of disease. Am J Surg Pathol 1992;16:130–137.

Zukerberg LR, Ferry JA, Southern JF, Harris NL. Lymphoid infiltrates of the stomach. Evaluation of the histologic criteria for the diagnosis of low-grade gastric lymphoma on endoscopic biopsy specimens. Am J Surg Pathol 1990;14:1087–1099.

Wotherspoon AC, Pan L, Diss TC, Isaacson PG. A genotypic study of low grade B-cell lymphomas, including lymphomas of mucosa associated lymphoid tissue (MALT). J Pathol 1990;162:135–140.

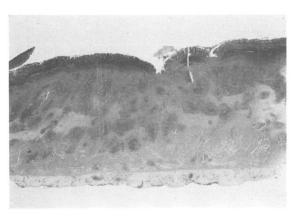

Figure 8–7. MALToma with a zone of surface lymphoid infiltrate and lymphoid aggregates extending into the muscularis propria.

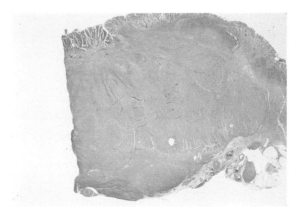

Figure 8–8. Full-thickness gastric wall involvement by small cell lymphoma.

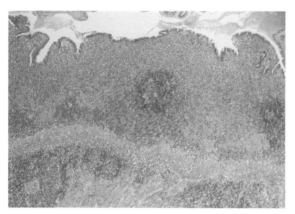

Figure 8–9. Bandlike infiltrate of lymphoma cells in upper portion of mucosa. The residual lymphoid follicles present are reactive.

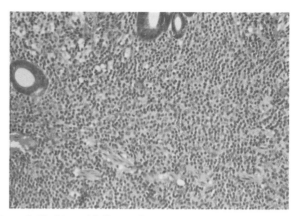

Figure 8–12. Mucosal infiltrate of monomorphic small lymphocytes.

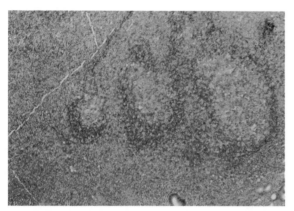

Figure 8–10. The reactive follicle on the left is surrounded by a monotonous infiltrate of small cleaved cells. The follicle on the right shows partial "colonization" by lymphoma cells.

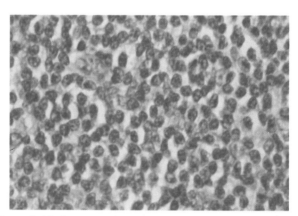

Figure 8–13. Centrocyte-like (CCL) cells with predominantly small "cleaved" nuclei.

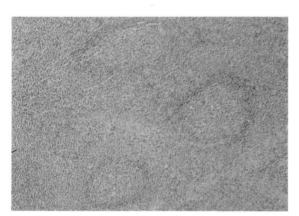

Figure 8–11. Follicles in a dense small cell infiltrate that are colonized by MALToma cells.

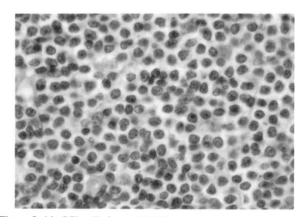

Figure 8–14. CCL cells from a MALToma.

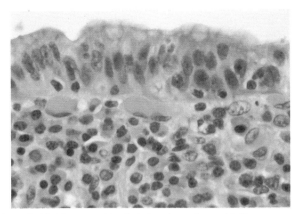

Figure 8–15. Plasmacytoid cells below the surface epithelium.

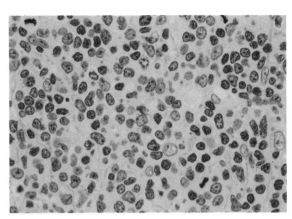

Figure 8–18. Mantle zone lymphoma.

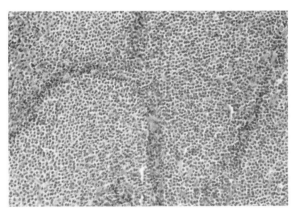

Figure 8–16. CCL cells replacing follicles.

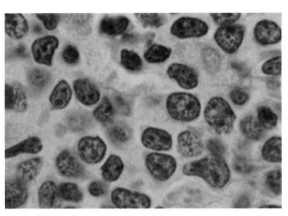

Figure 8–19. Mantle zone lymphoma with irregular nuclear outlines and densely staining nuclei.

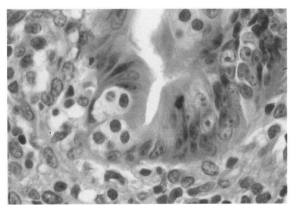

Figure 8–17. Lymphoepithelial lesion.

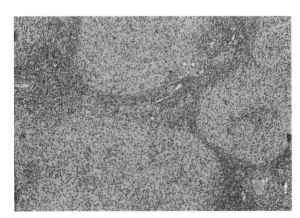

Figure 8–20. Follicular center cell (FCC) lymphoma.

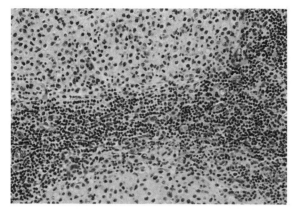

Figure 8–21. Edge of neoplastic follicle in FCC lymphoma.

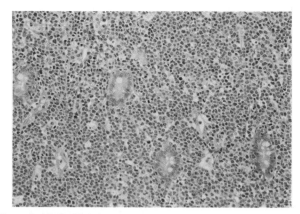

Figure 8–24. Burkitt's lymphoma infiltrating small bowel mucosa. Note the starry-sky pattern.

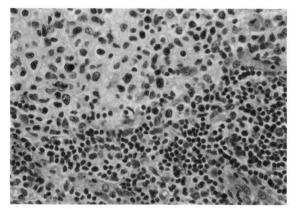

Figure 8–22. FCC lymphoma consisting mainly of large cleaved cells.

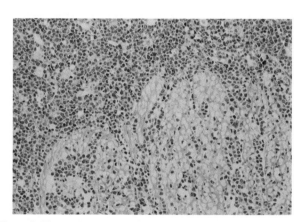

Figure 8–25. Burkitt's lymphoma infiltrating muscularis propria.

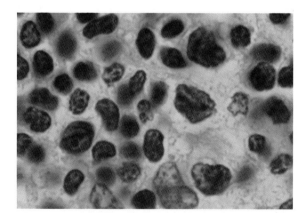

Figure 8–23. FCC lymphoma with large and small cleaved cells.

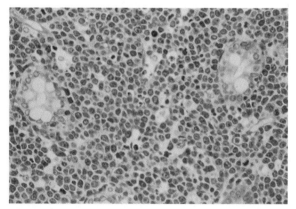

Figure 8–26. Burkitt's lymphoma showing a monotonous pattern of non-cleaved cells.

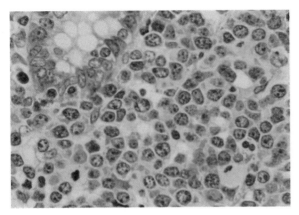

Figure 8–27. Burkitt's lymphoma.

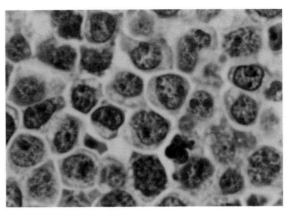

Figure 8–28. Burkitt's lymphoma. The cells are intermediate in size and noncleaved. Small amounts of bluish vacuolated cytoplasm are present.

LARGE CELL LYMPHOMAS

Biology of Disease

- Both T- and B-cell lymphomas may occur as primary gastrointestinal large cell lymphomas.
- Large cell lymphoma is the most common type of gastrointestinal lymphoma.
- Most gastrointestinal large cell lymphomas involve the stomach. The small bowel is the next most frequent site.
- Most gastric large cell lymphomas are of B-cell origin. Some arise de novo, and others originate from a low-grade MALToma that has transformed.
- Large cell lymphomas of the small bowel may arise against a background of celiac disease. These are frequently T cell in origin.
- Some large cell lymphomas show immunoblastic differentiation. There may be a superficial resemblance to Hodgkin's disease, but it is generally considered that primary Hodgkin's disease does not occur in the gastrointestinal tract.
- Multifocal pleomorphic B-cell lymphomas may occur in immunosuppressed individuals (AIDS patients or organ transplant recipients).
- Intestinal large cell lymphomas occur predominately in middle aged or elderly patients.

Clinical Features

- Gastric large cell lymphomas may present with symptoms indistinguishable from a carcinoma. There may be weight loss, early satiety, and gastric outlet obstruction.
- Intestinal large cell lymphomas usually present with obstruction. If the lymphoma occurs against a background of celiac disease, the symptoms of malabsorption can be exacerbated.

Gross Pathology

- Large cell lymphomas are usually high grade. In the stomach they tend to be bulky exophytic masses, resembling intestinal adenocarcinomas. However, they can also have a flat infiltrative pattern, similar to diffuse carcinomas. Occasionally, this may manifest as prominent rugal folds.
- Most intestinal lymphomas are bulky and exophytic, but they too can be more diffuse, producing segmental thickening of the bowel wall.

Microscopic Pathology

- Large cell lymphomas grow in a sheetlike pattern, often sparing normal epithelial structures like crypts and glands.
- Lymphoma cells are noncohesive and usually monomorphic.
- As with all lymphomas, the tumor cells may be mixed with some reactive non-neoplastic cells.
- The nuclei are vesicular with prominent nucleoli and nuclear membranes.
- A moderate amount of amphophilic cytoplasm may be present. This will vary with the degree of immunoblastic differentiation.
- Lymphomas associated with celiac disease are of T-cell lineage and can be pleomorphic with some of the pleomorphic cells resembling Reed-Sternberg cells. Some pleomorphic T-cell lymphomas may be Ki-1 positive.
- Some small bowel lymphomas may be accompanied by prominent local tissue eosinophilia.
- Lymphomas associated with immunosuppression are generally pleomorphic and have prominent immunoblastic features.
- In the Keil classification, most large cell lymphomas would be categorized as centroblastic (subtypes include

classical, polymorphic, centrocytoid, and multilobated variants).

- Lymphoblastic lymphoma is composed of intermediate-sized cells that have an irregular nuclear outline, stippled nuclear chromatin, and indistinct nucleoli. This type accounts for 8% of small bowel lymphomas and is high grade.

Special Techniques

- Fresh tissue should be frozen for immunologic techniques. Other tissue should be fixed in Bouin's fluid or a mercury-based fixative, such as B-5.
- Immunostains for cytokeratin and carcinoembryonic antigen are negative.
- Immunostains for leukocyte common antigen (LCA) are usually positive. B-cell lymphomas will express L-26, while T-cell lesions will be positive for UCHL-1. Anaplastic large cell lymphomas may express BERH2 (Ki-1) and, paradoxically, epithelial membrane antigen.

Differential Diagnosis

Diffuse adenocarcinoma (for gastric lymphomas), metastatic tumors (for intestinal lymphomas).

Carcinomas tend to destroy normal structures as they infiltrate. Lymphomas may spare and infiltrate around glands and pits.

A PAS/Diastase stain may reveal intracellular mucus in carcinomas. Lymphomas are mucin negative.

Some gastric lymphomas can have a signet-ring morphology, but they are always mucin negative.

The immunostains listed above can be exceedingly useful. Evidence of monoclonality is best based on analysis of frozen or fresh material.

References

Brooks JJ, Enterline HT. Primary gastric lymphomas: a clinico-pathologic study of 58 cases with long term follow-up and literature review. Cancer 1983;51:701–711.

Castro CJ, Klimo P, Worth A. Multifocal aggressive lymphoma of the gastrointestinal tract in a renal transplant patient treated with cyclosporin A and prednisone. Cancer 1985;55:1665–1667.

Domizio P, Owen RA, Shepherd NA, et al. Primary lymphoma of the large intestine: A clinicopathological study of 119 cases. Am J Surg Pathol 1993;17:429–442.

Hernandez JA, Sheahan WW. Lymphomas of the mucosa associated lymphoid tissue: signet ring lymphomas presenting in mucosal lymphoid organs. Cancer 1985;32:592–597.

Ioachim HL, Weinstein A, Robbins RD, et al. Primary anorectal lymphoma: a new manifestation of the acquired immune deficiency syndrome (AIDS). Cancer 1987;60:1449–1453.

Isaacson PG, O'Connor NJ, Spencer J, et al. Malignant histiocytosis of the intestine: a T-cell lymphoma. Lancet 1985;2:688–691.

Nash JR, Gradwell E, Day DW. Large-cell intestinal lymphoma occurring in celiac disease: morphological and immunohistochemical features. Histopathology 1986;10:195–205.

Shepherd NA, Blackshaw AJ, Hall PA, et al. Malignant lymphoma with eosinophilia of the gastrointestinal tract. Histopathology 1987; 11:115–120.

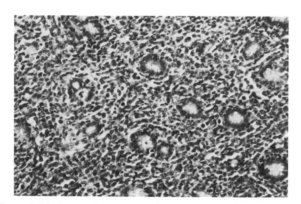

Figure 8–29. Large cell lymphoma infiltrating the lamina propria and separating rather than destroying existing pits.

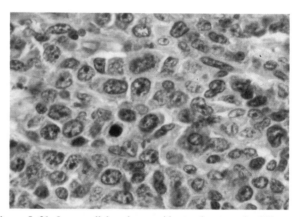

Figure 8–31. Large cell lymphoma with prominent amphophilic cytoplasm.

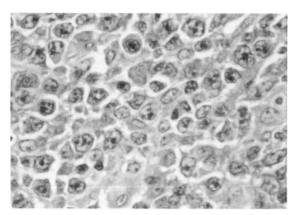

Figure 8–30. Large cell lymphoma with vesicular nuclei containing prominent nucleoli.

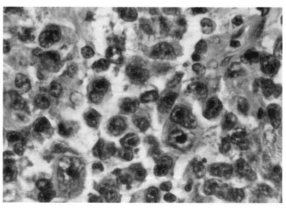

Figure 8–32. Large cell lymphoma arising in celiac disease. Note the nuclear pleomorphism.

IMMUNOPROLIFERATIVE SMALL INTESTINAL DISEASE

Biology of Disease

■ When originally described, immunoproliferative small intestine disease (IPSID) was identified in individuals living near the Mediterranean Sea, who had an unusual type of lymphoma. The term *Mediterranean lymphoma* was coined. However, it is now recognized that the disease can occur in a variety of developing countries and demonstrates a wide spectrum of immunoproliferation. Lymphoma is present in less than half the cases.

■ About 30 to 50% of IPSID cases produce a paraprotein consisting of alpha heavy chains. This occurs in patients with and without a complicating lymphoma and has been called alpha heavy chain disease.

■ Most cases occur in individuals who are malnourished, have poor personal hygiene, and are subject to intestinal infections. Typically, young adult males are affected.

■ There is a strong correlation with HLA-AW19 and HLA-12.

Clinical Features

■ Patients present with malabsorption, growth retardation, weight loss, abdominal pain, and clubbing of the fingers or toes.

Gross Pathology

■ Resected small bowel may show diffusely thickened mucosal folds.

■ When lymphoma develops, there may be a cobblestone pattern of small nodules or discrete tumor masses.

Microscopic Pathology

■ Three distinct patterns are recognized, which are considered to be equivalent to clinical stages of progression.

■ Initially, there is an infiltrate into the lamina propria of mature-appearing plasma cells. This may produce a wide separation of crypts with a variable degree of villous flattening.

■ Later, the plasma cell infiltrate shows occasional atypical cells (dystrophic plasma cells). These may be binucleate and contain a variable number of cells resembling immunoblasts.

■ Later still, a multifocal malignant lymphoma develops. This is of the large cell immunoblastic type and is polymorphous with cells resembling Reed-Sternberg cells. A background of small cleaved cells is present.

■ These changes primarily involve the jejunum, although other parts of the small bowel, as well as the stomach and colon, may be affected to a lesser extent.

■ In the majority of cases, nodular lymphoid hyperplasia is also present, but gradually diminishes as the disease becomes more obviously lymphomatous.

■ In the later stages of the disease, immunoblasts begin to infiltrate the epithelium, submucosa, and mesenteric nodes.

Special Techniques

■ Serologic work-up for alpha heavy chains should be done.

■ Immunohistochemistry provides evidence of IgA secretion and monoclonality.

Differential Diagnosis

Celiac disease, non-IPSID lymphoma (Western lymphoma).

The infiltrate in celiac disease is not as heavy as in IPSID, and plasma cells and lymphocytes are not atypical. Epithelial infiltration by lymphocytes is seen in celiac disease.

Western lymphomas lack any associated plasma cell infiltrates. Typically, they involve the stomach and ileum, rather than the jejunum.

References

Asselah F, Slavin G, Sowter G, Asselah H. Immunoproliferative small intestinal disease in Algerians: light microscopic and immunohistochemical studies. Cancer 1983;52:227–237.

Cammonn M, Jaafoura H, Tabbane F, Halphen M. Immunoproliferative small intestinal disease without alpha-chain disease. A pathological study. Gastroenterology 1989;96:750–763.

Isaacson P. Middle East lymphoma and alpha chain disease. Am J Surg Pathol 1979;3:431–441.

Isaacson P, Al-Dewachi HS, Mason DY. Middle Eastern intestinal lymphoma: a morphological and immunohistochemical study. J 1983; 36:489–498.

Khojasteh A, Haghshenass M, Haghighi P. Immunoproliferative small intestinal disease: a "third world lesion". N Engl J Med 1983; 308:1401–1405.

Salem P, El-Hashimi L, Anaissie E, et al. Primary small intestinal lymphoma in adults. A comparative study of IPSID versus non-IPSID in the Middle East. Cancer 1987;59:1670–1676.

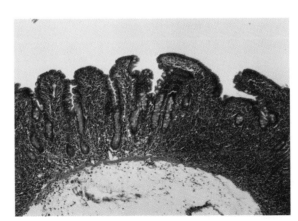

Figure 8–33. Immunoproliferative small intestine disease (IPSID). Note the dense infiltrate in the lamina propria and modest flattening of the villi.

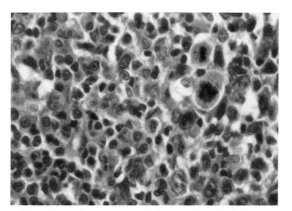

Figure 8–34. Medium-power view to show dense infiltrate of plasma cells with smaller numbers of atypical lymphoid cells.

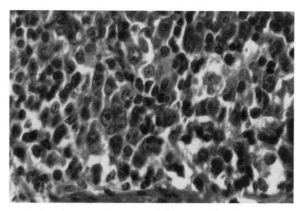

Figure 8–35. Area of developing lymphoma showing a predominance of larger cells with vesicular nuclei and prominent nucleoli.

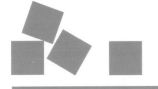

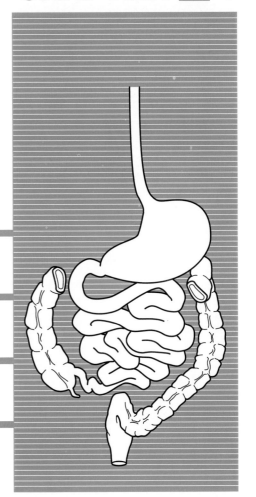

CHAPTER ■ 9

STROMAL LESIONS
AND NEOPLASMS

INFLAMMATORY FIBROID POLYPS

Biology of Disease

■ These polyps are found throughout the gastrointestinal tract, but are most common in the stomach.
■ They may occur at any age, but the mean age is 50 years.
■ The sex incidence is equal.
■ The polyps are generally considered to be reactive not neoplastic in nature. The underlying cell of origin is a fibroblast or a myofibroblast.
■ There are no systemic features.
■ The polyps are usually single.

Clinical Features

■ Most polyps smaller than 3 cm diameter are incidental findings.
■ Larger tumors may cause pyloric or small bowel obstruction.
■ Ileal tumors can cause intussusception.

Gross Pathology

■ Smaller polyps are sessile with a smooth, lobulated surface that may be ulcerated at the tip.
■ Larger polyps may be pedunculated.
■ Polyps may involve the muscularis propria and can also extend to the subserosal fat.
■ The polyp base is usually poorly delineated and merges in an irregular fashion with adjacent normal tissue.

Microscopic Pathology

■ Polyps are predominately composed of a hypocellular myxoid stroma that is highly vascular. The vessels are thin walled and tortuous or may be surrounded by a sclerotic or concentric condensation of stroma.
■ The stromal cells are stellate with small amounts of amphophilic cytoplasm. Usually, there is no pleomorphism.
■ There is a light scattering of inflammatory cells throughout the stroma, usually lymphocytes and eosinophils.
■ Larger tumors may be more sclerotic.
■ Mitotic activity is generally sparse.

References

Johnstone JM, Morson BC. Inflammatory fibroid polyp of the intestinal tract. Histopathology 1978;2:349–361.

Navas-Palacios JJ, Colina-Ruizdelgada F, Sanchez-Larrea MD, Cortez-Cansino J. Inflammatory fibroid polyps of the gastrointestinal tract: an immunohistochemical and electron microscopic study. Cancer 1983; 51:1682–1690.

Shimer GR, Helwig EB. Inflammatory fibroid polyps of the intestine. Am J Clin Pathol 1984;81:708–714.

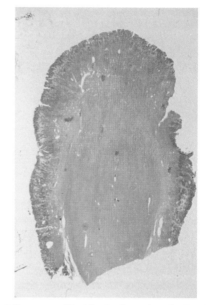

Figure 9–2. Inflammatory fibroid polyp located predominantly in the submucosa. In this small polyp, the overlying mucosa is intact.

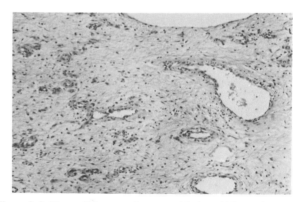

Figure 9–3. Hypocellular area of stroma with sinusoidal vessels.

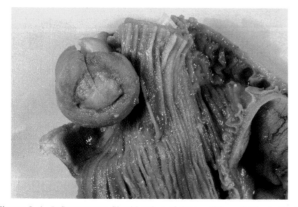

Figure 9–1. Inflammatory fibroid polyp of the small bowel. The lesion is ulcerated on the surface.

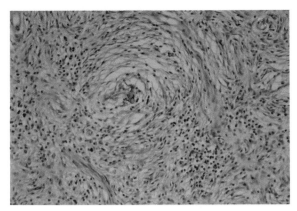

Figure 9–4. Fibrous tissue growing in a concentric fashion around small vessels.

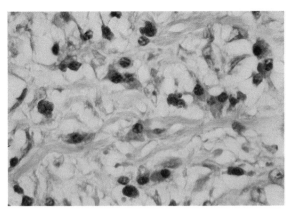

Figure 9–6. Mixed stromal inflammatory cells. Note the small number of eosinophils.

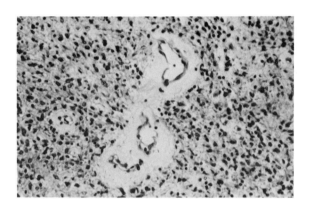

Figure 9–5. Vessels surrounded by a zone of sclerosis.

STROMAL AND SMOOTH MUSCLE TUMORS

Biology of Disease

■ The histogenesis of gastrointestinal smooth muscle tumors is controversial. By ultrastructural and immunohistochemical examination, only a minority show clear cut evidence of smooth muscle or neural origin. The majority are either undifferentiated or show equivocal smooth muscle differentiation. For routine diagnosis, these special techniques are not critical, since the clinical behavior is governed by light microscopic appearances, not histogenesis.

■ If special techniques have been performed and evidence concerning histogenesis is available, then it is reasonable to label a neoplasm as a schwannoma, leiomyoma, leiomyosarcoma, etc. Otherwise, the terms *benign* and *malignant stromal tumor* are appropriate.

■ Sixty percent of all clinically significant gastrointestinal stromal tumors occur in the stomach. The small bowel is the next most common site. Esophageal and large bowel stromal tumors are unusual. Stromal tumors less than 1

cm in diameter are a frequent finding at autopsy if a thorough search is made. Since these are of no clinical significance, they are excluded from the discussion.

■ Determining whether stromal tumors will behave in a benign or malignant fashion is not straightforward. Classification into one of four categories of clinical behavior is recommended: benign, low malignant potential, high malignant potential, and malignant.

■ The term *leiomyoblastoma* has now been replaced by *epithelioid stromal tumor*. It is now accepted that tumors with a mixture of spindle and epithelioid cells may occur, but that the presence of epithelioid features does not influence prognosis.

Clinical Features

■ Stromal tumors occur at all ages, but are most frequent in patients 40 to 80 years of age. The sex incidence is equal.

■ In the stomach, they may be discovered incidentally, or may cause nausea, anorexia, and bleeding.

■ In the small bowel, they may produce obstruction with abdominal pain and bleeding.

- Malignant tumors may cause weight loss.
- Esophageal tumors, which can cause dysphagia, occur at all levels of the esophagus. Sarcomas are quite uncommon at this site.
- Stromal tumors of the large bowel fall into two distinct clinicopathologic groups. Small tumors (<2 cm) are discovered incidentally at endoscopy as smooth-surfaced polyps. Large tumors (>5 cm) act and look like carcinomas. In spite of a "benign" histologic appearance, they behave in a malignant fashion.
- Carney's triad consists of the combination of gastric stromal tumor, pulmonary chondroma, and functioning extra-adrenal paraganglioma (pheochromocytoma).

Gross Pathology

- Most stromal tumors are well demarcated and are round or lobulated. Occasionally, they may have a dumbbell shape, as a result of growth on either side of the muscularis propria.
- Malignant tumors may have an outline irregular and infiltrate adjacent structures.
- The tumors protrude into the gut lumen as dome-shaped structures that may have surface ulceration.
- Particularly in the larger neoplasms, there may be central areas of necrosis, degeneration, cyst formation, or myxoid change.
- Tumors that metastasize or invade other organs are considered unequivocally malignant.
- Tumor size is closely related to malignant potential, as follows:

Stomach

<5.5 cm diameter	1% metastasize	Benign
5.5–10.0 cm diameter	15–30% metastasize	Low malignant potential
Diameter >10 cm	60% metastasize	High malignant potential

Small Bowel

<4.5 cm diameter	Rarely metastasize	Benign
4.5–10.0 cm diameter	50% metastasize	Low malignant potential
Diameter >10 cm	70% metastasize	High malignant potential

- Factors such as surface ulceration and central necrosis are not independent variables of malignancy but rather are related to tumor size.

Microscopic Pathology

- Most gastrointestinal stromal tumors are composed of spindle cells. These have elongated cigar-shaped nuclei and abundant eosinophilic cytoplasm. The growth pattern is fascicular or occasionally palisaded.
- A minority of tumors have abundant epithelioid cells. These have a sheetlike growth pattern and are composed of polygonal cells with central rounded nuclei and cytoplasm that may be eosinophilic or clear. Cleared cytoplasm is generally regarded as a fixation artifact due to retraction. This type of tumor may have nuclei containing prominent nucleoli.
- Both types of tumor may show foci of hyalinization, myxoid change, calcification, or hemorrhage. However, these features are not useful in determining biologic behavior.

- Frank sarcomas are highly cellular lesions with a mitotic count frequently in excess of 10 per 10 high power fields (hpfs). They often have large areas of necrosis.
- The most useful microscopic feature in estimating malignant potential in stromal tumors is the mitotic count. Increasing cellularity also makes a tumor more likely to behave in a malignant fashion but is a less useful feature than the mitotic count, partly because it is so subjective. In the stomach, tumors with no mitoses are considered benign. Tumors with one to five mitoses per 50 hpfs are considered to have a low malignant potential. Between five and ten mitoses per 50 hpfs, tumors have a high malignant potential. Above 10 mitoses per 50 hpfs, all tumors are considered to be malignant. In the small bowel, the presence of any mitoses indicates a high malignant potential. Generally, the mitotic count correlates well with the malignant potential of the neoplasm as determined by gross size.

Special Techniques

- By immunohistologic analysis, 50 to 60% of tumors are desmin positive, and 60 to 70% are smooth muscle actin positive. Only 5% are neuron-specific enolase (NSE) positive (presumed neural origin).
- Flow cytometric analysis of DNA content has shown that aneuploidy may occur in both benign and malignant tumors. Fifty to 75% of malignant tumors and 20 to 25% of benign tumors are aneuploid. The significance of aneuploidy as a prognostic indicator is as yet unclear.

Differential Diagnosis

Inflammatory pseudotumor, glomus tumor.

Myofibroblastic pseudotumors may have prominent fibroblastic features with an admixture of chronic inflammatory cells. They tend to have an irregular outline and be firmly attached to adjacent structures and fat. Stromal tumors are generally relatively sharply circumscribed, although microscopically malignant neoplasms have an infiltrating border. Most stromal tumors contain only small numbers of inflammatory cells.

Glomus tumors are composed of uniform boxlike cells with dark staining nuclei. They have a characteristic vascular pattern.

References

Appelman HD. Smooth muscle tumors of the gastrointestinal tract. What we now know that Stout didn't know. Am J Surg Pathol 1986;10 (Suppl):83–89.

Appelman HD, Helwig EB. Cellular leiomyomas of the stomach in 49 patients. Arch Pathol Lab Med 1977;101:373–377.

Appelman HD, Helwig EB. Gastric epithelioid leiomyoma and leiomyosarcoma (leiomyoblastoma). Cancer 1976;38:708–728.

Appelman HD, Helwig EB. Sarcomas of the stomach. Am J Clin Pathol 1977;67:2–10.

Carney JA. The triad of gastric epithelioid leiomyosarcoma, pulmonary chondroma and functioning extra-adrenal paraganglioma: a 5 year review. Medicine 1983;62:159–169.

Evans HL. Smooth muscle tumors of the gastrointestinal tract. A study of 56 cases followed for a minimum of 10 years. Cancer 1985;56:2242–2250.

El-Naggar AK, Ro JY, McLemore D, et al. Gastrointestinal stromal tumors:

DNA flow-cytometric study of 58 patients with at least 5 years follow up. Mod Pathol 1989;2:511–515.

Hjermstad BM, Sobin LH, Helwig EB. Stromal tumors of the gastrointestinal tract: myogenic or neurogenic? Am J Surg Pathol 1987;11:383–386.

Ma CK, Amin MB, Kintanar E, et al. Immunohistologic characterization of gastrointestinal stromal tumors: a study of 82 cases compared with 11 cases of leiomyomas. Mod Pathol 1993;6:139–144.

Ranchod M, Kempson RL. Smooth muscle tumors of the gastrointestinal tract and retroperitoneum. Cancer 1977;39:255–262.

Saul SH, Rast ML, Brooks JJ. The immunocytochemistry of gastrointestinal stromal tumors: evidence supporting an origin from smooth muscle. Am J Surg Pathol 1987;11:464–473.

Shiu MH, Farr GH, Papachristou DN, Hadju SI. Myosarcomas of the stomach: natural history, prognostic factors and management. Cancer 1982;49:177–187.

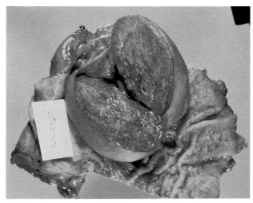

Figure 9–7. Gastric leiomyoma. Note the beefy-red appearance of the cut surface. The mucosa is not ulcerated and is stretched smoothly over the surface.

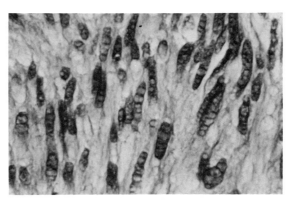

Figure 9–10. Spindle cell leiomyoma with blunt, cigar-shaped nuclei.

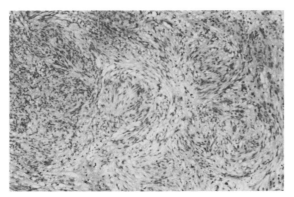

Figure 9–8. Spindle cell leiomyoma. The lesion is variably cellular and is growing in a whorled fashion.

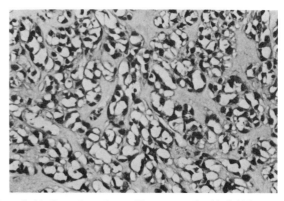

Figure 9–11. Stromal neoplasm with pronounced epithelioid features.

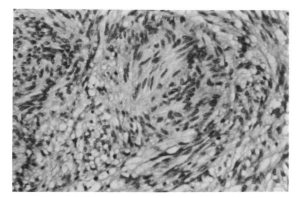

Figure 9–9. Poorly developed palisading in a leiomyoma.

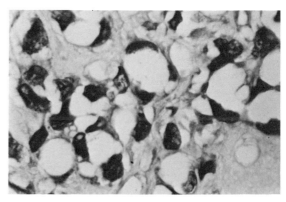

Figure 9–12. At high power, this stromal tumor has signet-ring–like cells.

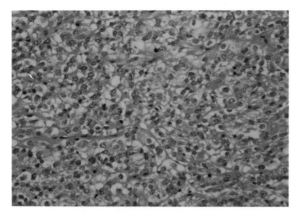

Figure 9–13. Epithelioid leiomyoma.

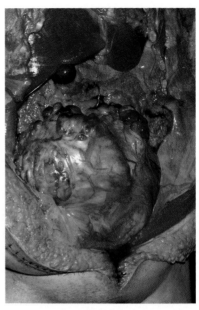

Figure 9–15. Leiomyosarcoma arising from ascending colon.

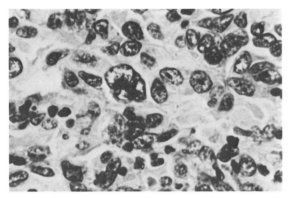

Figure 9–14. Stromal tumor with pleomorphic nuclei. With this degree of abnormality, it is usual to find a high mitotic count.

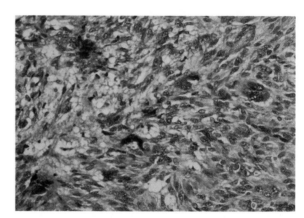

Figure 9–16. Sarcoma with pleomorphism and high cellularity.

NEUROGENIC TUMORS

Biology of Disease

■ Neurogenic tumors include schwannoma, neurofibroma, gangliocytic paraganglioma (see Chapter 3), and ganglioneuromatosis.

■ These lesions are almost invariably benign. Only exceedingly rare examples of malignant schwannomas are described.

■ Most tumors occur as isolated lesions. Neurofibromas are seen predominately in von Recklinghausen's disease. Ganglioneuromatosis may occur in association with von Recklinghausen's disease, multiple endocrine neoplasia type IIB, Hirschsprung's disease, Cowden's syndrome, and familial adenomatous polyposis.

■ Solitary schwannoma can be distinguished from other gastrointestinal stromal tumors only on the basis of electron microscopy or immunohistochemistry.

■ Ganglioneuromatosis is a diffuse disease and may consist of solitary or plexiform neurofibromas and ganglioneuromas in the submucosa.

Clinical Features

■ Information specifically relevant to isolated schwannomas is sparse. Most appear to be benign. Otherwise, there are no obvious differences from other types of stromal tumor.

■ Most patients with gastrointestinal neurofibromas have von Recklinghausen's disease.

■ Patients with ganglioneuromatosis may present with abdominal pain, melena, and intussusception. Occasionally, occult bleeding producing anemia may result.

Gross Pathology

■ Schwannomas resemble leiomyomas and cannot be distinguished from them by gross inspection.
■ Neurofibromas are unencapsulated lesions. They are generally firm in consistency and are present in a submucosal location.
■ Ganglioneuromatosis is characterized by focal non-encapsulated neoplasms and a diffuse irregular submucosal thickening. On closer examination, this thickening can be seen to consist of enlarged nerves trapped by fibrous proliferation.

Microscopic Pathology

■ Schwannomas are distinguishable from other stromal tumors only by ultrastructural and immunohistochemical examination. Palisading is not a reliable criterion of nerve sheath differentiation. These tumors are composed of elongated spindle cells, and sometimes the stroma may be densely hyalinized.
■ Neurofibromas are identical to schwannomas except that they are nonencapsulated.
■ Ganglioneurofibromatosis consists of neurofibromas and plexiform neurofibromas containing interspersed ganglion cells.

References

Barwick KW. Gastrointestinal manifestations of multiple endocrine neoplasia, type IIB. J Clin Gastroenterol 1983;5:83–87.

Daimaru Y, Kido H, Hashimoto H, Enjoji M. Benign schwannoma of the gastrointestinal tract. Hum Pathol 1988;19:257–264.

Hochberg FH, Dasilva AB, Galdabini J, Richardson EP. Gastrointestinal involvement in von Recklinghausen's neurofibromatosis. Neurology 1974;24:224–251.

Lashner BA, Riddell RH, Winans CS. Ganglioneuromatosis of the colon and extensive glycogenic acanthosis in Cowden's syndrome. Dig Dis Sci 1986;31:213–216.

Weidner N, Flanders DJ, Mitros FA. Mucosal ganglioneuromatosis associated with multiple colonic polyps. Am J Surg Pathol 1984;8:779–786.

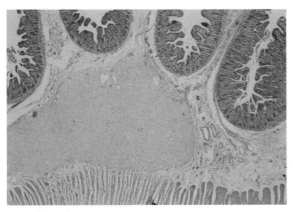

Figure 9–17. Plexiform neurofibroma of the small bowel, from a case of von Recklinghausen's disease.

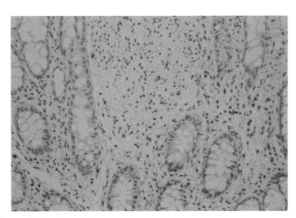

Figure 9–19. Neurofibromatous component.

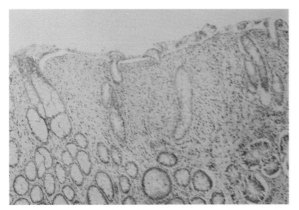

Figure 9–18. Ganglioneurofibroma of colon showing intramucosal growth.

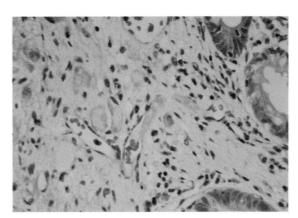

Figure 9–20. Ganglion cell component.

GLOMUS TUMORS

Biology of Disease

■ These benign tumors occur mainly in the gastric antrum but occasionally develop at other sites.
■ They are similar to glomus tumors of the skin and are regarded as proliferations of pericapillary cells.
■ Glomus tumors occur with equal frequency in both sexes. The mean age of incidence is the sixth decade.

Clinical Features

■ Most gastric glomus tumors are either discovered incidentally or present with peptic ulcer–like symptoms, such as abdominal pain and bleeding.

Gross Pathology

■ The tumors are usually between 1 and 4 cm in diameter.
■ Consistency varies from soft to firm. Very occasionally, they may be calcified.
■ Surface ulceration is present in about one third of tumors.
■ The tumors are circumscribed, but not encapsulated.

Microscopic Pathology

■ The tumors generally grow within the muscularis propria. They are divided into lobules by fine trabeculae extending inward from the muscularis.
■ Many thin-walled vessels are present.
■ The tumor is composed of uniform round or boxlike cells with central darkly staining nuclei. Small amounts of cytoplasm are present, which is either palely eosinophilic or clear. Mitotic activity is not seen.
■ Ultrastructurally, there are features of smooth muscle derivation, namely, basement membrane, pinocytotic vesicles, and cytoplasmic dense bodies.

References

Almagro UA, Schulte N, Norback DH, Turcott J. Glomus tumor of the stomach: histologic and ultrastructural features. Am J Clin Pathol 1981; 75:415–419.

Appelman HD, Helwig EB. Glomus tumors of the stomach. Cancer 1969;23:203–213.

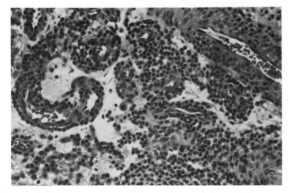

Figure 9–21. Glomus tumor showing relationship of cells to vessels.

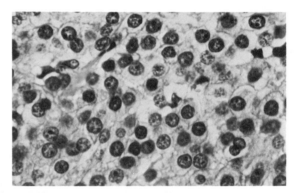

Figure 9–22. Boxlike regular glomus cells.

INDEX

Note: Page numbers in *italics* refer to illustrations.

Abetalipoproteinemia, 106–107
  small bowel lesions in, 107, *107*
Abscess, appendiceal, 124, *125*
  eosinophilic, *Anisakis* larvae and, 202, *203*
Absorption defects, ulcer with, duodenojejunoileitis
  and, 77. See also *Jejunoileitis, ulcerative.*
Acanthosis, glycogenic, 2
Achalasia, 7, *8*
Acute appendicitis, 124, *124*, *125*
Acute erosive gastritis, 25, *25*, *26*
Adenocarcinoid (crypt cell carcinoma, goblet cell
    carcinoid), of appendix, 128, 129, *130*
  vs. adenocarcinoma, 128
Adenocarcinoma, of ampulla of Vater, 117
  of anus, 192, *192*, 193
  of appendix, 127–128, *128*
    pseudomyxoma peritonei associated with, 126,
      128
    vs. adenoma, 126, 128
    vs. carcinoid tumor, 128, 129
    vs. cecal adenocarcinoma, 128
  of cecum, vs. appendiceal carcinoma, 128
    with lymphatic spread to small bowel, *116*
  of colon, 177–178, *179*, *180*. See also *Adenocarci-*
    noma, of rectum.
    development of, adenoma and, 173, 174, *175*,
      176, 177, 178
      ulcerative colitis and, 146, 147
    small cell carcinoma arising in, 181, *182*
    ulceration and obstruction proximal to, 151, *152*
    vs. adenoma, 174
    vs. hyperplastic polyp, 168
    vs. metastatic disease, 179
    vs. pseudoinvasive lesions, 178
  of esophagus, 15, *16*, 17
    Barrett's epithelium and, 11, 15, *16*
    vs. dysplasia, 15
    vs. trapped glands, 15
  of prostate, invasive, vs. rectal adenocarcinoma,
    178–179, *180*
  of rectum, *168*, 177–178. See also *Adenocarci-*
    noma, of colon.
    vs. carcinoid tumor, 178
    vs. endometriosis, 179, *180*
    vs. invasive prostate cancer, 178–179, *180*
  of small bowel, 116, *116*
    vs. adenoma, 116
    vs. carcinoid tumor, 116
    vs. gangliocytic paraganglioma, 114
    vs. metastatic disease, 116, 118

Adenocarcinoma (*Continued*)
  of stomach, 50–51, *51*, *52*
    development of, polyps and, 42, 45
    vs. adenoma, 45–46, 50
    vs. diffuse carcinoma, 51
    vs. early gastric cancer, 50
    vs. peptic ulcer, 51
    vs. xanthelasma, 23
Adenoma, of ampulla of Vater, 117, *117*
  of appendix, 126, *127*
    vs. adenocarcinoma, 126, 128
    vs. hyperplastic polyp, 125, 126
  of colon, 169, 173–174, *174–176*
    cancer arising in or associated with, 173, 174,
      175, 177, 178, 181, *182*
    cancer invading stalk of, 174, *176*
    coincidental development of, in ulcerative coli-
      tis, 147
    dysplasia in, 174, *175*
    familial syndrome marked by, 173, *175*
    flat, 173, 174
    Gardner's syndrome and, 173
    goblet cell–rich, 169
    mixed with hyperplastic polyp, 168, 169, *169*
    residual stalk of, 176, *177*
    serrated, 168, 169, *169*
    squamous metaplasia in, 174, *175*
    tubular, 173, 174, *174*, *175*
      vs. juvenile polyp, 170
    tubulovillous, 173
    villous, 173
      cancer arising in, *175*
    vs. adenocarcinoma, 174
    vs. hyperplastic polyp, 168, 174
    vs. inflammatory polyp, 171
    vs. juvenile polyp, 170
  of duodenum, *115*
  of small bowel, 115, *115*
    vs. adenocarcinoma, 116
    vs. Peutz-Jeghers polyp, 111
  of stomach, 45–46, *46*
    cancer risk associated with, 45
    vs. adenocarcinoma, 45–46, 50
    vs. dysplasia, 46, 55
    vs. non-neoplastic polyps, 42, 46
Adenomatous polyps. See *Adenoma.*
Adenomyoma, vs. heterotopic pancreatic tissue, 69
Adenosquamous carcinoma, of stomach, 57, *58*
Adenovirus infection, of small bowel, 89, *90*
Adult cecal volvulus, 137

Large bowel (*Continued*)
chronic granulomatous disease of, 136, *136*
vs. melanosis coli, 140
Crohn's disease of, 144–145, *145, 146.* See also *Crohn's disease, of colon.*
vs. Behçet's syndrome, 163
vs. diverticular disease, 138
vs. lymphogranuloma venereum, 161
disorders of, 133–183, *135–184*
diverticular disease of, 138, *139*
dysplasia in, neuronal, 134
ganglion cells of, absence of, 133–134, *135*
graft versus host disease involving, 199, 200, *201*
granulomatous disease of, chronic, 136, *136*
vs. melanosis coli, 140
gross anatomy of, 132
hemorrhage in, diverticula and, 138, *139*
hemosiderin deposition in, vs. melanosis coli, 140
Hirschsprung's disease of, 133–134, *135*
hyperplasia in, lymphoid, 216
polyp-like, 168
vs. dysplasia, 147
hyperplastic polyps of. See *Colon, hyperplastic polyps of.*
hypoganglionosis of, 134
impacted feces in, ulcers associated with, 164
infection of, 152–163, *155–163.* See also *Infectious colitis* and specific pathogen sub-entries under *Colon.*
inflammatory diseases of, 141–162, *141–162.* See also *Colitis.*
ischemia of, *204.* See also *Ischemia, colonic.*
vs. stercoral ulcer, 164
lymphoid follicles of, 132
lymphoid hyperplasia in, 216
malignant tumors of. See *Colon, carcinoma of; Rectum, carcinoma of.*
metaplastic polyps of. See *Colon, hyperplastic polyps of.*
microscopic features of, 132, *133*
mucosa of, 132, *133*
prolapse of, polypoid, in diverticular disease, *139*
neuronal dysplasia in, 134
Peutz-Jeghers polyps of, 111, 170
polyp-like hyperplasia in, 168
vs. dysplasia, 147
polypoid mucosal prolapse in, diverticular disease and, *139*
polyps of. See *Colon, polyps of; Rectum, polyps of.*
prolapsed mucosa in, and polyp formation in diverticular disease, *139*
pseudo-obstruction of, vs. diverticular disease, 138
self-limited infection of. See *Infectious colitis.*
skip-segment Hirschsprung's disease of, 134
spirochetosis of, 162–163, *163*
stercoral ulcers of, 164, *164*
stromal tumors of, 230
submucosa of, 132, *133*
tumors of, malignant. See *Colon, carcinoma of; Rectum, carcinoma of.*
ulcer of. See also *Ulcer(s), colonic; Ulcer(s), rectal.*
Behçet's syndrome and, 163
graft versus host disease and, *201*
stercoral, 164, *164*
volvulus of, 137, *137*
zonal aganglionosis of, 134
Large cell lymphoma, 223–224, *224*
Laxative abuse, 140
and melanosis coli, 140, *140*
Leiomyoma, epithelioid, 232
gastric, *231*
vs. pyloric stenosis, 22
spindle cell, *231*

Leiomyosarcoma, colonic, *232*
Linitis plastica, diffuse gastric carcinoma and, 52, *53*
Lipid island (xanthelasma, xanthoma), gastric, 23, *23*
Lipid storage disease(s), vs. Whipple's disease, 87
Lipofuscin, melanin-like, colonic accumulation of, 140, *140*
Lipoma, colonic, 172–173, *173*
Lipoprotein deficiencies, 106–107, 109–110
small bowel lesions in, 107, *107,* 109, 110, *110*
Lower esophageal sphincter, 2
idiopathic hypertrophy of, 7
incomplete relaxation of, 7
Lung, small cell carcinoma of, visceral neuropathy secondary to, 120
Lymphangiectasia, intestinal, 104–105, *105*
vs. local or normal lymphatic dilation, 105
vs. lymphangiectatic cyst, 106
vs. macroglobulinemic enteropathy, 108
Lymphangiectatic cyst (chylous cyst), of small bowel, 105–106, *106*
Lymphangioma, cystic, of mesentery of small bowel, 105–106, *106*
Lymphatics, dilated, in small bowel mucosa, 104, 105, *105, 106*
macroglobulinemia and, 107, *108*
Lymphoblastic lymphoma, 224
Lymphocytes, in colon, 132
increase in, 149, *150*
in esophagus, 2, *2*
in stomach, 38. See also *Lymphocytic (varioliform) gastritis.*
Lymphocytic colitis (microscopic colitis), 149–150, *150*
Lymphocytic gastritis (varioliform gastritis), 38–39, *39*
vs. acute erosive gastritis, 25
vs. atrophic gastritis, 38
vs. gastric lesions in Zollinger-Ellison syndrome, 47
vs. *Helicobacter pylori* gastritis, 38
vs. lymphoma, 38–39
vs. Menetrier's disease, 39, 49
Lymphogranuloma venereum, 161
Lymphoid follicles. See also *Lymphoid hyperplasia.*
of large bowel, 132
hyperplasia of, 216
of small bowel, 62, *63*
hyperplasia of, 216, *217*
hypogammaglobulinemia and, 109, *109,* 217
membranous enterocytes on, 62, 63
Lymphoid follicular proctitis, *143,* 151
Lymphoid hyperplasia, 216, *217*
of appendix, 216
of colon, 216
of duodenum, in hypogammaglobulinemia, 109, *109*
of large bowel, 216
of rectum, 216, *217*
of small bowel, 216, *217*
in hypogammaglobulinemia, 109, *109,* 217
of terminal ileum, 216, *217*
vs. lymphoma, 216, 219
vs. MALToma, 216
Lymphoid tissue, diseases of, 216–225, *217–226.* See also *Lymphoid hyperplasia* and *Lymphoma.*
mucosa-associated, lymphoma arising in. See *MALToma.*
Lymphoma, 218–224, *219–224*
Burkitt's, 219, *222, 223*
celiac disease and, 223, *224*
eosinophilic infiltration of GI tract due to, 202
follicular, 218–219
follicular center cell, 219, *221, 222*
gastric, 218, *219,* 223
vs. carcinoma, 53, 224

Small bowel (*Continued*)
  Gaucher's disease affecting, vs. Whipple's disease, 87
  giardiasis of, 78–79, *79*, *80*
  goblet cells in, 62
  graft versus host disease involving, 199, 200, *200*
  granuloma in, Crohn's disease and, 98, *101*
    histoplasmosis and, 98
    tuberculosis and, 94, *94*
  granulomatous disease of, chronic, vs. Crohn's disease, 98
  gross anatomy of, 62. See also specific parts: *Duodenum*; *Ileum*; *Jejunum*.
  hemorrhage in, necrotizing clostridial infection and, 96, *97*
  heterotopic tissue in. See *Small bowel, gastric mucosa in*; *Small bowel, pancreatic tissue in*.
  histoplasmosis of, 198
    vs. Crohn's disease, 98
    vs. Whipple's disease, 87
  hyperinfection of, by *Strongyloides stercoralis*, 85
  hyperplasia of crypts in, celiac disease and, 75, *76*
  hyperplasia of lymphoid tissue in, 216, *217*
    hypogammaglobulinemia and, 109, *109*, *217*
  hypogammaglobulinemia affecting, 108–109, *109*, *217*
  ileal portion of. See *Ileum*.
  immunodeficiency syndromes affecting, 108, 109
    vs. celiac disease, 75
  immunoproliferative disease of, 225, *225*, *226*
  infection of, 78–96, *79–97*
  inflammatory fibroid polyp of, *228*
  intussusception of, 71, *71*
  ischemia of, vs. radiation enteropathy, 207
  ischemic necrosis of, 96
  ischemic stricture in, 98, 204, *206*
  isosporiasis of, 83–84, *84*
    vs. microsporidiosis, 82, 84
  jejunal portion of. See *Jejunum*.
  Kaposi's sarcoma of, *212*
  lipid storage diseases affecting, vs. Whipple's disease, 87
  lipoprotein deficiencies affecting, 107, *107*, 109, 110, *110*
  lymphangiectasia of, 104–105, *105*
    vs. local or normal lymphatic dilation, 105
    vs. lymphangiectatic cyst, 106
    vs. macroglobulinemic enteropathy, 108
  lymphangiectatic (chylous) cyst of, 105–106, *106*
  lymphoid follicles in, 62, *63*
    hyperplasia of. See *Small bowel, lymphoid hyperplasia of*.
    membranous enterocytes on, 62, 63
  lymphoid hyperplasia of, 216, *217*
    hypogammaglobulinemia and, 109, *109*, *217*
  lymphoma of, 223, *224*
    immunoproliferative disease and, 225, *226*
    vs. melanoma, 119
    vs. ulcerative duodenojejunoileitis, 77
  macroglobulinemia affecting, 107–108, *108*
    vs. lymphangiectasia, 108
    vs. *Mycobacterium avium-intracellulare* infection, 108
    vs. Whipple's disease, 87, 108
  macrophages in, Tangier disease and, 110, *110*
    Whipple's disease and, 87, *88*
  malignant tumors of. See *Small bowel, cancer of* and specific tumor sub-entries.
  melanoma of, 119, *119*
  membranous enterocytes in, 62, 63
  mesentery of, 62
    cystic lymphangioma of, 105–106, *106*
  metastatic (secondary) tumors in, 118, *118*, 119, *119*
    vs. primary tumors, 116, 118

Small bowel (*Continued*)
  microscopic features of, 62–63, *63*, *64*
  microsporidiosis of, 82, *83*
    vs. isosporiasis, 82, 84
  microvilli of, *64*
  microvillus inclusion disease of, 76
  mucosa of, 62, *63*, *64*
    crypts in, 62, *63*
      destruction of, in Crohn's disease, 98, *101*
      egg deposition in, in strongyloidiasis, 85, *86*
      fate of, in graft versus host disease, 200, *200*
      hyperplasia of, in celiac disease, 75, *76*
    dilated lymphatics in, 104, 105, *105*, *106*
      macroglobulinemia and, 107, *108*
    flat. See *Small bowel, flat mucosa of*.
    villi in. See *Small bowel, villi of*.
  Mycobacterium avium-intracellulare infection of, 95, *95*, *96*, 212–213, *213*
    vs. macroglobulinemic enteropathy, 108
    vs. Tangier disease, 110
    vs. tuberculosis, 95, 213
    vs. Whipple's disease, 87, 95, 213
  Mycobacterium tuberculosis infection of, 93–94, *94*
    vs. Crohn's disease, 94, 98
    vs. *Mycobacterium avium-intracellulare* infection, 95, 213
    vs. yersiniosis, 92, 94
  myenteric plexus (Auerbach's plexus) in, 62
    lesions of, 120
  myopathy of, 121
  necrotizing disease of, clostridial toxins and, 96, *97*
    ischemia and, 96
  neuroendocrine carcinoma of, 113, *113*
  neurofibroma of, *233*
  neuropathy of, 120
    vs. alimentary tract lesions in Chagas' disease, 120
    vs. cytomegalovirus infection, 120
    vs. visceral myopathy, 121
  normal, 62–63, *63*, *64*
  Norwalk virus infection of, 89, *90*
  NSAID-induced disease of, 102, *103*
    vs. Crohn's disease of jejunum, 102
    vs. ulcerative duodenojejunoileitis, 77
  obstruction of, gallstones and, 72, *72*
  pancreatic tissue in, 68–69, *69*
    vs. adenomyoma, 69
    vs. ectopic gastric mucosa, 69, 70
  Paneth cells in, 62, *63*
  paraganglioma of, gangliocytic, 114, *114*
  paraneoplastic neuropathy of, 120
  parvovirus-like infection of, *90*
  Peutz-Jeghers polyps of, 111, *111*, *112*
  Peyer's patches in, 63, *63*
    ulcers of, *Salmonella typhi* infection and, 91, *91*, *92*
    yersiniosis and, 93, *94*
  pneumatosis of, 166, *167*
  polyps of, adenomatous. See *Small bowel, adenoma of*.
    Cowden's disease and, 176
    inflammatory fibroid, *228*
    Peutz-Jeghers, 111, *111*, *112*
  primary hypogammaglobulinemia affecting, 108–109, *109*, *217*
  primary tumors in. See specific tumor sub-entries, e.g., *Small bowel, carcinoma of*.
  pseudo-obstruction of, 120, *122*
  rotavirus infection of, 88, *90*
  salmonellosis of, 91, *91*, *92*
  sarcoma of, Kaposi's, *212*
  secondary (metastatic) tumors in, 118, *118*, 119, *119*
    vs. primary tumors, 116, 118